Early Detection and Treatment
of Head & Neck Cancers

Rami El Assal
Dyani Gaudilliere
Stephen Thaddeus Connelly

Editors

Early Detection and Treatment of Head & Neck Cancers

Practical Applications and Techniques for Detection, Diagnosis, and Treatment

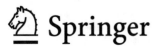 Springer

Editors
Rami El Assal
Canary Center at Stanford for Cancer Early Detection
Stanford University School of Medicine
Palo Alto, CA
USA

Dyani Gaudilliere
Division of Plastic & Reconstructive Surgery, Department of Surgery
Stanford University School of Medicine
Palo Alto, CA
USA

Stephen Thaddeus Connelly
Department of Oral and Maxillofacial Surgery
University of California, San Francisco
San Francisco, CA
USA

ISBN 978-3-030-69861-4   ISBN 978-3-030-69859-1   (eBook)
https://doi.org/10.1007/978-3-030-69859-1

This Springer imprint is published by the registered company Springer Nature Switzerland AG
The registered company address is: Gewerbestrasse 11, 6330 Cham, Switzerland

This book is dedicated to the late Professor Sam Gambhir of Stanford.

Sam was the pioneer in the foundation of cancer early detection. He dedicated his life to developing methods of early disease detection, ushering in a new era of molecular imaging and nanotechnologies to flag signals of disease in its nascent stages. Dr. Gambhir was the Virginia and D.K. Ludwig professor of cancer research and chair of radiology at Stanford University School of Medicine. He was the founding director of the Canary Center at Stanford for Cancer Early Detection, Precision Health and Integrated Diagnostics Center at Stanford, and the director of the molecular imaging program at Stanford.

The editor-in-chief, Dr. Rami El Assal, would like to express his gratitude for the selfless devotion of Dr. Gambhir, a kind and honest man. Dr. El Assal commented, "In our last meeting while I was transitioning out of Stanford, Dr. Gambhir demonstrated the care and support to me at multi-level including stating that 'if you wanted to come back to Stanford, just let me know.'"

Dr. El Assal added, "I still remember that in the 2015 Department of Radiology Retreat, Sam stated, 'I want to make an impact on human health even if it is not recognized in my lifetime.'" *"And I believe he did,"* Dr. El Assal said.

Foreword

It is with great pleasure that I write this foreword for the first edition of *Early Detection and Treatment of Head and Neck Cancer* (HNC). The fields of early detection and early treatment in cancer biology are advancing rapidly as both the concept and practical applications have entered clinical practice.

The recent release of the most comprehensive genomic HNC data to date (Nature, 2015) from The Cancer Genome Atlas, a project funded by the National Institute of Health to characterize cancer genomes, is enabling scientists to refine their list of candidate biomarkers and to identify new ones for early detection of HNCs. Such an expanding body of knowledge is essential given that roughly two-thirds of HNCs present at advanced stages, and the prognosis remains poor. Therefore, new approaches are urgently needed for early HNC detection to improve treatment outcomes. For example, circulating DNA has shown great promise as a non-invasively obtained biomarker in a number of HNC cohorts. Using the known mutational signatures of HNC to identify tumor DNA in body fluids has demonstrated the potential for detecting tumors at early stages and for monitoring tumor relapse and response to treatment.

In the era of precision health and medicine, there are opportunities to select treatment plans that are most likely to succeed based on an individual's personal data. HNC can be monitored and treated more efficiently by taking multiple forms of medical data into consideration and by implementing more effective methodologies that are currently being validated, including liquid biopsy, salivary biomarkers, imaging, and treatments, including gene therapy, immunotherapy, surgery, radiotherapy, and many others.

Early detection is an evidence-based field in which we have come a long way, but it is still in its infancy. We have discovered many of the fundamental principles but still need to develop, translate, and improve detection and diagnostics as well as treatment standards to, hopefully, prevent cancer, including HNC.

Here, I would like to invite readers to enjoy the carefully and expertly prepared material by the authors of this book series (Volumes I and II), which are based on solid scientific evidence and diverse clinical experience achieved through many years of professional practice.

R. Bruce Donoff, DMD, MD
Dean of Harvard School of Dental Medicine (1991–2019)
Boston, MA, USA

Dean Emeritus R. Bruce Donoff in Few Words

Dr. R. Bruce Donoff served as dean of Harvard School of Dental Medicine (HSDM) from 1991 to 2019. He was born in New York City and attended Brooklyn College as an undergraduate. He received his DMD from HSDM in 1967 and his MD from Harvard Medical School in 1973. Dr. Donoff's professional career has centered on Harvard's Faculty of Medicine and the Massachusetts General Hospital's Department of Oral and Maxillofacial Surgery. He began as an intern in 1967, served as chairman and chief of service from 1982 through 1993, and continues to see patients today.

In addition to leading HSDM as its dean, Dr. Donoff has made major contributions in research to the specialty of oral and maxillofacial surgery with interest in oral and head and neck cancers. He has published over one hundred papers, authored textbooks, and lectured worldwide. He recently helped launch the HSDM Initiative – Integrating Oral Health and Medicine, a project of great importance to him.

Dr. Donoff served 12 years on the board of the Oral and Maxillofacial Surgery Foundation and is former president of the Friends of the National Institute of Dental and Craniofacial Research. He is editor of the *MGH Manual of Oral and Maxillofacial Surgery* and a member of the editorial board of the *Journal of Oral and Maxillofacial Surgery* and the *Massachusetts Dental Society Journal*.

Dr. Donoff has received numerous honors during his academic career, including the American Association of Oral and Maxillofacial Surgeons Research Recognition Award, the William J. Gies Foundation Award for Oral and Maxillofacial Surgery, Fellow of the American Association for the Advancement of Science, the Alpha Omega Achievement Award, and the Distinguished Alumni and Faculty Awards from HSDM. In 2014, he was a Shils-Meskin awardee for leadership in the dental profession.

Acknowledgments

A Historic Perspective

I shall be telling this with a sigh somewhere ages and ages hence;
Two roads diverged in a wood, and I took the road less traveled by,
And that has made all the difference.

– The Road Not Taken by Robert Frost, 1916

I would like to acknowledge first and foremost my family:

To my mother who endured this long process with me, always offering support and for whom grace is all in her steps, heaven in her eye, in every gesture dignity and love. Everything I am or ever hope to be, I owe to my angel mother.

To my wife, Somayeh, and my son, Adam, you all are my world and reason for being. My gratitude for your understanding that my career being of service to others often entails long hours. Thank you for your patience and compassion.

To my sister, Lina, who always supported and guided me all the way, and my devoted brother-in-law, Ghiath, and my elegant nieces, Sana, Maria, Naya, and Zeina.

To my brother, Shadi, who was always there for me.

I can never forget my father, who was a blend of strength (may he rest in peace).

To my cousin, Hussein, whose friendship and support I treasure.

To my wife's family: my father- and mother-in-law; brother-in-law, Wahid; and my sisters-in-law, Susan, Samira, Sudaba, and Saeeda.

To my close friends whom I consider part of my family. They helped shape my education and supported me throughout my academic and professional journey.

Additionally, I would like to thank my friends and co-editors, Dyani and Thaddeus; without their help, this book would not have come to fruition. I am so proud of you and wish to let you know that your friendship touches me deeply. I know we will continue to work closely in the future and support one another's ideas and projects.

I would like to express my sincere gratitude to all authors who contributed to these two volumes; this project would not be possible without their contribution.

I feel a deep sense of gratitude to Emeritus Dean R. Bruce Donoff, who kindly wrote the foreword to this book series.

To all of my past teachers, mentors, and fellow students, I hope this book is worthy of the many contributions you have given me.

I am very grateful to all my colleagues and friends around the world.

Lastly, to head and neck cancer (HNC) patients, my respectful and gentle gratitude goes to you all. As a part of our commitment to service HNC patients, I recently co-founded with Thaddeus an "Early Disease Detection & Treatment Fund" to translate innovations from research labs, bringing them close to patients. We are proud to have partnered and invested with visionary entrepreneurs who are tackling head and neck cancers.

Palo Alto, CA, USA   Rami El Assal

Preface

Head and neck cancer (HNC) is a heterogeneous group of cancers that, if combined, represent one of the most common cancer types. Patients with HNC suffer significant morbidity and mortality due to the importance of the structures involved. Over two-thirds of these patients are diagnosed at a late stage, leading to a poor prognosis. Therefore, advancements in early detection and treatment of HNC are crucial.

With the emerging fields of precision health and precision medicine, treatment of HNC is undergoing a paradigm shift to become more proactive instead of predominantly reactive. There is extensive literature to support early detection and early treatment, which has made a significant impact, not only in the field of HNC, but in the management of cancer overall.

Volume I begins with a general overview, including the industry landscape, of HNC detection, diagnosis, and treatment. Next, it covers the applications of innovative technologies such as microfluidics, nanotechnology, and deep learning to early detect as well as study HNC. For example, studying the cellular features at a single-cell level became possible with the advancement of technologies such as mass cytometry or specifically, Cytometry by Time Of Flight Mass Spectrometry (CyTOF), which has revolutionized the way we can study complex human diseases such as HNC. Finally, the last few chapters are dedicated to describing the standard of care of HNC.

The Head and Neck Cancer Early Detection and Treatment book series is highly pertinent to the next generation of interdisciplinary clinicians, scientists, residents, and students who are particularly interested in HNC and in the translation of early detection methods, technologies, and research to clinical practice.

This series is the joint work of many healthcare enthusiasts who share a common vision towards advancing the field of cancer early detection and early treatment. We thank all those individuals who contributed to this book, without whom this effort to fight HNC would not have been possible.

Finally, the editors and contributing authors of this book humbly thank our readers for taking this journey to gain essential knowledge, to refine skills, to inform future research directions, and, above all, to treat our patients suffering from HNC.

Palo Alto, CA, USA   Rami El Assal
Palo Alto, CA, USA   Dyani Gaudilliere
San Francisco, CA, USA   Stephen Thaddeus Connelly

Contents

Contributors

Rafiullah Bashiri Department of Prosthodontics, Division of Comprehensive Oral Health, The University of North Carolina, Adams School of Dentistry, Chapel Hill, NC, USA

Laura Bianciardi Exosomics Spa, Siena, Italy

Karl C. Bruckman Division of Plastic & Reconstructive Surgery, Department of Surgery, Stanford University School of Medicine, Stanford, CA, USA

Deborah J. Chute Department of Pathology, Cleveland Clinic, Cleveland, OH, USA

Claudio Corallo Exosomics Spa, Siena, Italy

Mattia Criscuoli Exosomics Spa, Siena, Italy

Vasu Divi Division of Plastic & Reconstructive Surgery, Department of Surgery, Stanford University School of Medicine, Stanford, CA, USA

Mehdi Ebrahimi Prince Philip Dental Hospital, The University of Hong Kong, Sai Ying Pun, Hong Kong

Jakob F. Einhaus Stanford University School of Medicine, Department of Anesthesia, Stanford, CA, USA
Eberhard Karls University of Tübingen, Tübingen, Germany

Diogo Fortunato Exosomics Spa, Siena, Italy

Brice Gaudilliere Stanford University School of Medicine, Department of Anesthesia, Stanford, CA, USA

Dyani Gaudilliere Division of Plastic & Reconstructive Surgery, Department of Surgery, Stanford University School of Medicine, Palo Alto, CA, USA

Christopher C. Griffith Department of Pathology, Cleveland Clinic, Cleveland, OH, USA

Julien Hedou Stanford University School of Medicine, Department of Anesthesia, Stanford, CA, USA

Andrew Janowczyk Department of Biomedical Engineering, Case Western Reserve University, Cleveland, OH, USA

Maryam Khalili Department of Restorative Dentistry, Temple University Maurice H. Kornberg School of Dentistry, Philadelphia, PA, USA

Nagarjun Konduru Department of Cellular and Molecular Biology, University of Texas Health Science Center at Tyler, Tyler, TX, USA

Can Koyuncu Department of Biomedical Engineering, Case Western Reserve University, Cleveland, OH, USA

Shilpa Kusampudi Department of Cellular and Molecular Biology, University of Texas Health Science Center at Tyler, Tyler, TX, USA

James S. Lewis Jr. Vanderbilt University Medical Center, Department of Pathology, Microbiology and Immunology, Nashville, TN, USA

Cheng Lu Department of Biomedical Engineering, Case Western Reserve University, Cleveland, OH, USA

Anant Madabhushi Department of Biomedical Engineering, Case Western Reserve University, Cleveland, OH, USA

Louis Stokes Cleveland Veterans Administration Medical Center, Cleveland, OH, USA

David Perrault Division of Plastic & Reconstructive Surgery, Department of Surgery, Stanford University School of Medicine, Stanford, CA, USA

Ryan Spitler Stanford University, School of Medicine, Stanford, CA, USA

Amy S. Tsai Stanford University School of Medicine, Department of Anesthesia, Stanford, CA, USA

University of California, Davis School of Medicine, Sacramento, CA, USA

Eileen Tsai Stanford University School of Medicine, Department of Anesthesia, Stanford, CA, USA

Ohio State University College of Medicine, Columbus, OH, USA

Hongjun Wang Department of Biomedical Engineering, Stevens Institute of Technology, Hoboken, NJ, USA

Saul Weiner Department of Restorative Dentistry, Rutgers School of Dental Medicine, Newark, NJ, USA

Department of Biomedical Engineering, Stevens institute of Technology, Hoboken, NJ, USA

Robin T. Wu Division of Plastic & Reconstructive Surgery, Department of Surgery, Stanford University School of Medicine, Stanford, CA, USA

Yamin Yang Department of Biomedical Engineering, Nanjing University of Aeronautics and Astronautics, Nanjing, Jiangsu, China

Natasa Zarovni Exosomics Spa, Siena, Italy

Davide Zocco Exosomics Spa, Siena, Italy

Chapter 1
Overview of Early Detection, Diagnosis, and Treatment of Head and Neck Cancers

Ryan Spitler

Introduction

Cancer is the second most common cause of death in the United States [11]. Often, symptoms are not specific or present, until tumors have already metastasized. Head and neck cancers (HNCs) include all malignancies from nasal and oral cavities, pharynx, larynx, and the paranasal sinuses with smoking and alcoholism being known predisposing factors. HNCs make up 3% of all cancer cases in the United States each year with over 90% of HNCs arising from squamous cell carcinomas and head and neck squamous cell carcinoma (HNSCC), which is the sixth common cause of cancer mortality globally [38]. When compared to other cancers such as breast or colorectal cancer, the five-year survival rate of HNSCC after diagnosis is significantly lower and with little to no improvement in mortality rates even with ongoing research efforts [40]. Failure in early diagnosis and insufficient effectiveness of therapeutic modalities lead to poor clinical outcomes [36]. Thus, the ability to diagnose cancer at an early stage is critically important, since the predominant cause of mortality is regional and/or distal metastatic spreading of tumor cells from the primary site. There is a significant need for rapid, highly accurate, and noninvasive tools for cancer screening, early detection, diagnostics, and prognostics. Screening methodologies should have high sensitivity and specificity, be noninvasive, and be inexpensive to allow widespread applicability. Even though molecular alteration precedes clinical symptoms and detection by imaging or histopathology-based diagnosis, many disorders remain undiagnosed until an advanced stage, which is often irreversible, and treatment is inefficient/ineffective. However, there have been many recent developments that are beginning to demonstrate promise.

R. Spitler (✉)
Precision Health and Integrated Diagnostics (PHIND) Center,
Stanford University School of Medicine, Palo Alto, CA, USA
e-mail: rspitler@stanford.edu

© Springer Nature Switzerland AG 2021
R. El Assal et al. (eds.), *Early Detection and Treatment of Head & Neck Cancers*, https://doi.org/10.1007/978-3-030-69859-1_1

In the era of precision health and medicine, there are opportunities to diagnose cancers early and to select treatment plans that are most likely to succeed based on an individual's personal data. Importantly, cancers originating from different parts of the body have different characteristics and require different diagnoses and treatment approaches [51]. In order to address this need, HNCs can be monitored and treated more efficiently taking into consideration multiple forms of medical data and implementing more effective methodologies that are currently being validated including liquid biopsy, salivary biomarkers, imaging, and treatments including gene therapy, immunotherapy, surgery, radiotherapy, and many others [1, 7, 10, 12, 15, 37]. In this review, recent developments in diagnostics and treatment management for HNCs are described.

Big Data in HNC

A large part of being able to detect and treat cancers "precisely" is having sufficient data available to make informed and actionable clinical decisions. HNCs represent an opportunity to explore "big data" applications in oncology. In the era of growing big data and artificial intelligence capabilities, there exists tremendous potential to implement computational strategies to better understand molecular mechanisms and complex biological systems, identify prognostics and predictive biomarkers, and for the discovery and monitoring of treatment. Big data may assist with broad applications including driving and sustaining guideline recommendations, expediting the period between research and clinical practice, monitoring guideline applications and quality assurance, and helping work toward a personalized healthcare decision support system [42]. Aggregating and sharing research data can be particularly useful in the case of rare cancers. However, even with great promise, there are still many challenges that exist to implement big data strategies.

Researchers tend to use many different platforms to store and analyze data, which present significant challenges for handling large volumes of data. Moreover, researchers often do not have access to raw or primary data sources and lack the necessary infrastructure. One potential solution has been to use "data clouds" to better integrate and improve overall access to data. However, even if these resources become accessible, there is still the question of how best to protect patient privacy and share data while keeping it de-identified. As efforts continue to increase in this area and with some patience and the right know-how, these mountains of data can significantly contribute to our understanding of cancer's inner workings.

Diagnostics and Early Detection

It is known that the chance of survival and quality of life in HNC is directly related to the size of the primary tumor at detection. One challenge is that most patients, even those at risk (smokers), will likely not participate in screening programs until they present with symptoms. In order to have a significant impact on early detection, primary (measures that prevent the onset of disease) and secondary prevention (measures for early diagnosis and treatment of disease) will need to be improved. Screening for cancer can be population-based, opportunistic, or targeted, but ultimately, patients have to elect to participate. Some community-based screening has shown value in reducing oral cancers in high-risk groups. The most powerful tools in early detection for HNC are medical history, risk factors, and clinical examination [19]. Recent advances in early cancer detection methods have improved clinician's ability for early diagnoses, such as using saliva specimens to identify asymptomatic patients at cancer risk. For oral cancers, visual examination remains the primary initial screen method. Additionally, there is a need to further examine cost-effectiveness for cancer screening and early detection methods. HNCs are diagnosed most often among people over the age of 50. Common symptoms of HNCs include a lump or sore that does not heal, sore throat that does not go away, difficulty swallowing, and hoarseness. Other symptoms may include discoloration of the lining of the mouth, swelling of the jaw, trouble breathing, trouble hearing, blocked sinuses, and paralysis of the muscles in the face [18]. Yet once symptoms present, the likelihood for successful treatment outcomes greatly diminishes.

Liquid Biopsy and Circulating Tumor Cells

HNC remains one of the leading causes of death, which is why early detection is critically important [53]. Liquid biopsy has emerged as a promising tool for detecting and monitoring disease status at all stages. Analyses of circulating tumor DNA (ctDNA), circulating tumor cells (CTCs), and exosomal miRNAs have paved the way for precision health and medicine approaches. Circulating biomarkers have demonstrated efficacy for detection, treatment, and monitoring response as well as prognosis assessment [41]. While these new biomarkers may have broad clinical application, no validated circulating biomarkers have been integrated into clinical practice in the context of HNC. However, there is great potential for the clinical utility of these biomarkers from multiple body fluids. In general, ctDNA in the plasma could be useful for the early detection of HNC [2]. CTCs released from metastatic lesions can be analyzed for surface expression of drug targets including EGFR and PD-L1 for planning therapeutic interventions [54, 55]. Additional information can be gained from biomarkers such as exosomal miRNAs, and the ability to target multiple types of biomarkers may improve the specificity and sensitivity of cancer diagnosis [43]. Analyzing biomarkers from multiple body fluids in conjunction with other measures could enable better delivery of personalized medicine approaches (Fig. 1.1).

Of particular interest for screening purposes is saliva, which is a mixture of secretions from major and minor salivary glands. These secretions contain proteins, microorganisms, and cellular debris. The use of whole saliva is an attractive diagnostic method since it is relatively easy to work with, is noninvasive, and can

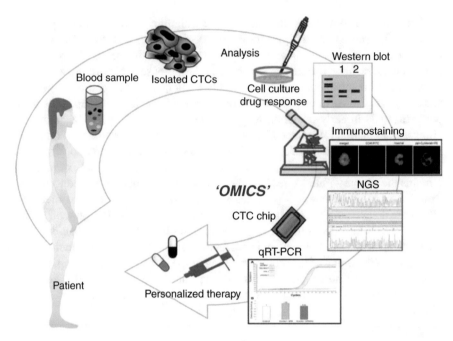

Fig. 1.1 Overview of analysis of patient-derived CTCs. CTCs are isolated from a patient's blood sample and analyzed using methods such as immunostaining, Western blotting, NGS, CTC-chip analysis, and qRT-PCR. The results can then be used to develop better precision health and medicine approaches. (Figure reproduced with permission from [23])

provide informative diagnostic information regarding disease state. Moreover, a unique subset of exosomes from tumors appear to be present in saliva and are highly variable even in patients with the same tumor types and stages [54, 55]. More work is needed toward the creation of simple and affordable technologies to screen for circulating biomarkers; however, further characterization will be required in order for implementation to be possible.

There is a significant demand for simple less invasive blood tests to determine disease state. Standard clinical diagnostics, such as imaging, often lack the sensitivity to enable the detection of CTCs. Techniques are also required for molecular characterization to better enable understanding of the underlying biology, which could then lead to improved tumor targeting capabilities. The ability to identify high-risk patients prior to disease presentation or metastasis could significantly improve rates of survival. Current methods are limited by specificity and sensitivity. However, nanotechnology-based methods could improve efficiency, sensitivity, specificity, and accuracy [23].

Salivary Biomarkers

Saliva has emerged as a potential source of cancer biomarkers including proteins, DNA, mRNA, and metabolites [54, 55]. It is composed of secretions from the major and minor salivary glands and is extensively in the lining of the mouth and throat. Saliva is simple to collect and process, is cost-effective, and does not cause patient discomfort. Unlike other bodily fluids, saliva tends to have a lower background of inhibitory substances and materials when compared with blood [48]. Saliva for the screening of oral cancer has great potential, due to the shed of cancer cells in the oral cavity. Several salivary biomarkers for clinical use have been discovered using ELISA, quantitative PCR, microarrays, immunoblot, and LC/MS. Some of these biomarkers could be used to monitoring for cancer diagnosis and cancer risk prediction using differences in the expression of proteins, genes, RNA, and/or inflammatory cytokines [22]. While most of these biomarkers have limitations in clinical diagnosis, one notable example is interleukin (IL)-8 and melanoma-associated genes, which have demonstrated good sensitivity and specificity [25]. Similarly, IL-8 and IL-1ß have been found to be elevated in HNSCC patients as well as having a significantly different microbial environment compared to healthy controls [52]. Further, advanced stages of oral cavity squamous cell carcinoma (OSCC) have shown higher levels of proteins complement factor H (CFH), fibrinogen alpha chain (FGA), and alpha-1-antitrypsin (SERPINA1) [8]. Overall, these predictive and prognostic markers can hopefully one day be used as therapeutic targets to treat HNCs including HNSCC.

Imaging

Many optical tools are being used to enhance diagnostics and treatment beyond the clinician's trained eye. Approaches such as chromoendoscopy and autofluorescence can help identify altered mucosal areas. While hyperspectral imaging can be used to discover suspicious lesions, optical coherence tomography and confocal endomicroscopy can be used to better identify structural abnormalities or when subcellular resolution is needed [9]. For the head and neck area with complex lymph drainage, it is important to be as exact as possible with functional imaging techniques (e.g., positron emission tomography/computed tomography (PET/CT) scanning) [35]. This is especially important during the early stages of tumor development, so that the resection margin is minimized to preserve the organ. This type of imaging is also important after a treatment and during the recovery phase.

Surgery still remains the first-line choice for treating HNC patients. However, surgeons must often balance between extensive cancer resection and a better quality of life, given the complicated anatomy in the head and neck region. To improve clinical outcomes, early diagnosis and treatment of premalignancies are necessary. Moreover, many real-time imaging approaches can be used for *in vivo* detection of surgical margins to better identify cancers and minimize the resection of normal tissues. Such approaches include autofluorescence imaging, targeted fluorescence imaging, high-resolution microendoscopy, narrow-band imaging, and Raman spectroscopy [56]. Another approach is to combine new approaches with existing ones, such as using imaging guidance and a surgical robot [33]. However, even with decades of research in this area, still many challenges exist. For instance, Raman spectrometers are generally not as commercially available or portable and as such are generally not used for routine clinical procedures. Additionally, more clinical trials are needed to demonstrate benefits beyond diagnostic accuracy.

For early-stage cancers, typically a single modality, usually contrast-enhanced CT, is sufficient for adequately staging. However, it is often desirable for the management of advanced cancers (stage III/IV) to use a combined modality approach (PET/CT with or without contrast-enhanced CT or MRI). This combines the advantages of both modalities providing improved cross-sectional anatomical details and superior soft-tissue contrast, both especially important in the context of head and neck squamous cell carcinoma (HNSCC). Multidisciplinary treatment is often required and includes surgery, radiotherapy, and chemotherapy [49]. One such probe that has proven especially useful for these patients is fludeoxyglucose F 18 PET/CT [16].

Extracellular Vesicles

Extracellular vesicles (EVs) are heterogeneous membrane-enclosed vesicles, which play a key role in intercellular communication for processes such as proliferation, metastasis, angiogenesis, and immune regulation [58]. Studies have shown that tumor-derived EVs, mainly exosome and microvesicles, transfer oncogenic cargo such as proteins, lipids, messenger RNAs, microRNA, noncoding RNAs, and DNAs that may influence the tumor microenvironment (TME) and impact tumor progression [57]. While the molecular mechanisms and clinical applications of EVs in HNC still require further investigation, the ability to better understand this complex signaling network in mediating tumor progression, angiogenesis, and cancer drug resistance, as well as immune regulation, could be very valuable. EVs can be sampled and assessed from saliva and circulating blood diagnostics and have the potential for early screening, monitoring, and risk assessment of HNCs. EVs may also be useful for creating more precise anti-tumor treatments for individual therapy due to their inherent biocompatibility, being modifiable, and low immunogenicity [21]. An example is EVs derived from nasopharyngeal carcinoma, which have been reported to facilitate proliferation, metastasis, and immune escape [6]. These EVs could serve as biomarkers as well as therapeutic targets, given their unique nucleic acid and protein content profiles.

Multiplexed Biomarker Profiling

We have discussed a number of potential diagnostic tools that are actively being implemented for early cancer detection and intervention. While these tools can be implemented on an individual basis, there is often also the possibility of enhanced diagnostic power through the combination of biomarkers. For instance, in the context of immune-based biomarkers, panels have been used that consist of multiple cytokines, chemokines, growth factors, and other relevant tumor biomarkers [27]. Additionally, immune profiling of HNSCC patients using a multiplex immunofluorescence panel has produced evidence to suggest that p16 tumors could be immunosuppressed through increased expression of PD-L1, while CD8+ cells cannot infiltrate the tumor [20]. Another study used an electrochemiluminescence multiplex assay and was able to classify OSCC versus normal subgroups using IL2, IL_1R_a, and macrophage inhibitory factor (MIF) with a sensitivity of 0.96 and specificity of 0.92 [28]. It is likely that combinations of biomarkers will become used more frequently, which are expected to improve clinical outcomes.

Treatment and Cancer Management

Great care must be given to the treatment of HNCs especially due to the potential toxicity of treatment proximity to critical structures [30]. This is also why it is important to initially exhaust noninvasive and/or lower-morbidity approaches prior to performing more invasive procedures. Optimal treatment should also include (i) early detection of recurrence or residual disease and (ii) minimalization of toxicity and morbidity and (iii) should be cost-effective for the healthcare system and the patient. Posttreatment surveillance is critically important, such as the use of imaging modalities including PET-CT. However, in the context of imaging, there is no consensus guidelines on the frequency and modality (i.e., CT, ultrasound, MRI, and PET-CT) used for posttreatment imaging [59]. More work is needed to improve the current guidelines as well as to come up with individualized surveillance plans that better address patient's needs.

Gene Therapy

Gene therapy can be a viable approach for HNC as there is a current lack of systemic options, there are many potential targets, and tumor tissue is accessible. There are multiple types of gene therapy used for HNCs including corrective, cytoreductive, and gene editing [10]. While gene therapy has been an emerging area, most patients will still require the inclusion of standard therapy methods such as surgery, radiation, and chemo- or immunotherapy. In order to successfully deliver gene therapy, it is essential to first understand a patient's unique genetic profile. For example, in the case of HNSCC, patients' common mechanisms to target include oncogenes, EGFR receptor, p53 gene correction, prodrugs for suicide gene therapy, and immunomodulatory strategies [45]. Some of these approaches will be generalizable between cancer types, whereas others will be patient-/cancer-specific in order to improve successful outcomes. This is yet another example of how precision medicine is already beginning to shape cancer care.

Cancer Immunotherapy

Cancer immunotherapy is driven by the body's ability to recognize tumor cells as a foreign antigen, thereby triggering the activation of the immune system. One potential advantage of immunotherapy over cytotoxic chemotherapy is possible durable response of memory T cells, with induction of T cell immunity being a critical step to success [5]. This field is already seeing great progress with FDA-approved anti-PD-1 antibodies including nivolumab and pembrolizumab showing efficacy in clinical trials [47]. However, there are still challenges for clinicians to better understand when to use immunotherapy and in which clinical setting in order to provide improved clinical benefit. Additionally, cancers such as HNSCC are known for their immunosuppressive character, reducing the effectiveness of immune-based approaches. Moreover, many patients generate immune responses to the presented antigen, but they still do not respond to conventional treatment or immunotherapy [44]. Yet patients with preexisting endogenous immune response have better outcomes than those lacking an activated phenotype. To advance the field of immunotherapy, more robust markers of treatment efficacy must be developed as well as an increased understanding of patient immune responsiveness and how to best leverage combined therapies (Fig. 1.2).

Robotic Surgery

Many minimally invasive approaches for head and neck surgery now incorporate robotic surgery. Transoral robotic surgery has been used for resecting oropharyngeal, hypopharyngeal, and laryngeal tumors [17]. Other applications include transaxillary, transoral, and retroauricular robotic approaches for the neck and thyroid also exist. Important factors to consider are safety, cost, availability, and outcomes when considering the utility of robotic surgery. It is also necessary to have a skilled operator. Fortunately, many new surgeons have been receiving formal training in robotic surgery. It is anticipated that minimally invasive robotic head and neck surgery will continue to be pioneered and lead to more positive clinical outcomes.

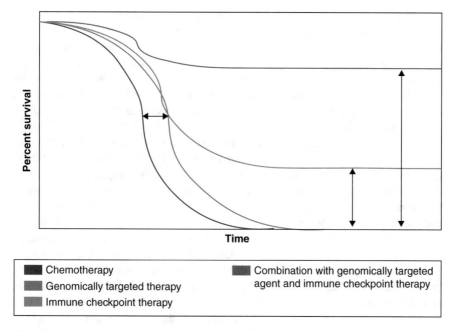

Fig. 1.2 The potential of immunotherapy. The Kaplan-Meier curve tail demonstrates how the combination of complementary approaches used in conjunction with other immunotherapies could lead to better outcomes. (With permission from [46])

Radiotherapy

In general, patients with early-stage HNCs limited to the site of origin are good candidates for radiation therapy or surgery. The treatment plan and behavior of the cancer is dependent on the primary site of origin. A "simulation" of the particular treatment plan can be generated using scans such as X-rays and CTs. Based on these data, the ideal medical physics can be determined. Much care must be taken based on the cancer location with the side effects of treatment dependent on the site and extent of cancer. Definitive radiotherapy or adjuvant management has been demonstrated to be a reasonable treatment for early- and late-stage cancers such as non-melanoma skin cancers and Merkel cell carcinoma [32]. Altered fractionation radiotherapy has been shown to improve survival in patients with HNSCC. When comparing different types of altered radiotherapy, evidence suggests that hyperfractionation provides the greatest benefit [1].

Molecular Diagnostics for Personalized Treatment

In order to develop personalized treatment plans, it is necessary to have biomarkers that are effective for predicting therapeutic response and large-scale molecular profiling to identify subgroups for particular prognostics. While next-generation sequencing is readily being used for genetic profiling, this technique is still limited by cost, interpretation of data, and validation of results. There are, however, a number of statistical techniques that have been developed to address the challenge of interpreting large data sets. Microarray analysis has also been used but has challenges such as the use of different platforms, experimental protocols, and other variables. Functional genomics is also adding to the possibilities of discovery and implementation. Some examples of how this can be implemented are described.

At present, only the site and stage of tumor are used for treatment planning of HNSCC [31]. Both molecular profiling and SLNB are promising tools to optimize lymph node staging and adequate management of HNC. Prognosis of HNSCC improved only moderately during the last decades. This improvement may relate to a steady increase in oropharyngeal cancers caused by human papillomavirus (HPV) that have a very favorable prognosis. Detection of residual cancer cells may provide early discovery of recurrent disease and tailoring of postoperative radiation or chemoradiation therapy but is hampered by sampling error. Detection of premalignant fields by molecular markers reliably predicts malignant transformation. Noninvasive diagnostics may further enhance clinical implementation. At present, two clinically relevant molecular subgroups are recognized: HPV-positive tumors and HPV-negative tumors. Personalized treatment of HPV-positive tumors is within reach, but accurate detection of HPV in formalin-fixed paraffin-embedded specimens is still challenging. A third molecular subgroup is emerging, which is characterized by few chromosomal aberrations, wild-type TP53, and a favorable prognosis. Other molecular subgroups of HNSCC have been established with gene expression profiling, but the clinical relevance still remains to be established.

Cancer Tumor Cells and Cancer Stem Cells

CTCs represent a subset of cells that escape the primary tumor and enter the bloodstream and can be an important point of early cancer detection given that even high-resolution PET/CT and MRI are currently unable to detect the early spread of tumor cells. Moreover, even with improvement in current treatment approaches, there is still up to 50–60% local-regional recurrence and/or distant metastasis [39]. CTCs can form metastatic deposits and can sometimes reestablish themselves at the primary cancer site. These cells tend to be more aggressive and accumulate genetic alterations, due to additional modifications acquired when in circulation [24]. Liquid biopsy is an emerging technology to create a reliable method for minimally invasive analysis (i.e., genotyping) of small-volume blood samples. The data can then be applied beyond early detection as well as developing treatments, treatment monitoring, and assessing mutational changes in cancer resistance and radiation sensitivity. While this is a promising new area, there is currently limited guidance in utilizing CTC data. The true prognostic value of CTCs is still to be determined and will require a deeper understanding of the complex interplay at the cellular level.

The growth of cancer is maintained by a population of cancer stem cells (CSCs), which have an unlimited self-renewal potential and can continue to induce tumor growth if this population of cells is not completely eliminated by therapy. Thereby, CSCs can be a target for treatment as well as used as a cancer biomarker of treatment efficacy [3]. The prognostic and predictive potential can be determined by measuring the number of CSCs present, if any, after treatment [50]. Clinical outcomes can potentially improve using CSC-targeted strategies, especially to sensitize resistant tumor cells. However, there can be strong side effects resulting from this type of treatment as stem cell targeting strategies also affect common stem cell signaling mechanisms. While this approach has shown some potential, further clinical validation is necessary before this approach can be implemented, and more preclinical model validation is also necessary. There is significant work already underway to develop effective methods of engineering individualized therapies to improve patient's response.

Epigenetic Modifications

Progression of oral carcinogenesis results from a complex interplay of epigenetic alternations including DNA methylation, histone covalent modifications, chromatin remodeling, and noncoding RNAs [4]. These pathways can also play a role in cancer resistance to therapy. Epigenetic alterations occur as part of the aberrant transcriptional machinery and give a selective advantage to tumor cells. The modifications also contribute to cellular plasticity during tumor progression and can lead to the formation of CSCs. Thus, understanding epigenetic modifications and markers associated with HNC may lead to new strategies for therapy. These novel therapies can also be used in combination with conventional therapies to increase the potential for treatment effectiveness. This is still a research area that requires further exploration.

Recurrent and Metastatic Cancers

While recurrent and metastatic HNC is usually incurable, precision oncology, using tools such as molecular profiling, is improving our ability to better understand molecular alternations and better manage treatment-resistant HNCs. By identifying more actionable alterations, there will be a larger portion of patients that can have earlier diagnosis and guide treatment of rare and advanced cancers. For instance, the molecular profile of recurrent and metastatic tumors is quite distinct from primary tumors (Fig. 1.3) [34]. However, one challenge is that many HNCs tend to be understudied due to how rare they are. In order for a precision-based approach to be possible, it will be necessary to sequence recurrent and metastatic tumors. Unfortunately,

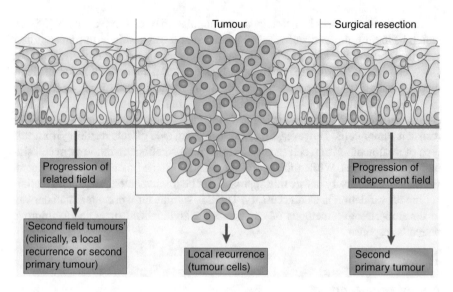

Fig. 1.3 Local relapse: three sources of recurrent disease. (i) Local recurrence resulting from cells left behind after tumor resection, (ii) a second tumor resulting from a premalignant cell and clonally related to the original tumor, and (iii) a second tumor from unrelated premalignant cells. Molecular analysis must be used to distinguish between local recurrence and second field tumors. (Reproduced with permission [26])

in the last decades, the overall survival rate has only improved marginally. This has come about because cancer was only detected after an advanced clinical stage of diagnosis and this is associated with a high rate of treatment failure. Other issues as described in previous sections are cancer cells left behind after surgical resection and more aggressive cancers (oftentimes more than the primary site) resulting from CTCs. Outcomes are slowly improving with more effective screening and treatment approaches.

Conclusion

HNCs can lead to rapid deterioration of the patient due to the proximity of the tumor in the human body and other associated issues such as malnutrition and disability associated with disease. Similarly, careful consideration must be given towards treatment plans and doses to improve the quality of life as well as extend the life of the patient, if a cure is not possible. While many challenges still exist, the fields of precision health [13], precision medicine [14], and digital health [29] hold much promise to addressing these still unmet needs. The emerging technologies enable earlier detection of disease, which should result in better clinical outcomes, especially if more efforts are put towards prevention and early detection in addition to treatment approaches. Additional clinical data is being generated at an ever-increasing rate, and the digital health revolution is now allowing physicians and scientists to start taking advantage of these data-driven approaches. Some key issues to address will be providing access to these approaches at a population level, adjusting screening, and guidance documents for new capabilities, as well as presenting data to be best utilized by the physician while also empowering the patient. The era of precision head and neck oncology has arrived and is already becoming implemented.

References

1. Baujat B, Bourhis J, Blanchard P, Overgaard J, Ang KK, Saunders M, Le Maître A, Bernier J, Horiot JC, Maillard E, Pajak TF, Poulsen MG, Bourredjem A, O'Sullivan B, Dobrowsky W, Andrzej H, Skladowski K, Hay JH, Pinto LH, Fu KK, Fallai C, Sylvester R, Pignon JP, Audry H, Bourhis J, Bolla M, Duchateau L, Hill C, Pignon JP, Sylvester R, Syz N, Ang KK, Bernier J, Dische S, Eschwege F, Fu KK, Horiot JC, Overgaard J, Parmar MKB, Ang KK, Awwad HK, Baerg B, Benhamou E, Bernier J, Bourhis J, Collette L, Cummings BJ, Dische S, Dobrowsky W, Denham JW, Fallai C, Fu KK, Grau C, Hansen HS, Hay JH, Hliniak A, Horiot JC, Jacskon SM, Kraszewska E, Lotayef M, Maciejewski B, Olmi P, O'Sullivan B, Overgaard J, Pajak TF, Parmar MKB, Pintilie M, Pinto LHJ, Poulsen MG, Saunders M, Skladowski K, Tandon N, Torri V, Widder J, Baujat B, Blanchard P, Bourredjem A. Hyperfractionated or accelerated radiotherapy for head and neck cancer. Cochrane Database Syst Rev. 2010;12:CD002026.
2. Bellairs JA, Hasina R, Agrawal N. Tumor DNA: an emerging biomarker in head and neck cancer. Cancer Metastasis Rev. 2017;36:515–23.
3. Bhaijee F, Pepper DJ, Pitman KT, Bell D. Cancer stem cells in head and neck squamous cell carcinoma: a review of current knowledge and future applications. Head Neck. 2012;34:894–9.
4. Castilho RM, Squarize CH, Almeida LO. Epigenetic modifications and head and neck cancer: implications for tumor progression and resistance to therapy. Int J Mol Sci. 2017;18:1506.
5. Chanana R, Noronha V, Joshi A, Patil V, Prabhash K. Evolving role of immunotherapy in head-and-neck cancers: a systemic review. J Head Neck Physicians Surg. 2018;6:2–11.
6. Cheng S, Li Z, He J, Fu S, Duan Y, Zhou Q, Yan Y, Liu X, Liu L, Feng C, Zhang L, He J, Deng Y, Sun L-Q. Epstein–Barr virus noncoding RNAs from the extracellular vesicles of nasopharyngeal carcinoma (NPC) cells promote angiogenesis via TLR3/RIG-I-mediated VCAM-1 expression. Biochim Biophys Acta Mol basis Dis. 2019;1865:1201–13.
7. Cheng Y-S, Rees T, Wright J. A review of research on salivary biomarkers for oral cancer detection. Clin Transl Med. 2014;3:3.
8. Chu HW, Chang KP, Hsu CW, Chang IYF, Liu HP, Chen YT, Wu CC. Identification of salivary biomarkers for oral cancer detection with untargeted and targeted quantitative proteomics approaches. Mol Cell Proteomics. 2019;18:1796–806.
9. Deutsche Gesellschaft für Hals-Nasen-Ohrenheilkunde KH, Deutsche Gesellschaft für Hals-Nasen-Ohrenheilkunde KHJ n.d. GMS current topics in otorhinolaryngology, head and neck surgery. Deutsche Gesellschaft für Hals-Nasen-Ohren-Heilkunde, Kopf- und Hals-Chirurgie.
10. Farmer ZL, Kim ES, Carrizosa DR. Gene therapy in head and neck cancer. Oral Maxillofac Surg Clin North Am. 2019;31:117–24.
11. FastStats – Leading Causes of Death [WWW Document] n.d. URL https://www.cdc.gov/nchs/fastats/leading-causes-of-death.htm. Accessed 6.11.19.
12. Ferris RL. Immunology and immunotherapy of head and neck cancer. J Clin Oncol. 2015;36:6061.
13. Gambhir SS, Ge TJ, Vermesh O, Spitler R. Toward achieving precision health. Sci Transl Med. 2018;3612:1–6.

14. Gameiro G, Sinkunas V, Liguori G, Auler-Júnior J. Precision medicine: changing the way we think about healthcare. Clinics. 2018;73:e723.
15. Garg A, Dwivedi RC, Sayed S, Katna R, Komorowski A, Pathak KA, Rhys-Evans P, Kazi R. Robotic surgery in head and neck cancer: a review. Oral Oncol. 2010;46:571–6.
16. Goel R, Moore W, Sumer B, Khan S, Sher D, Subramaniam RM. Clinical practice in PET/CT for the management of head and neck squamous cell cancer. Am J Roentgenol. 2017;209:289–303.
17. Gorphe P. A contemporary review of evidence for transoral robotic surgery in laryngeal cancer. Front Oncol. 2018;8:121.
18. Head and Neck Cancer: Symptoms and Signs | Cancer.Net [WWW Document], n.d. URL https://www.cancer.net/cancer-types/head-and-neck-cancer/symptoms-and-signs. Accessed 6.8.19.
19. Iyer S, Thankappan K, Balasubramanian D. Early detection of oral cancers: current status and future prospects. Curr Opin Otolaryngol Head Neck Surg. 2016;24:110–4.
20. De La Iglesia J, Martin L, Van Veen T, Song F. Immune profiling of head and neck squamous cell carcinoma (HNSCC) by a multiplex immunofluorescence (mIF) panel using multispectral microscopy. J Clin Oncol. 2018;36:6061.
21. Jabalee J, Towle R, Garnis C. The role of extracellular vesicles in cancer: cargo, function, and therapeutic implications. Cells. 2018;7:93.
22. Khurshid Z, Zafar MS, Khan RS, Najeeb S, Slowey PD, Rehman IU. Role of salivary biomarkers in oral cancer detection. Adv Clin Chem. 2018;86:23–70.
23. Künzel J, Gribko A, Lu Q, Stauber RH, Wünsch D. Nanomedical detection and downstream analysis of circulating tumor cells in head and neck patients. Biol Chem. 2019;400:1465–79.
24. Lambert AW, Pattabiraman DR, Weinberg RA. Emerging biological principles of metastasis. Cell. 2017;168(4):670–91.
25. Lee K-D, Lee H-S, Jeon C-H. Body fluid biomarkers for early detection of head and neck squamous cell carcinomas. Anticancer Res. 2011;31:1161–7.
26. Leemans CR, Braakhuis BJM, Brakenhoff RH. The molecular biology of head and neck cancer. Nat Rev Cancer. 2011;11:9–22.
27. Linkov F, Lisovich A, Yurkovetsky Z, Marrangoni A, Velikokhatnaya L, Nolen B, Winans M, Bigbee W, Siegfried J, Lokshin A, Ferris RL. Early detection of head and neck cancer: development of a novel screening tool using multiplexed immunobead-based biomarker profiling. Cancer Epidemiol Biomark Prev. 2007;16:102–7.
28. Liu KYP, Lu XJD, Zhu YS, Le N, Kim H, Poh CF. Plasma-derived inflammatory proteins predict oral squamous cell carcinoma. Front Oncol. 2018;8:585.
29. Mathews SC, McShea MJ, Hanley CL, Ravitz A, Labrique AB, Cohen AB. Digital health: a path to validation. npj Digit Med. 2019;2:38.
30. McKeever MR, Sio TT, Gunn GB, Holliday EB, Blanchard P, Kies MS, Weber RS, Frank SJ. Reduced acute toxicity and improved efficacy from intensity-modulated proton therapy (IMPT) for the management of head and neck cancer. Chinese Clin Oncol. 2016;5:54.
31. Mes SW, Leemans CR, Brakenhoff RH. Applications of molecular diagnostics for personalized treatment of head and neck cancer: state of the art. Expert Rev Mol Diagn. 2016;16:205–21.
32. Mierzwa ML. Radiotherapy for skin cancers of the face, head, and neck. Facial Plast Surg Clin North Am. 2019;27:131–8.
33. Morinière S. Transoral robotic surgery in head and neck cancer. In: Head and neck cancer: multimodality management. 2nd ed. New York, NY: Springer; 2016.
34. Morris LGT, Chandramohan R, West L, Zehir A, Chakravarty D, Pfister DG, Wong RJ, Lee NY, Sherman EJ, Baxi SS, Ganly I, Singh B, Shah JP, Shaha AR, Boyle JO, Patel SG, Roman BR, Barker CA, McBride SM, Chan TA, Dogan S, Hyman DM, Berger MF, Solit DB, Riaz N, Ho AL. The molecular landscape of recurrent and metastatic head and neck cancers: insights from a precision oncology sequencing platform. JAMA Oncol. 2017;3(2):244–55.
35. Müller-Richter UDA, Gesierich A, Kübler AC, Hartmann S, Brands RC. Merkel cell carcinoma of the head and neck: recommendations for diagnostics and treatment. Ann Surg Oncol. 2017;24:3430–7.

36. Neal RD, Tharmanathan P, France B, Din NU, Cotton S, Fallon-Ferguson J, Hamilton W, Hendry A, Hendry M, Lewis R, Macleod U, Mitchell ED, Pickett M, Rai T, Shaw K, Stuart N, Tørring ML, Wilkinson C, Williams B, Williams N, Emery J. Is increased time to diagnosis and treatment in symptomatic cancer associated with poorer outcomes? Systematic review. Br J Cancer. 2015;112 Suppl 1(Suppl 1):S92–107.
37. Nonaka T, Wong DTW. Liquid biopsy in head and neck cancer: promises and challenges. J Dent Res. 2018;97:701–8.
38. Overview of Head and Neck Cancer – American Head & Neck Society [WWW Document], n.d. URL https://www.ahns.info/patient-information/understanding-head-neck-cancer/overview/. Accessed 6.8.19.
39. Perumal V, Corica T, Dharmarajan A, Sun Z, Dhaliwal S, Dass C, Dass J. Circulating tumour cells (CTC), head and neck cancer and radiotherapy. Cancers (Basel): Future Perspectives; 2019.
40. Pulte D, Brenner H. Changes in survival in head and neck cancers in the late 20th and early 21st century: a period analysis. Oncologist. 2010;15:994–1001.
41. Rapisuwon S, Vietsch EE, Wellstein A. Circulating biomarkers to monitor cancer progression and treatment. Comput Struct Biotechnol J. 2016;14:211–22.
42. Resteghini C, Trama A, Borgonovi E, Hosni H, Corrao G, Orlandi E, Calareso G, De Cecco L, Piazza C, Mainardi L, Licitra L. Big data in head and neck cancer. Curr Treat Options in Oncol. 2018;19:62.
43. Salehi M, Sharifi M. Exosomal miRNAs as novel cancer biomarkers: challenges and opportunities. J Cell Physiol. 2018;233:6370–80.
44. Saussez S, Duray A, Demoulin S, Hubert P, Delvenne P. Immune suppression in head and neck cancers: a review. Clin Dev Immunol. 2010;2010:701657.
45. Sharafinski ME, Ferris RL, Ferrone S, Grandis JR. Epidermal growth factor receptor targeted therapy of squamous cell carcinoma of the head and neck. Head Neck. 2010;32:1412–21.
46. Sharma P, Allison JP. Immune checkpoint targeting in cancer therapy: toward combination strategies with curative potential. Cell. 2015;161:205–14.
47. Sim F, Leidner R, Bell RB. Immunotherapy for head and neck cancer. Oral Maxillofac Surg Clin North Am. 2019;31:85–100.
48. Tiwari M. Science behind human saliva. J Nat Sci Biol Med. 2011;2:53–8.
49. Varkey P, Liu Y-T, Tan NC. Multidisciplinary treatment of head and neck cancer. Semin Plast Surg. 2010;24:331–4.
50. Ventola CL. Cancer immunotherapy, part 3: challenges and future trends. P T. 2017;42(8):514–21.
51. Verma M. Personalized medicine and cancer. J Pers Med. 2012;2:1–14.
52. Vesty A, Gear K, Biswas K, Radcliff FJ, Taylor MW, Douglas RG. Microbial and inflammatory-based salivary biomarkers of head and neck squamous cell carcinoma. Clin Exp Dent Res. 2018;4:255–62.
53. Vigneswaran N, Williams MD. Epidemiologic trends in head and neck cancer and aids in diagnosis. Oral Maxillofac Surg Clin North Am. 2014;26:123–41.
54. Wang H, Stoecklein NH, Lin PP, Gires O. Circulating and disseminated tumor cells: diagnostic tools and therapeutic targets in motion. Oncotarget. 2017;8:1884–912.
55. Wang X, Kaczor-Urbanowicz KE, Wong DTW. Salivary biomarkers in cancer detection. Med Oncol. 2017;34:7.
56. Wu C, Gleysteen J, Teraphongphom NT, Li Y, Rosenthal E. In-vivo optical imaging in head and neck oncology: basic principles, clinical applications and future directions review-article. Int J Oral Sci. 2018;10:10.
57. Xie C, Ji N, Tang Z, Li J, Chen Q. The role of extracellular vesicles from different origin in the microenvironment of head and neck cancers. Mol Cancer. 2019;18:83.
58. You B, Shan Y, Bao L, Chen J, Yang L, Zhang Q, Zhang W, Zhang Z, Zhang J, Shi S, You Y. The biology and function of extracellular vesicles in nasopharyngeal carcinoma (review). Int J Oncol. 2018;52:38–46.
59. Zhao X, Rao S. Surveillance imaging following treatment of head and neck cancer. Semin Oncol. 2017;44:323–9.

Chapter 2
Emerging Technologies in Markets for the Early Detection of Head and Neck Cancer

Laura Bianciardi, Claudio Corallo, Mattia Criscuoli, Diogo Fortunato, Natasa Zarovni, and Davide Zocco

Introduction

Head and neck cancer (HNC) is a heterogeneous group of cancers that, if combined, represent one of the most common cancer types and a leading cause of death worldwide. HNCs are often associated with risk factors such as tobacco and alcohol use or viral infections, including human papillomavirus (HPV) and Epstein-Barr virus (EBV) [1]. Over two-thirds of patients with HNC are currently diagnosed with advanced cancer and lymph node metastases, often leading to poor clinical outcomes. Therefore, it has become apparent that anticipating the time of HNC diagnosis has the potential to radically change the clinical management of these patients, who currently lack effective therapeutic options especially when the cancer is diagnosed at later stages [2].

Identifying risk factors and at-risk groups, as well as health and cost benefits reported in early diagnosis of HNC, supports the need for early detection. While conceptually sound, no screening programs for HNC have been set in place in clinical practice yet, partially because the available screening options are still based on invasive clinical exams and/or time-consuming and expensive radiological tests. New screening and early diagnosis tools for cancers have been introduced in clinical trials over the last decade and promise to boost early detection of early-stage primary tumors and HNC micrometastases [3].

In this chapter, we describe two major approaches (i.e., liquid biopsy and imaging) for early detection of HNC and systematically map current and technologies highlighting key metrics, such as performance and cost-effectiveness, that will play a role in their clinical adoption.

L. Bianciardi · C. Corallo · M. Criscuoli · D. Fortunato · N. Zarovni · D. Zocco (✉)
Exosomics, S.p.A, Siena, Italy
e-mail: dzocco@exosomics.eu

© Springer Nature Switzerland AG 2021
R. El Assal et al. (eds.), *Early Detection and Treatment of Head & Neck Cancers*, https://doi.org/10.1007/978-3-030-69859-1_2

Liquid Biopsy

Liquid biopsy has been dubbed as the cornerstone of future precision medicine and one of the breakthrough technologies of the twenty-first century [4]. In essence, liquid biopsy is an approach that exploits the use of body fluids to identify biomarkers for patient stratification, disease monitoring (e.g., minimal residual disease), and therapy monitoring and selection. Several observational studies have shown the benefit of using liquid biopsy to complement molecular analyses from tissue biopsies or to provide molecular insights when the diseased tissue is no longer available (e.g., monitoring post-surgery disease recurrence); however, interventional clinical studies are ongoing to fully integrate this approach into clinical practice (Fig. 2.1).

Most recently, start-up companies such as Grail (Menlo Park, CA, USA) and Thrive Earlier Detection (Cambridge, MA, USA) have been established to develop liquid biopsy tests for screening and early detection of multiple cancers [5, 6]. These companies rely on deep, next-generation sequencing and proteomics platforms supported by powerful algorithms and machine learning to fish out cancer-specific molecular signatures from blood. Their initial large multicenter observational

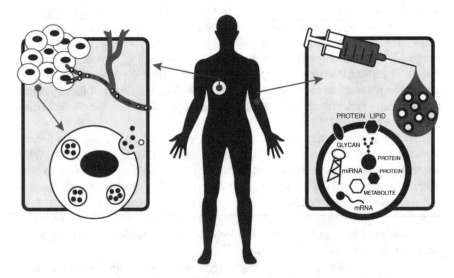

Fig. 2.1 How do tumor biomarkers end up in biofluids? All cells and tissues require vascularization to grow and maintain their functions. Due to their especially high energy requirements, tumor cells often stimulate vascularization in their surroundings, thereby increasing their nutrient supply. As the exchanges between tumor cells and blood increase, so does the presence of tumor-derived biomolecules and potentially relevant biomarkers. The same can happen in other biofluids, where, for instance, oral squamous cell carcinoma (OSCC) cells are in direct contact with saliva. These biomolecules can be released in their native state, in homo- or heterocomplexes, or even incorporated in bigger macromolecular structures such as extracellular vesicles, depicted on the right side of the figure. Extracellular vesicles (EVs) encapsulate and protect tumor-derived material, which could otherwise undergo fast turnover rates when present isolated in circulating biofluids, limiting their isolation and downstream analysis

studies showed impressive diagnostic performances in patients with advanced cancers, but not in those with early-stage cancer (Stage I/II). Two recent studies published by Grail showed that tests based on deep sequencing of DNA lesions or targeted methylation of circulating tumor DNA (ctDNA) have an average sensitivity of 54% that drops to 18% for Stage I cancers [5]. In another study published by Thrive Earlier Detection, 10,000 women with no prior history of cancer were screened with the company's test, which raised the average sensitivity of standard-of-care test from 25% to 52% in cancers where screening tests are available [6]; however, the average sensitivity of Thrive Earlier Detection's test across all cancers was 27.1% [6]. Several factors, such as cancer type, small tumor size ($<1cm^3$), and limited biomarker availability in the early stage [7], may contribute to the poor sensitivity of liquid biopsy tests in early-stage cancers.

In this section, we outline two steps of the diagnostic workflow (i.e., pre-analytics and analytical platforms) that may benefit from new technologies in the quest to improve the detection of early-stage HNC (Fig. 2.2).

Pre-analytics

Sample collection, processing, and biomarker enrichment are collectively called pre-analytical steps or pre-analytics. These steps play essential roles in the success of the diagnostic procedure, especially when rare biomarkers are sought after. Many promising biomarkers have failed to reach the clinic due to lack of "standardization" of pre-analytical steps during validation [8]. Therefore, only a handful of biomarkers are currently used for cancer screening but none of them for HNC.

Sample Collection and Processing

In HNC, three body fluids—(i) blood, (ii) saliva, and (iii) exhaled breath condensate (EBC)—are considered to be potential sources of biomarkers for screening and early detection. The following sections give an overview of the current pre-analytical steps required for these three body fluids, the factors that contribute to sample variability, and the new technologies that may promote sample standardization.

Blood

Blood is the most used body fluid for cancer biomarker detection. Most of the clinically validated screening tests (e.g., Prostate-Specific Antigen (PSA) and Cancer Antigen 125 (CA-125)) and future pan-cancer screening tests (e.g., Grail or Thrive Earlier Detection tests) are based on the use of blood-derived products (i.e., plasma or serum) as the biomarker source. To obtain plasma or serum suitable for biomarker detection, blood is usually drawn through venipuncture with a syringe or a

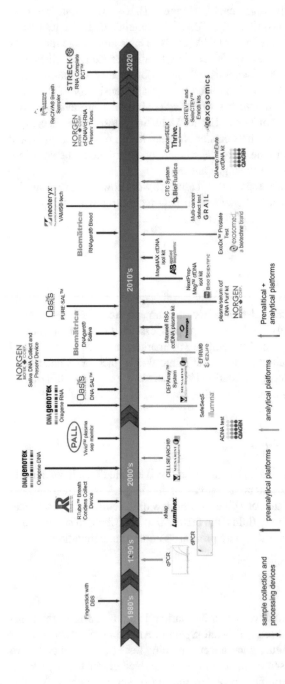

Fig. 2.2 Timeline of key platforms applied in sample collection, pre-analytical and analytical processing for liquid biopsy approaches. The development of PCR-based techniques in the 1990s completely revolutionized research and the techniques were swiftly adapted to routine clinical practices. The first report on the detection of circulating nucleic acids can be dated back to the late 1940s, and the introduction of PCR opened a wide range of possibilities for cell-free DNA (cfDNA) analysis. Entering the 2000s, CELLSEARCH became the first Food and Drug Administration (FDA)-approved device to be used in peripheral blood for the isolation of circulating tumor cells (CTCs), which were first discovered in 1869. Alongside rose the need for optimization of standardized sample collection and preservation strategies, and thus, the 2000s kicked off the race to explore the liquid biopsy field. With that, an exponential increase of research and clinical efforts took place in the 2010s, which consequently led to an explosion of state-of-the-art liquid biopsy-targeted sample collection and processing devices, pre-analytical tools, or analytical platforms. Noteworthily, EV research was actively propelled, shifting the attention of many researchers looking for the potential of combining biosources for early-stage cancer detection. Still, in the 2010s, the discovery of tumor-educated platelets (TEPs) and the validation of their potential as a source of tumor biomarkers proved to be a high-value asset in cancer diagnostics. Access to multiple biosources from various biofluids enabled the development of novel platforms and massive large-scale studies such as the Grail and Thrive projects

butterfly system by a trained phlebotomist and collected into tubes that contain anti-coagulants (e.g., K2-EDTA Vacutainer™ tubes (BD, Franklin Lakes, NJ, USA) for plasma) and/or biomarker preservatives. After collection, the blood is centrifuged once or twice at 1000–2000 relative centrifugal force (RCF) for 10–20 minutes at room temperature. This step separates blood cellular components from plasma, which can then be easily transferred into a new tube for the following analyses. While seemingly straightforward, this procedure is affected by several pre-analytical variables that should be tightly controlled to ensure sample standardization. These pre-analytical steps have been extensively discussed elsewhere [9, 10], but in recent years, several new technologies have been proposed to reduce sample variability, as summarized in Table 2.1.

Fingerstick with dried blood spotting (DBS) and the newer volumetric absorptive microsampling technology (VAMS®; Neoteryx®, Torrance, CA, USA) enable

Table 2.1 Established and new technologies for blood collection/processing

Blood (plasma/serum)	Established technology	Challenges	New technologies
Collection method	Venipuncture with syringe/butterfly system; anticoagulant for plasma as K2-EDTA, citrate (CTAD), P100 and heparin (VacutainerTM; BD Biosciences)	Discomfort, requires trained clinical staff, not ideal for pediatric patients. Hemolysis and platelet activation due to mechanical stress	Fingerprick with dried blood spotting (DBS) Volumetric absorptive microsampling (VAMS®) technology (Neoteryx®)
Biomarker preservatives	Cell-Free DNA BCT® (Streck) PAXgene Blood ccfDNA Tube (CE-IVD) (PreAnalytiX)	Lack of preservatives for new classes of biomarkers (CTCs, RNA, exosomes)	RNA Complete BCT™ (Streck) cf-DNA/cf-RNA Preservative Tubes (Norgen Biotek) LBgard® Blood Tubes (Biomatrica) RNAgard® Blood (Biomatrica) PAXgene Blood RNA Tube (IVD; PreAnalytiX) CellSave Preservative Tubes (Menarini Silicon Biosystems)
Sample processing	One- or two-step centrifuge protocol	Hemolysis and platelet activation due to mechanical stress Centrifuge affects sample standardization	Filtration with Vivid plasma separation membrane (Pall) Acoustic wave separation Microfluidic device [11]

ccfDNA circulating cell-free DNA, *CTCs* circulating tumor cells, *cf-DNA* cell-free DNA, *cf-RNA* cell-free RNA the collection of small amounts of blood in a less invasive way than standard veni-puncture. Furthermore, these procedures do not require trained clinical staff and are ideal for pediatric patients; however, whether these technologies allow the collection of a sufficient amount of blood for the detection of early-stage cancer biomarkers is still unclear.

Preservatives for new classes of biomarkers potentially suitable for early detection, such as microRNAs, have also been recently launched in the market. Products such as cell-free DNA (cfDNA)/cell-free RNA (cfRNA) Preservative Tubes (Norgen Biotek, Thorold, ON, Canada) or RNAgard® Blood (Biomatrica, San Diego, CA, USA) preserve both cfDNA and cfRNA, allowing the detection of both biomarkers. The RNA Complete BCT™ from Streck (La Vista, NE, USA) has been developed to preserve both circulating RNAs and extracellular vesicles (EVs), another promising biomarker for early cancer detection. The use of these preservatives is poised to become a gold standard as it allows sample handling and shipping at room temperature, reducing the cost of the diagnostic procedure, and enabling molecular analyses to be performed in centralized labs where standardization can be better enforced.

Centrifuge-free production of plasma is also a major technological breakthrough in sample standardization. There is still a lack of consensus regarding which centrifugation protocol should be used for liquid biopsy, and there is evidence to suggest that small protocol variations may introduce significant sample biases [12]. Filtration-based protocols, such as Vivid plasma separation membrane™ (Pall, Port Washington, NY, USA), have been proposed due to their low cost and ease of use; however, they have not been further developed into medical devices. The use of more technologically complex systems, such as microfluidic devices and acoustic wave separation devices, has been limited to academic research at this point [11, 13], though companies like AcouSort (Lund, Sweden) are developing promising prototypes for clinical use [14].

Saliva

Saliva is an easily accessible body fluid and one of the most promising sources of biomarkers for HNC. Saliva is collected after passive drooling at 2600 RCF for 15 minutes at 4 °C followed by aspiration from the pellet to obtain a salivary supernatant suitable for biomarker discovery [15]. Salivary biomarkers, such as ctDNA or cancer cells, can also be obtained from buccal swabs, though their concentrations are typically lower than that in saliva after drooling. As for blood, standardization of saliva collection and processing is key for diagnostic applications, and several low-cost devices have been produced to fulfill this need (Table 2.2).

The Oragene DNA device (DNA Genotek, Kanata, ON, Canada) is the market-leading technology for the collection of salivary DNA [15]. Patients expectorate into the device until a volume of 2 mL is reached; the lid is then closed, letting the stabilizing buffers flow into the saliva, stabilizing the sample for up to 1 year at

Table 2.2 Established and new technologies for saliva collection/processing

Saliva	Established technology	Challenges	New technologies
Collection method	Passive drooling Buccal swab	Sample volume variability, lack of standardization	Oragene DNA/RNA device (DNA Genotek) DNA·SAL™/RNA·ProSAL™ device (Oasis Diagnostics®) Pure·SAL™ device (Oasis Diagnostics®) Saliva DNA/RNA Collection and Preservation Device (Norgen Biotek) DNAgard® Saliva device (Biomatrica) iSWAB-DNA Isolation Kit (Mawi technologies) Isohelix DNA Buccal Swab kit (Isohelix)
Biomarker preservatives	None	Lack of preservatives	
Sample processing	One-step centrifugation [15]	Centrifuge affects sample standardization	

room temperature. The Saliva DNA Collection and Preservation Device (Norgen Biotek) and the DNAgard® Saliva (Biomatrica) are like the Origene device, where patients expectorate into a tube through a removable funnel until a "fill mark" is reached [15]. The DNA·SAL™ device (Oasis Diagnostics®, Vancouver, WA, USA) is a raking/scraping tool that collects cells from the inside of the oral cavity with a stabilizing rinse solution after mild raking of the buccal mucosa.

Devices for salivary RNA biomarkers have also been developed, such as the Oragene RNA device, that contain specific stabilizers for RNA molecules and have a fill mark for saliva volume. Of note, the Pure·SAL™ (Oasis Diagnostics®) has been used for the isolation of cfRNA, cfDNA, and exosomes from the same saliva sample [15]. Taken together, these devices provide an inexpensive solution to saliva sample standardization and will play a key role in the validation of salivary biomarkers of HNC.

Exhaled Breath Condensate (EBC)

EBC is the exhalate from breath that has been condensed by cooling with a collection device. EBC contains volatile organic compounds (VOCs) such as DNA, proteins, and ions. A recent report suggests that VOCs, such as aldehydes, found in the EBC can be used as biomarkers for oral cancer [16]. Devices for the collection of EBC such as the RTube™ Breath Condensate Collection Device (Respiratory Research, Inc., Charlottesville, VA, USA) and the ReCIVA® Breath Sampler (Owlstone Medical, Cambridge, UK) are currently under evaluation for cancer detection via analysis of VOCs or other macromolecules [17].

Liquid Biopsy and Biomarker Enrichment for Early-Stage Cancer Diagnosis

Tumor-derived materials from early-stage cancer are often scarce and highly diluted by much more abundant biomolecules coming from healthy tissues or circulating non-tumor cells. Therefore, pre-analytical workflows that enrich for tumor-derived biomarkers are key to increase the sensitivity of analytical platforms, ultimately reducing the percentage of false negatives from the diagnostic procedure.

Circulating tumor cells (CTCs), EVs, cfDNA/ctDNA, and, more recently, tumor-educated platelets (TEPs) have been proposed as potential biosources of tumor biomarkers for early-stage cancer detection. However, several reports suggest that their abundance can be exceedingly low even in late-stage cancer [18–22]. For instance, in metastatic cancer patients, CTC counts range from 1 to 10 per mL of whole blood [18], resulting in a ratio of CTCs to healthy cells of one to billions. Similarly, it is estimated that tumor-derived EVs may represent less than 1% of the total vesicular content in plasma [19]. As for ctDNA, certain patients with cancer show a very low tumor mutational burden, which falls under the sensitivity of analytical platforms. In many cases, mutated alleles derived from tumor cells are less than 0.01% of the total wild-type cfDNA content [20, 21]. This discrepancy is further exacerbated in patients with early-stage cancer that may carry only one mutated DNA copy per mL of blood [22].

Enrichment strategies for these rare biomarkers rely on two major principles: (i) selection of the body fluid in which the biomarker is more likely to be found at an early disease stage and (ii) affinity-based isolation techniques to at least partially separate these biomarkers from background molecules or cells (Fig. 2.3).

Tumor-derived EVs are relatively abundant, stable, and present in virtually all biofluids, including blood and saliva. They show the highest potential for enrichment-based methodologies, although, due to their heterogeneous nature, selective tumor-derived EV isolation strategies can be challenging. For instance, confounding particles from plasma – such as lipoproteins – are often co-purified with EVs, as they share similar physical properties with EVs and far exceed them in number [23]. Instead, saliva is an optimal biofluid for selective isolation of tumor-derived EVs as there are no confounding, similar-sized nanoparticles present nor the high protein content found in plasma that interferes with the performance of affinity-based methodologies. As observed in other biofluids, salivary EV size and concentration increase in oral squamous cell carcinoma (OSCC). Furthermore, these EVs show differential expression of the classical tetraspanins CD9, CD63, and CD81 [24]. Proteomic analysis of salivary EVs found 44 differentially expressed proteins, most of them downregulated, between healthy individuals and patients with OSCC. Looking at the whole salivary proteome, researchers were able to identify proteins present exclusively in early-stage OSCC or advanced OSCC, pinpointing their functions and potential roles [25].

EV enrichment technologies, such as SoRTEV™ and SeleCTEV™ Enrichment kits (Exosomics Spa, Siena, Italy), enrich for tumor-derived EVs from plasma by affinity isolation. The SoRTEV™ Enrichment kit allows selective purification of exosomal RNA following affinity isolation of EVs with proprietary antibodies

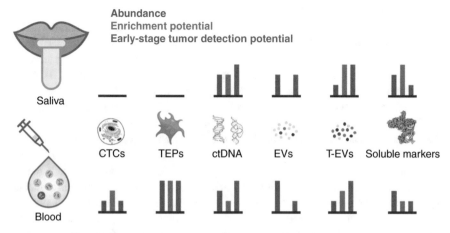

Fig. 2.3 Biosource availability in saliva and blood. From the biosources depicted, circulating tumor cells and tumor-educated platelets can exclusively be found in blood, whereas circulating tumor DNA (ctDNA), EVs, tumor-derived EVs (T-EVs), and soluble markers are carried not only in blood but also in saliva. Selective isolation strategies for enrichment are affected by the increasing complexity in the composition of each biofluid. Often, the efficiency of such affinity-based enrichment methodologies is limited in plasma, due to a richer and more diversified content, when compared with saliva. Represented by illustrative bar charts, columns in blue show the relative abundance of biosources in each biofluid. Pink columns indicate the potential for complete biosource enrichment from biofluids. Red columns convey how much relevant information each biosource could provide for early-stage tumor detection. Missing columns mean the absence of biosource or not applicable in the context

targeting metabolic biomarkers based on the Warburg effect, a hallmark of cancer [26, 27]. Instead, the SeleCTEV™ Enrichment kit is based on a proprietary affinity peptide that allows for the purification of both cfDNA and tumor-derived exosome DNA from 0.5 to 2 mL of plasma [28]. Another emerging technology that isolates EVs by affinity isolation, though not specifically tumor-derived EVs, is the ExoDx™ Prostate Test (Biotechne, Minneapolis, MN, USA/Exosome Dx, Waltham, MA, USA). This test combines DNA and RNA analysis for the detection of prostate cancer-specific biomarkers from urine, which are highly expressed during tumor growth. Then, a validated algorithm calculates a score that estimates the risk of an individual having aggressive prostate cancer, helping doctors decide whether to proceed with further treatments [29].

Platelets are highly abundant and readily available in blood, but not in saliva. Platelet count and size alone may suffice to indicate the presence of cancer [30]. TEPs carry not only valuable tumor RNA biomarkers [31] but also fundamental proteins responsible for tumor development and progression [32]. TEPs can be isolated relatively easily by centrifugation without enrichment steps, though technologies already used for CTC enrichment may be exploited for their selective isolation.

CTCs have, in our opinion, less potential to become biosources for early HNC detection; however, multiple enrichment platforms have been reported over the last two decades. The CELLSEARCH® System (Menarini Silicon Biosystems, Castel Maggiore, Bologna, Italy) is the first and only clinically validated FDA (Food and

Drug Administration)-cleared system for the identification, isolation, and enumeration of CTCs from a simple blood test. This technique detects and enumerates CTCs of epithelial origin (CD45$^-$, EpCAM$^+$, and cytokeratins 8$^+$, 18$^+$, and/or 19$^+$) from 7.5 mL of blood, combining immunomagnetic and fluorescence imaging technology. A positive correlation between the frequency of CELLSEARCH® CTCs and patient survival has been demonstrated for HNC [33], metastatic breast cancer [34], and metastatic prostate cancer [35]. From enriched CELLSEARCH® samples, the DEPArray platform (Menarini Silicon Biosystems, Castel Maggiore, Bologna, Italy) also allows the isolation of single CTCs and characterization of them at the molecular level using Ampli1 WGA and Ampli1 LowPass Kit for mutation detection and copy number aberration by NGS analysis. However, not all CTCs derive from EPCAM$^+$ epithelial cells. Indeed, during cancer progression, there is a phenotypic reassessment due to the epithelial-mesenchymal transition (EMT) process [36]. Thus, an EPCAM-based approach may have limitations in some cancer types. To circumvent this challenge, the ADNA test technology (Qiagen, Venlo, Netherlands) uses a combination of antibodies for prostate and breast CTC selection in 5 mL of whole blood [36]. Another emerging technology based on selective capture of CTCs is the BioFluidica's platform (San Diego, CA, USA) that uses 1 mL of whole blood to capture and release CTCs for downstream analysis. BioFluidica's CTC system is equipped with a CTC capture surface, comprised of 50–500 sinusoidally shaped channels, where chemically immobilized antibodies specifically isolate CTCs from whole blood. Clinical data enables the detection of multiple myeloma, leukemia, lung, and breast cancer [37].

cfDNA/ctDNA is often found highly fragmented, and it is not very stable either in plasma or in saliva. As is true for other cancer types, ctDNA is more abundant in the plasma of patients with late-stage HNC [22]. Usually, cfDNA is purified without an enrichment step for ctDNA. Commercial kits such as the plasma/serum cell-free circulating DNA Purification Midi kit (Norgen Biotek), QIAamp MinElute ccfDNA mini kit (Qiagen), Maxwell RSC ccfDNA plasma kit (Promega, Madison, WI, USA), MagMAX cell-free DNA isolation kit (Applied Biosystems, Waltham, MA, USA), and NextPrep-Mag cfDNA isolation kit (Bioo Scientific, Austin, TX, USA) allow the recovery of fragmented DNA from biological samples such as plasma, serum, urine, and saliva, using magnetic bead-based technologies. Total nucleic acid kits that allow the co-isolation of cfDNA and cfRNA from the same plasma sample may also improve biomarker detection [38, 39]. In addition to integrating the analysis of various biosources, pooling tumor-derived material of the same nature obtained from different biofluids has proven to be a valid approach [40]. Notably, combined analysis of ctDNA from both saliva and plasma enabled the detection of cancer in 96% of the patients enrolled in this study, making it a proof of principle for the added value of a multi-biosource/biofluid approach to drastically increase sensitivity, without compromising on specificity [40]. In the same study, disease recurrence was directly linked to the presence of ctDNA, which was detected months before relapses were observed following established clinical practices [40].

Metabolites and soluble circulating markers have been proposed for decades as potential biomarkers for early cancer detection; however, very few of them reached clinical adoption due to poor diagnostic performances and limited reproducibility.

Indeed, these biomarkers can be very promiscuous and hardly represent the high molecular heterogeneity of complex diseases such as HNC. Notably, soluble CD44 has been proposed as a candidate as an early-stage HNC detection and screening tool, reaching a sensitivity of 80% and a specificity of 65.5% in patients with benign diseases, in populations in which 60% were smokers [41]. Soluble proteins such as carcinoembryonic antigen, squamous cell carcinoma antigen, immunosuppressive acidic protein, and Cyfra provided moderate sensitivity and specificity for OSCC detection [42, 43]. Nonetheless, more recently, soluble protein biomarkers have been successfully combined with other biosources, such as ctDNA, to increase the sensitivity of the diagnostic test; this method provides the basis for Thrive Earlier Detection technology [6, 44].

Analytical Platforms

This section provides an overview of the most relevant analytical platforms either that have been proposed for early diagnosis of HNC so far or that could potentially revolutionize this field in the future. Several technologies have already been tested in clinical trials for the early detection of HNC, but none of them has been granted FDA approval yet (Table 2.3).

Quantitative real-time PCR (qPCR) is one of the most established technologies for sensitive and specific detection of DNA and RNA biomarkers [45, 46]. It uses

Table 2.3 Validated platforms for early detection in HNC

Analytical platform	Analyte (biofluid)	Target	Application	Sensitivity/ specificity	FDA-approved
qPCR	cfDNA (blood)	EBV DNA	NPC [46]	Sensitivity of 97.1%; specificity of 98.6%	no
RT-qPCR	miRNA (saliva)	miR-125a and miR-200a/ miR-139-5p/ miR-let-7a-5p and miR-3928/miR-31	OSCC, TSCC, HNSCC [47–50]	n/a	no
dPCR + Safe-SeqS	cfDNA (blood/ saliva)	HPV DNA and somatic mutations	HNSCC [52]	Sensitivity of 96%	no
Luminex Multianalyte Profiling (xMAP)	Proteins (saliva, serum)	IL-8 and IL-1beta/ Abs to HPV16 proteins/expanded panel of protein biomarkers	OSCC, OPC, SCCHN [55–57]	Sensitivity of 75–84.5%; specificity of 80–98%	no

qPCR quantitative PCR, *cfDNA* cell-free DNA, *EBV* Epstein-Barr virus, *NPC* nasopharyngeal carcinoma, *RT-qPCR* real-time quantitative PCR, *OSCC* oral squamous cell carcinoma, *TSCC* tongue squamous cell carcinoma, *HNSCC* head and neck squamous cell carcinoma, *dPCR* digital PCR, *OPC* Oropharyngeal Cancer, *SCCHN* squamous cell carcinoma of the head and neck

fluorescence chemistries (DNA-intercalating agents or fluorogenic probes) to monitor the amplification of the target sequence after each PCR cycle [45, 46]. The intensity of the fluorescence signal after each cycle is proportional to the quantity of the
starting target molecule in the reaction. The increase in fluorescence during the PCR
reaction is monitored by a modified thermocycler and plotted in an amplification
plot [45, 46]. In a landmark study enrolling 20,000 asymptomatic participants, EBV
DNA, a known HNC biomarker, was detected by qPCR and correlated with cancer
diagnosis in 34 individuals, representing 11% of the total EBV-positive tests that
underwent further examination [47]. Reverse transcription qPCR has been widely
used to detect microRNA biomarkers in blood and saliva from patients with HNC
[48–51].

Digital PCR (dPCR) provides a precise and accurate absolute quantification of
the target molecule, partitioning the input sample in a large number of compartments in which the amplification reaction takes place individually [52]. After amplification, each compartment is scanned for fluorescence signal following a binary
system, absence (0) or presence (1) of fluorescence, to calculate the concentration
of the target molecule using Poissons' statistics [52].

An integrated approach using ctDNA from plasma and saliva showed that the
combined use of several biomarkers (HPV DNA and somatic mutations in genes
commonly altered in Head and Neck Squamous Cell Carcinoma - HNSCC) on
diverse body fluids can help achieve higher sensitivity in cancer detection. The
tumor-specific alteration was detected in at least one bodily fluid in 96% of patients
in whom both plasma and saliva were available; in early-stage disease, tumor-
specific DNA was detected in the plasma or saliva of 100% of patients, with saliva
being a more sensitive predictor of the early stage for many cancer types [40, 53].
The screening of HPV was performed using dPCR [53], while somatic mutations
were detected with Safe-Sequencing System (Safe-SeqS, Illumina, San Diego, CA,
USA), an NGS-based system to detect rare variants [54].

One of the most interesting platforms for multiplex analysis of protein biomarkers is the Luminex (Austin, TX, USA) Multianalyte Profiling (xMAP). The xMAP
is a flexible bioassay platform that allows simultaneous analysis of up to 500
molecular targets. Different sets of microspheres with different dye concentrations
are coupled to specific capture molecules so that one specific microsphere type is
coupled to one specific capture molecule [55]. Once the microspheres are added to
the reaction, the analyte binds to its capture molecule, and then, a reporter molecule binds to the complex. During analysis, the specific microsphere bearing the
analyte of interest is detected and identified, allowing the characterization of the
coupled biomolecule [55]. The xMAP has been exploited to quantify salivary proteins IL-8 and IL-1β in patients with early HNC [56], to detect serum antibodies
against HPV16 proteins [57], or to use a multiplexed panel of ad hoc serum biomarkers [58].

Electric Field Induced Release and Measurement (EFIRM®) by EZLife Bio,
Inc. (Northridge, CA, USA) is a technology with great potential in early biomarker
detection, since it allows rapid and sensitive analyte testing without sample lysis

and DNA/RNA extraction. This platform is based on a multiplexible electrochemical sensor with a conduction polymer upon which specific capture probes/antibodies are coated. In the case of hybridization with a target, an HRP-labeled detector probe and a reporter enzyme added to the reaction trigger the electrochemical signal transduction to the sensor [59, 60]. The resulting signal is proportional to the concentration of the target copies detected by the system [61]. The molecular hybridization between target and capture molecule is enhanced by the application of a cyclic square wave (csw) [60] that also causes temporary pore formation in exosomes, resulting in biomolecule release [59]. This allows rapid and sensitive analysis of encapsulated analytes (DNA, RNA, and proteins), not only those freely present in the biofluid, reducing extraction-associated data bias and sample loss. For the moment, this technique has not been employed in HNC, but it has been successfully used in cancer fields to detect epidermal growth factor receptor (EGFR) mutations in plasma and saliva from non-small cell lung cancer (NSCLC) samples [60, 62] and in plasma of patients with early-stage NSCLC [63].

However, none of the abovementioned technologies have received FDA approval or clearance at this point, despite initial promising studies. As of today, Epi proColon® (Epigenomics AG, Berlin, Germany) is the only liquid biopsy platform for early diagnosis and screening in cancer that received FDA approval for the screening of colorectal cancer (CRC) by real-time qPCR [64].

Analytical platforms for the early diagnosis of several cancers with one single test have recently entered the FDA Breakthrough Devices Program. Among them, GRAIL launched a multi-cancer early detection test that could detect more than 50 types of cancer with a single blood draw. It is a methylation-based technology (whole-genome bisulfite sequencing, WGBS) with bisulfite conversion of plasma cfDNA. After library preparation and next-generation sequencing (NGS), methylation patterns are analyzed to determine cancer/non-cancer status and tissue of origin (TOO) localization [5]. HNC was included among the 12 deadly cancer types in the training-validation substudy of the Circulating Cell-free Genome Atlas (CCGA) study. TOO accuracy for HNC was 71% (on a total of 65 samples) and 83% (on a total of 18 samples) in the training and validation sets, respectively [5].

CancerSEEK (Thrive Earlier Detection) is another platform that entered the FDA Breakthrough Devices Program. It is designed for the early detection of multiple types of cancers from a simple blood draw combining the analysis of mutations on cfDNA with established protein biomarkers [6]. The test was able to detect cancer in 26 women (10 different types of cancer), including 17 early-stage tumors that had not yet spread. On the other hand, the test gave 101 false-positive results and missed the detection of 24 patients who were diagnosed by conventional screening; 46 additional women were negative for both approaches (CancerSEEK and conventional screening) but then turned out to have cancer instead. Despite these initial shortcomings, multi-cancer screening platforms hold the greatest potential of being adopted as a means for the early identification of many types of cancers, including HNC, in a noninvasive and cost-effective manner.

Imaging: State-of-the-Art Imaging Methods in HNCs

Imaging technologies are critical to the state-of-the-art management of patients with cancer, while their overall use and impact can differ in different phases (diagnosis, staging, and treatment) and in different cancer types. In HNCs, imaging methods are part of an initial clinical evaluation that supports current therapeutic paradigms [65]. Two early interventions that employ imaging in HNC assessment to date are diagnostic imaging and targeted visual resection. The most common imaging modalities in routine clinical use for cancer diagnostics and staging are computed tomography (CT), magnetic resonance imaging (MRI), and positron emission tomography (PET). Out of these, CT and MRI are based on pathological morphological features that can be contrast-enhanced, while PET relies on a disease-driven tracer accumulation. Other emerging modalities involve innovative technologies featuring either optical imaging or the use of novel contrast agents that boost spatial resolution, signal-to-background ratio, and overall sensitivity and specificity, thus converting conventional imaging to the detection of metabolic or molecular alterations.

In terms of "value for money," imaging methods are typically costly and unlikely to be broadly applied across a population. The high cost is mostly caused by high total costs of ownership, with a yearly cost of $1 M for PET, MRI, or CT, as well as limited throughput (one instrument/operator limits to 8–13 exams per day). The average per-examination cost is around $500–1000 [66]. Given the prevalence of cancers, one can expect that imaging will find cancerous tumors in less than 2% of the non-symptomatic population. However, it can still deliver effective health benefits to well-defined subjects/groups. Today, in HNC practice, imaging is in use for pre- and post-therapy planning, staging, and restaging of symptomatic and already diagnosed patients. The use of imaging in a very early setting, rather than contemplated for large population sectors, could be targeted to high-risk groups (such as HPV-positives, heavy smokers, or alcohol consumers), in which the benefits would be more striking.

The key requirement of imaging to ensure a meaningful impact on early cancer diagnosis is the tumor-to-background ratio. The goal of cancer imaging should be to detect tumors before the angiogenic switch at the 10^5 cell stage. The present detection threshold of conventional imaging for solid tumors (including micrometastases) is approximately 10^9 cells (1 g or 1 cm^3). Today, a negative scan means there could be between zero and 10^9 malignant cells in the patient's body [67]. The other side of the coin is a scarce overall specificity, which also raises concerns; some small, 1cm^3 tumors detected by scans are actually indolent and would either disappear or would never cause problems within the patient's life. Scarce sensitivity and specificity may necessitate further diagnostic evaluations, increasing the costs and time-to-therapy. Besides the costs, CT, PET, and contrast-enhanced MRI comprise radiation exposure risk that is 40–1000 times higher than the exposure from a plain X-ray. Therefore, these modalities, though traditionally indicated as noninvasive, are not indicated as a close interval screening in non-symptomatic subjects nor as serial monitoring options.

To increase the sensitivity, exogenous contrast agents, either nontargeted or targeted, may be used. Nontargeted exogenous contrast fluid is routinely used in CT and MRI, to indirectly detect tumors, but it still provides only anatomical insight and does not significantly enhance the tumor-to-background ratio. On the other hand, molecular imaging uses tracer agents targeting malignant cells or their products. The most common molecular imaging used as part of the state of care for HNCs is FDG-PET [65]. FDG is a glucose mimetic that is taken up by metabolically active cells and trapped inside due to phosphorylation by hexokinases. This technology exploits a hallmark of cancer, the Warburg effect [26]. However, FDG is not exclusively up taken by tumor cells. For instance, the bone marrow, uterus, or brain show high FDG uptake, which can also be increased by other non-cancer conditions such as inflammation. Indeed, FDG-PET, although it has been shown to have higher sensitivity and higher negative predictive value compared to CT or MRI, especially for the identification of small lymph nodes of the neck [65–68], has around 30% false-positive rate in the detection of HNCs. Although FDG-PET is informative and leads to a modification of treatment planning in approximately one-third of the patients with HNC but is still of no value as a first-line test for early diagnostics [68].

Tumor Targeted Imaging

Over the last decade, the influx of novel technologies and the emphasis on a paradigm of precision medicine incorporated novel, tumor-specific targeting strategies to improve diagnostic imaging while supporting multimodal therapeutic options. The field of molecular imaging is an intersection between physics, chemistry, and biology, not only combining new imaging agents with conventional instruments such as PET, MRI, and CT but also enabling the use of other techniques such as ultrasound, spectroscopy, optical imaging, and microscopy. Besides the development of targeting agents with high affinity and specificity for a tumor, another mechanism to further enhance the tumor-to-background signal is to leverage tumor cell- or tumor environment-specific mechanisms that enable trapping or activation of otherwise invisible agents. To this purpose, specific moieties are included in the "smart" tracer's composition, activated by low pH or activity of specific enzymes such as cathepsins, caspases, or metalloproteases [69].

There are several good examples of tumor target-specific strategies including tumor-targeting peptides and antibodies coupled to radioisotopes or to fluorescence dyes. Some of these have been tested in preclinical and clinical research settings in HNCs [70]. In the past few years, 30 clinical trials evaluated the utility of antibody-based PET tracers using FDA-approved and/or experimental antibodies in various cancer types. These probes target antigens that are also targets of monoclonal antibodies, which are either approved for state-of-care treatments or in drug development pipelines (cetuximab, bevacizumab, and trastuzumab). EGFR is one of the most ubiquitously overexpressed receptors in HNC with an increased expression level in more than 80% of cases. However, clinical visualization of EGFR has not been very successful due to EGFR expression in non-tumor tissues [65–70]. In contrast, the expression of CD44 v6 splicing variant in organs with distant metastases of HNC is negligible. Radiolabeled aCD44v6 antibody (U36) was shown to have high potential for in vivo targeting of HNSCC xenografts in mice as well as in human patients, and this further inspired radioimmunotherapy that was well-tolerated and displayed excellent targeting of tumor lesions [71]. Another important target for radioimaging in HNC is the carbonic anhydrase IX (CAIX) [72]. CAIX is widely expressed in solid tumors and not in normal tissues except for the gastrointestinal tract; it is, therefore, a promising biomarker and FDA-approved therapeutic target. CAIX-targeting radiotracers (girentuximab) are used in HNCs and other solid tumors to identify hypoxic and therapy-resistant tumor areas [72].

Synthetic peptides are an appealing alternative to the use of antibodies with advantages in terms of costs, immunoreactivity, ease of labeling, and tissue penetration. For instance, BIWA1 peptide is currently tested for CD44 binding, but other peptides have also been under preclinical and clinical investigation as agents for conventional nuclear medicine or coupled to optical surgical navigation systems in HNCs [65–70]. The HN-1 peptide is identified as an HNC lesion binding peptide without a known specific molecular target [65]. This peptide was first coupled to radioisotopes and tested in gamma-emitting or positron-emitting radioimaging. Subsequently, it was also employed in the context of novel optical detection systems that are used as navigators for real-time intraoperative fluorescence detection. In the latter case, it was coupled to near-infrared (NIR) fluorescent emission dyes such as NIR800 that are characterized by low tissue autofluorescence, better tissue penetration, and minimal in vivo toxicity. These features make it an appealing rival to more widely used fluorescent imaging contrast agents such as indocyanine green (ICG), a clinical-grade tracer for the identification of lymph nodes during surgical procedures in HNC and other cancers. Vascular targeting peptides such as integrin like cyclic RGD peptides have been studied as conjugates to NIR dyes, with particular appeal for use in highly vascularized tumors, such as HNCs [65]. In any case, there is a wide variety of FDA-approved fluorescence imaging systems for navigated surgical procedures and diagnostics (i.e., produced by Olympus, Zeiss, Leika, Karl Storz, and Novadaq).

Best of Both Worlds: Theranostics

Besides pure imaging or surgery guidelines, tumor-targeting peptides and antibodies can be adapted and used for both therapeutic and diagnostic purposes (i.e., theranostic). This is accomplished by conjugation of targeted moieties to both optical, fluorescent dyes or radioisotopes and small therapeutic molecules. Interestingly, dyes and radioisotopes themselves can also serve as therapeutic effectors. For instance, Cyanine fluorescent dyes can be used for concomitant imaging and photodynamic or photothermal therapy, by converting light energy to heat upon NIR irradiation and consequently ablating tumor cells [73]. Alternatively, antibodies or peptides, including those targeting HNC, have been studied as carriers of additional therapeutic molecules such as inhibitory PKCε peptide, diphtheria toxin, or anti-hRRM2 siRNAs [65]. Today, all of these agents have entered clinical trials, still facing hurdles for transition into clinical practice.

In recent years, various nanomaterials have emerged as exciting tools for cancer theranostic applications due to their multifunctional properties. The first generation of synthetic nanoparticles has raised high expectations but has delivered poorly, displaying several fundamental problems related to the cost, toxicity, and effectiveness. Bio-inspired nanoparticles mimicking natural body components have recently gained immense attention due to their ability to serve as alternative biocompatible drug delivery systems in cancer theranostics [74]. They claim biocompatibility and biodegradability, low cost, ease of synthesis, sustained release of the therapeutics, effortless penetration abilities, improved retention inside target (tumor) tissue, and low toxicity. The foremost advantage of these nanomaterials is that they are able to incorporate multiple functionalities and serve multiple applications. Several multi-functional nanosystems are presently clinically FDA approved and/or under clinical trials, and some of them have tested or explored for use in HNCs [75].

The latest frontiers of nanoengineering in theranostics feature particles that are not only inspired but are also produced by nature – exosomes. These liposome-like nanoparticles have intrinsic homing and pharmacological properties that depend on the cell source. They also lend themselves to both genetic and chemical engineering as well as loading with both hydrophilic and hydrophobic cargo that can redirect or enhance their targeting and/or functional properties. Their imaging or theranostic applications are still at the proof-of-concept stage, while huge investments are poured into "exosome companies" developing advanced diagnostics and therapy.

So, How About Early Diagnostics?

In the context of early diagnosis, imaging technologies face the challenge of the sensitivity and resolution, concerning not only the scale (from anatomical to molecular) or absolute detection limit (sub-millimeter and sub-nanomolar) but also the integration of information in multiplex and possibly automated platforms that can detect numerous markers or features and feed the test results into a diagnostic algorithm. Coupling of ultrasensitive imaging techniques (mostly optical imaging) to machine learning can expand the horizon of imaging technologies towards easy-to-handle, truly noninvasive, and affordable examinations that can be transferred into primary care as screening or triage tests.

Currently, physical examination with visual inspection is the mainstay of the diagnosis of oral cavity cancer, the most frequent tumor type among HNCs. Such an exam can be enhanced with contrast staining (for instance, with toluidine blue binding acidic groups, mostly of nuclear DNA and cytosolic RNA) and/or optical imaging (fluorescence, autofluorescence, contact endoscopy, and in vivo microscopy) that reveal abnormal tissue patterns indicative of malignant lesions. Such methods, if empowered by AI tools for image elaboration, may reach the incremental value required for a screening compliant test in high-risk groups.

Imaging and Artificial Intelligence

The concept of artificial intelligence (AI) was first described in 1956, and it encompasses the field of computer science in which machines are trained to learn from experience [76]. The field of AI is constantly growing and has the potential to affect many aspects of our lives, including healthcare [77]. Regarding the latter, the biggest revolution of AI in the health care field is the potential to diagnose diseases [78, 79]. Machine learning (ML) is a subset of AI, and it consists of employing mathematic models (e.g., statistical linear models and neural networks) to the computation of sample data sets [80, 81]. These models are designed to recognize different patterns and achieve complex computational tasks within a matter of minutes, often challenging human ability [82]. In fact, ML can increase efficiency by decreasing computation time with high precision with respect to human decision-making standards [83]. In the field of healthcare, AI and ML have already shown their potential to improve the interpretation of imaging, particularly in cancer [84]. Based on a set of images selected to represent a specific tissue or disease process, the computer can be trained to evaluate and recognize new and unique images from patients and facilitate a diagnosis, especially when early diagnosis becomes fundamental [85]. In fact, there are some tumor types, such as HNC, in which the impact of imaging on early diagnosis is crucial, especially when confirmatory biopsy is not an option for hard-to-reach tumors [86] or to reduce unnecessary neck dissections [87]. In this section, some examples of how AI applied to imaging could improve the early detection of HNC will be evaluated in a cost-benefit and healthcare-economics analysis based on statistical outcomes and on the feedback of the clinicians assessing the performance (Fig. 2.4).

Approximately 60,000 patients are diagnosed with HNSCC in the United States each year, with a death rate of about 13,000 patients per year [88]. Diagnosis, prognostic staging, and therapy selection for HNSCC are guided by routine diagnostic CT scan of the head and neck to identify tumor and lymph node characteristics [89]. Despite the innovative imaging techniques, there are still some radiographic features that remain difficult to detect, including the presence of lymph node metastasis (NM) and lymph node extranodal extension (ENE) [90]. In addition, ENE can only be reliably diagnosed from postoperative pathology evaluation, and the importance of its early identification is an indication for adjuvant treatment intensification with the addition of chemotherapy to radiation therapy [91]. Previous studies of radiologic ENE detection showed suboptimal performance (accuracies of 67–70%, sensitivities of 57–66%, and specificities of 76–81%), with the area under the curve (AUC) of the receiver operating characteristic plot ranging from 0.65–0.69 [92] associated to high intra-observer variability in the prediction of ENE from CT [93].

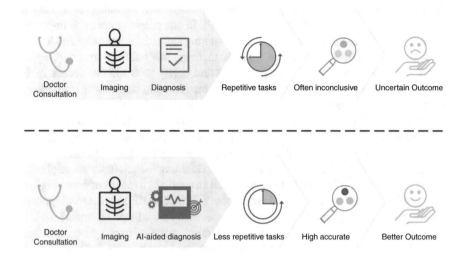

Fig. 2.4 Conventional diagnostics (top) vs AI-enabled diagnostics (bottom)

On the other hand, radiologic detection of NM on imaging for diagnostic purposes seems to be more reliable than ENE detection (average sensitivity: 0.77, average specificity: 0.85, AUC: 0.84), although room for improvement in this aspect is needed as well [94]. In this tumor type, the advantages of AI technology applied to imaging could help clinicians improve the diagnostic performance. In fact, deep learning neural networks (DLNNs) using convolutional layers have been shown to be promising in detecting ENE and NM in HNSCC patients based on diagnostic CT scans [95]. The DLNN model for ENE detection in HNSCC significantly improved the overall diagnostic performance statistics with AUC of 0.91 (95%CI: 0.85–0.97), average accuracy of 85.7%, average sensitivity of 88% (false-negative rate: 0.12), and average specificity of 85% (false-positive rate: 0.15) [95]. For NM prediction, the DLNN model demonstrated AUC of 0.91 (95%CI: 0.86–0.96), average accuracy of 85.5%, average sensitivity of 84%, and average specificity of 87%, thus statistically improving CT-based diagnostic performance [95]. Of note, these data from the DLNN model should be considered "dynamic" rather than "static" data, meaning they could change over time (e.g., increased sensitivity and increased specificity over time) if the DLNN model is adopted in various centers worldwide allowing it to learn and improve performance from experience. This is a classic example of how the cost-benefit analysis is in favor of adopting AI technology to aid imaging analysis to facilitate the diagnostic paradigm for HNSCC patients by supporting the clinicians with robust statistics in the decision-making process and by reducing inter- and intra-observer variability [96].

The early detection concept is not applied to diagnosis only, but more generally to screening procedures [97]. In this space, the recent development of AI solutions could be beneficial, such as in the case of oral cancer. Oral cancer is easily detectable by physical (self) examination [98]. However, many cases of oral cancer could not be detected early, causing unnecessary morbidity and mortality, especially in countries with limited access to healthcare [99]. In this case, the potential impact of AI technology could improve oral cancer screening and reduce mortality and health-care access inequalities worldwide. To date, there are few publications on the appli-cation of these techniques to imaging in the oral cavity [100]. In one recent study, the performance of a deep learning algorithm for detecting oral cancer from hyper-spectral images of patients with oral cancer was evaluated [101]. The investigators reported a classification accuracy of 94.5% for differentiating between images of malignant and healthy oral tissues [101]. These results were in accordance with another study that imaged human tissue specimens, highlighting the benefits of the AI applied method [102]. In a third study, deep learning techniques were applied to confocal laser endomicroscopy to analyze cell structure as a means of detecting oral and oropharyngeal squamous cell carcinoma (OPSCC) [103]. A mean diagnostic accuracy of 88.3% (sensitivity 86.6% and specificity 90%) was reported [103]. In another recent multicenter study, a low-cost, point-of-care, deep learning, smartphone-based oral cancer probe was developed specifically for screeners in high-risk populations in remote regions with limited infrastructure [104]. The deep learning algorithm was initially trained using 1000 data sets of images, risk factors, and matching histopathological diagnoses which showed 80.6% agreement with standard-of-care diagnosis [104]. After additional training, the algorithm was able to classify intraoral lesions with sensitivities, specificities, positive predictive val-ues, and negative predictive values ranging from 81% to 95% [104], meaning the more it learns, the better the accuracy.

A question arises: How is AI perceived by healthcare professionals, and how will this emerging technology change their way of working? A recent study reported the results of a nationwide online survey on AI among radiologist mem-bers of the Italian Society of Medical and Interventional Radiology (SIRM) [105]. The survey consisted of 13 questions about the perceived advantages and issues related to AI implementation in radiological practice and their overall opinion about AI [105]. Perceived AI advantages included a lower diagnostic error rate (73.0%) and optimization of radiologists' work (67.9%). On the other hand, the increased costs and workload due to AI system maintenance and data analysis (39.0%) were identified as potential issues [105]. Most radiologists stated that specific policies should regulate the use of AI (90.4%) and were not afraid of los-ing their job due to it (88.9%) [105]. Overall, 77.0% of respondents were in favor of the adoption of AI, whereas 18.0% were uncertain and 5.0% were unfavorable [105]. This survey anticipates the potential issues that could arise in the complex relationship between the human decision-making process and AI. In fact, despite the fact that novel imaging technologies could provide more complex information over time, the unaided human mind is unable to process and interpret such com-plex datasets without computational assistance. Therefore, to facilitate the integra-tion of AI into screening and diagnostics, the perception of the technology should change, meaning that it has to be clearly understood that it could not replace human judgment, but rather it has to guide clinicians to earlier and more accurate disease diagnosis.

Conclusions and Perspectives

Screening and early detection hold the potential to revolutionize the clinical management of patients with HNC. New disruptive technologies are emerging to solve critical challenges, such as standardization of sample collection and enrichment of tumor-derived material in liquid biopsy approaches, or to completely reimagine the diagnostic workflow, such as AI-enabled imaging platforms. Theranostic approaches may also be conceived to treat early disease in the most specific and targeted way. Pilot clinical validation of many of these technologies can be envisaged within the next 5 years, though their clinical adoption will certainly depend on health economics metrics.

References

1. Döbróssy L. Epidemiology of head and neck cancer: magnitude of the problem. Cancer Metastasis Rev. 2005;24:9–17.
2. Leemans CR, Braakhuis BJ, Brakenhoff RH. The molecular biology of head and neck cancer. Nat Rev Cancer. 2011;11(1):9–22.
3. Spector ME, Farlow JL, Haring CT, Brenner JC, Birkeland AC. The potential for liquid biopsies in head and neck cancer. Discov Med. 2018;25(139):251–7.
4. Sorbara L, Srivastava S. Liquid biopsy: a holy grail for cancer detection. Biomark Med. 2019;13(12):991–4.
5. Liu MC, Oxnardy GR, Klein EA, Swanton C, Seiden MV. & on behalf of the CCGA consortium. Sensitive and specific multi-cancer detection and localization using methylation signatures in cell-free DNA. Ann Oncol. 2020;06(31):745–59.
6. Lennon AM, Buchanan AH, Kinde I, Warren A, Honushefsky A, Cohain AT, Ledbetter DH, Sanfilippo F, Sheridan K, Rosica D, Adonizio CS, Hwang HJ, Lahouel K, Cohen JD, Douville C, Patel AA, Hagmann LN, Rolston DD, Malani N, Zhou S, Bettegowda C, Diehl DL, Urban B, Still CD, Kann L, Woods JI, Salvati ZM, Vadakara J, Leeming R, Bhattacharya P, Walter C, Parker A, Lengauer C, Klein A, Tomasetti C, Fishman EK, Hruban RH, Kinzler KW, Vogelstein B, Papadopoulos N. Feasibility of blood testing combined with PET-CT to screen for cancer and guide intervention. Science. 2020;369:eabb9601.
7. Parsons HA, Rhoades J, Reed SC, Gydush G, Ram P, Exman P, Xiong K, Lo CC, Li T, Fleharty M, Kirkner GJ, Rotem D, Cohen O, Yu F, Fitarelli-Kiehl M, Leong KW, Hughes ME, Rosenberg SM, Collins LC, Miller KD, Blumenstiel B, Trippa L, Cibulskis C, Neuberg DS, De Felice M, Freeman SS, Lennon NJ, Wagle N, Ha G, Stover DG, Choudhury AD, Getz G, Winer EP, Meyerson M, Lin NU, Krop I, Love JC, Makrigiorgos GM, Partridge AH, Mayer EL, Golub TR, Adalsteinsson VA. Sensitive detection of minimal residual disease in patients treated for early-stage breast cancer. Clin Cancer Res. 2020;26:2556–64.
8. Diamandis EP. Cancer biomarkers: can we turn recent failures into success? J Natl Cancer Inst. 2010;102(19):1462–7.
9. Risberg B, Tsui DWY, Biggs H, Ruiz-Valdepenas Martin de Almagro A, Dawson SJ, Hodgkin C, Jones L, Parkinson C, Piskorz A, Marass F, Chandrananda D, Moore E, Morris J, Plagnol V, Rosenfeld N, Caldas C, Brenton JD, Gale D. Effects of collection and processing procedures on plasma circulating cell-free DNA from cancer patients. J Mol Diagn. 2018;20(6):883–92.
10. Venturella M, Carpi FM, Zocco D. Standardization of blood collection and processing for the diagnostic use of extracellular vesicles. Current Pathobiol Rep. 2019;7:1–8.

11. Kuan DH, Wu CC, Su WY, Huang NT. A microfluidic device for simultaneous extraction of plasma, red blood cells, and on-chip white blood cell trapping. Sci Rep. 2018;8(1):15345.
12. Rikkert LG, van der Pol E, van Leeuwen TG, Nieuwland R, Coumans FAW. Centrifugation affects the purity of liquid biopsy-based tumor biomarkers. Cytometry A. 2018;93(12):1207–12.
13. Wu M, Ozcelik A, Rufo J, Wang Z, Fang R, Jun HT. Acoustofluidic separation of cells and particles. Microsyst Nanoeng. 2019;5:32.
14. Magnusson C, Augustsson P, Lenshof A, Ceder Y, Laurell T, Lilja H. Clinical-scale cell-surface-marker independent acoustic microfluidic enrichment of tumor cells from blood. Anal Chem. 2017;89(22):11954–61.
15. Slowey PD. Salivary diagnostics using purified nucleic acids. Methods Mol Biol. 2017;1537:3–15.
16. Bouza M, Gonzalez-Soto J, Pereiro R, de Vicente JC, Sanz-Medel A. Exhaled breath and oral cavity VOCs as potential biomarkers in oral cancer patients. J Breath Res. 2017;11(1):016015.
17. https://www.owlstonemedical.com/products/reciva/.
18. Miller MC, Doyle GV, Terstappen LW. Significance of circulating tumor cells detected by the cell search system in patients with metastatic breast colorectal and prostate cancer. J Oncol. 2010;2010:617421.
19. Brock G, Castellanos-Rizaldos E, Hu L, Coticchia C, Skog J Liquid biopsy for cancer screening, patient stratification and monitoring. Transl Cancer Res. 2015.
20. Li M, Diehl F, Dressman D, Vogelstein B, Kinzler KW. BEAMing up for detection and quantification of rare sequence variants. Nat Methods. 2006;3(2):95–7.
21. Diaz LA Jr, Bardelli A. Liquid biopsies: genotyping circulating tumor DNA. J Clin Oncol. 2014;32(6):579–86.
22. Bettegowda C, Sausen M, Leary RJ, Kinde I, Wang Y, Agrawal N, Bartlett BR, Wang H, Luber B, Alani RM, Antonarakis ES, Azad NS, Bardelli A, Brem H, Cameron JL, Lee CC, Fecher LA, Gallia GL, Gibbs P, Le D, Giuntoli RL, Goggins M, Hogarty MD, Holdhoff M, Hong SM, Jiao Y, Juhl HH, Kim JJ, Siravegna G, Laheru DA, Lauricella C, Lim M, Lipson EJ, Marie SK, Netto GJ, Oliner KS, Olivi A, Olsson L, Riggins GJ, Sartore-Bianchi A, Schmidt K, Shih LM, Oba-Shinjo SM, Siena S, Theodorescu D, Tie J, Harkins TT, Veronese S, Wang TL, Weingart JD, Wolfgang CL, Wood LD, Xing D, Hruban RH, Wu J, Allen PJ, Schmidt CM, Choti MA, Velculescu VE, Kinzler KW, Vogelstein B, Papadopoulos N, Diaz LA Jr. Detection of circulating tumor DNA in early- and late-stage human malignancies. Sci Transl Med. 2014;6(224):224ra24.
23. Sódar BW, Kittel Á, Pálóczi K, Vukman KV, Osteikoetxea X, Szabó-Taylor K, Németh A, Sperlágh B, Baranyai T, Giricz Z, Wiener Z, Turiák L, Drahos L, Pállinger É, Vékey K, Ferdinandy P, Falus A, Buzás EI. Low-density lipoprotein mimics blood plasma-derived exosomes and microvesicles during isolation and detection. Sci Rep. 2016;6:24316.
24. Zlotogorski-Hurvitz A, Dayan D, Chaushu G, Salo T, Vered M. Morphological and molecular features of oral fluid-derived exosomes: oral cancer patients versus healthy individuals. J Cancer Res Clin Oncol. 2016;142(1):101–10.
25. Winck FV, Prado Ribeiro AC, Ramos Domingues R, Ling LY, Riaño-Pachón DM, Rivera C, Brandão TB, Gouvea AF, Santos-Silva AR, Coletta RD, Paes Leme AF. Insights into immune responses in oral cancer through proteomic analysis of saliva and salivary extracellular vesicles. Sci Rep. 2015;5:16305.
26. Foroni C, Zarovni N, Bianciardi L, et al. When Less Is More: Specific Capture and Analysis of Tumor Exosomes in Plasma Increases the Sensitivity of Liquid Biopsy for Comprehensive Detection of Multiple Androgen Receptor Phenotypes in Advanced Prostate Cancer Patients. Biomedicines. 2020;8(5):E131. Published 2020 May 22. https://doi.org/10.3390/biomedicines8050131.
27. Warburg O. On the origin of cancer. Science. 1956;123(3191):309–14.
28. https://www.exosomics.eu/products/.
29. McKiernan J, Donovan MJ, O'Neill V, Bentink S, Noerholm M, Belzer S, Skog J, Kattan MW, Partin A, Andriole G, Brown G, Wei JT, Thompson IM Jr, Carroll P. A novel urine

exosome gene expression assay to predict high-grade prostate cancer at initial biopsy. JAMA Oncol. 2016;2(7):882–9.
30. Stone RL, Nick AM, McNeish IA, Balkwill F, Han HD, Bottsford-Miller J, Rupairmoole R, Armaiz-Pena GN, Pecot CV, Coward J, Deavers MT, Vasquez HG, Urbauer D, Landen CN, Hu W, Gershenson H, Matsuo K, Shahzad MM, King ER, Tekedereli I, Ozpolat B, Ahn EH, Bond VK, Wang R, Drew AF, Gushiken F, Lamkin D, Collins K, DeGeest K, Lutgendorf SK, Chiu W, Lopez-Berestein G, Afshar-Kharghan V, Sood AK. Paraneoplastic thrombocytosis in ovarian cancer. N Engl J Med. 2012;366(7):610–8.
31. Nilsson RJ, Balaj L, Hulleman E, van Rijn S, Pegtel DM, Walraven M, Widmark A, Gerritsen WR, Verheul HM, Vandertop WP, Noske DP, Skog J, Würdinger T. Blood platelets contain tumor-derived RNA biomarkers. Blood. 2011;118(13):3680–3.
32. Klement GL, Yip TT, Cassiola F, Kikuchi L, Cervi D, Podust V, Italiano JE, Wheatley E, Abou-Slaybi A, Bender E, Almog N, Kieran MW, Folkman J. Platelets actively sequester angiogenesis regulators. Blood. 2009;113(12):2835–42.
33. Nichols AC, Lowes LE, Szeto CC, Basmaji J, Dhaliwal S, Chapeskie C, Todorovic B, Read N, Venkatesan V, Hammond A, Palma DA, Winquist E, Ernst S, Fung K, Franklin JH, Yoo J, Koropatnick J, Mymryk JS, Barrett JW, Allan AL. Detection of circulating tumor cells in advanced head and neck cancer using the CellSearch system. Head Neck. 2012;34(10):1440–4.
34. Giuliano M, Giordano A, Jackson S, De Giorgi U, Mego M, Cohen EN, Gao H, Anfossi S, Handy BC, Ueno NT, Alvarez RH, De Placido S, Valero V, Hortobagyi GN, Reuben JM, Cristofanilli M. Circulating tumor cells as early predictors of metastatic spread in breast cancer patients with limited metastatic dissemination. Breast Cancer Res. 2014;16(5):440.
35. Bastos DA, Antonarakis. ES.CTC-derived AR-V7 detection as a prognostic and predictive biomarker in advanced prostate cancer. Expert Rev Mol Diagn. 2018;18(2):155–63.
36. Gorges TM, Tinhofer I, Drosch M, Röse L, Zollner TM, Krahn T, von Ahsen O. Circulating tumour cells escape from EpCAM-based detection due to epithelial-to-mesenchymal transition. BMC Cancer. 2012;12:178.
37. https://biofluidica.com/te_technology.html.
38. Zhang Y, Koneva LA, Virani S, Arthur AE, Virani A, Hall PB, Warden CD, Carey TE, Chepeha DB, Prince ME, McHugh JB, Wolf GT, Rozek LS, Sartor MA. Subtypes of HPV-positive head and neck cancers are associated with HPV characteristics, copy number alterations, PIK3CA mutation, and pathway signatures. Clin Cancer Res. 2016;22(18):4735–45.
39. Oreskovic A, Brault ND, Panpradist N, Lai JJ, Lutz BR. Analytical comparison of methods for extraction of short cell-free DNA from urine. J Mol Diagn. 2019;21(6):1067–78.
40. Wang Y, Springer S, Mulvey CL, Silliman N, Schaefer J, Sausen M, James N, Rettig EM, Guo T, Pickering CR, Bishop JA, Chung CH, Califano JA, Eisele DW, Fakhry C, Gourin CG, Ha PK, Kang H, Kiess A, Koch WM, Myers JN, Quon H, Richmon JD, Sidransky D, Tufano RP, Westra WH, Bettegowda C, Diaz LA Jr, Papadopoulos N, Kinzler KW, Vogelstein B, Agrawal N. Detection of somatic mutations and HPV in the saliva and plasma of patients with head and neck squamous cell carcinomas. Sci Transl Med. 2015;7(293):293ra104.
41. Franzmann EJ, Reategui EP, Pereira LH, Pedroso F, Joseph D, Allen GO, Hamilton K, Reis I, Duncan R, Goodwin WJ, Hu JJ, Lokeshwar VB. Salivary protein and solCD44 levels as a potential screening tool for early detection of head and neck squamous cell carcinoma. Head Neck. 2012;34(5):687–95.
42. Nagler R, Bahar G, Shpitzer T, Feinmesser R. Concomitant analysis of salivary tumor markers--a new diagnostic tool for oral cancer. Clin Cancer Res. 2006;12(13):3979–84.
43. Sridharan G, Ramani P, Patankar S, Vijayaraghavan R. Evaluation of salivary metabolomics in oral leukoplakia and oral squamous cell carcinoma. J Oral Pathol Med. 2019;48(4):299–306.
44. Cohen JD, Javed AA, Thoburn C, Wong F, Tie J, Gibbs P, Schmidt CM, Yip-Schneider MT, Allen PJ, Schattner M, Brand RE, Singhi AD, Petersen GM, Hong SM, Kim SC, Falconi M, Doglioni C, Weiss MJ, Ahuja N, He J, Makary MA, Maitra A, Hanash SM, Dal Molin M, Wang Y, Li L, Ptak J, Dobbyn L, Schaefer J, Silliman N, Popoli M, Goggins MG, Hruban RH, Wolfgang CL, Klein AP, Tomasetti C, Papadopoulos N, Kinzler KW, Vogelstein B, Lennon AM. Combined circulating tumor DNA and protein biomarker-

based liquid biopsy for the earlier detection of pancreatic cancers. Proc Natl Acad Sci U S A. 2017;114(38):10202–7.

45. Arya M, Shergill IS, Williamson M, Gommersall L, Arya N, Patel HR. Basic principles of real-time quantitative PCR. Expert Rev Mol Diagn. 2005;5(2):209–19.

46. Bustin SA, Benes V, Garson JA, et al. The MIQE guidelines: minimum information for publication of quantitative real-time PCR experiments. Clin Chem. 2009;55(4):611–22.

47. Chan KCA, Woo JKS, King A, et al. Analysis of plasma epstein-barr virus DNA to screen for nasopharyngeal cancer [published correction appears in N Engl J Med. 2018 Mar 8;378(10):973]. N Engl J Med 2017;377(6):513–522.

48. Park NJ, Zhou H, Elashoff D, et al. Salivary microRNA: discovery, characterization, and clinical utility for oral cancer detection. Clin Cancer Res. 2009;15(17):5473–7.

49. Duz MB, Karatas OF, Guzel E, et al. Identification of miR-139-5p as a saliva biomarker for tongue squamous cell carcinoma: a pilot study. Cell Oncol (Dordr). 2016;39(2):187–93. https://doi.org/10.1007/s13402-015-0259-z.

50. Fadhil RS, Wei MQ, Nikolarakos D, Good D, Nair RG. Salivary microRNA miR-let-7a-5p and miR-3928 could be used as potential diagnostic bio-markers for head and neck squamous cell carcinoma. PLoS One. 2020;15(3):e0221779.

51. Liu CJ, Lin SC, Yang CC, Cheng HW, Chang KW. Exploiting salivary miR-31 as a clinical biomarker of oral squamous cell carcinoma. Head Neck. 2012;34(2):219–24.

52. Kanagal-Shamanna R. Digital PCR: principles and applications. Methods Mol Biol. 2016;1392:43–50.

53. Ahn SM, Chan JY, Zhang Z, et al. Saliva and plasma quantitative polymerase chain reaction-based detection and surveillance of human papillomavirus-related head and neck cancer. JAMA Otolaryngol Head Neck Surg. 2014;140(9):846–54.

54. Kinde I, Wu J, Papadopoulos N, Kinzler KW, Vogelstein B. Detection and quantification of rare mutations with massively parallel sequencing. Proc Natl Acad Sci U S A. 2011;108(23):9530–5.

55. Reslova N, Michna V, Kasny M, Mikel P, Kralik P. xMAP technology: applications in detection of pathogens. Front Microbiol. 2017;8:55. Published 2017 Jan 25.

56. Arellano-Garcia ME, Hu S, Wang J, et al. Multiplexed immunobead-based assay for detection of oral cancer protein biomarkers in saliva. Oral Dis. 2008;14(8):705–12.

57. Anderson KS, Wong J, D'Souza G, et al. Serum antibodies to the HPV16 proteome as biomarkers for head and neck cancer. Br J Cancer. 2011;104(12):1896–905.

58. Linkov F, Lisovich A, Yurkovetsky Z, et al. Early detection of head and neck cancer: development of a novel screening tool using multiplexed immunobead-based biomarker profiling. Cancer Epidemiol Biomark Prev. 2007;16(1):102–7.

59. Wei F, Yang J, Wong DT. Detection of exosomal biomarker by electric field-induced release and measurement (EFIRM). Biosens Bioelectron. 2013;44:115–21.

60. Wei F, Lin CC, Joon A, Feng Z, Troche G, Lira ME, Chia D, Mao M, Ho CL, Su WC, Wong DT. Noninvasive saliva-based EGFR gene mutation detection in patients with lung cancer. Am J Respir Crit Care Med. 2014;190(10):1117–26.

61. Tu M, Wong MY, Sun X, Dai M, Huang R, Chen Y, Lin X, Yang A, Zheng Q, Liao W. Rapid PCR-free meat species mitochondrial DNA identification using Electric Field Induced Release and Measurement (EFIRM®). Anal Chim Acta. 2020;1099:68–74.

62. Pu D, Liang H, Wei F, Akin D, Feng Z, Yan Q, Li Y, Zhen Y, Xu L, Dong G, Wan H, Dong J, Qiu X, Qin C, Zhu D, Wang X, Sun T, Zhang W, Li C, Tang X, Qiao Y, Wong DT, Zhou Q. Evaluation of a novel saliva-based epidermal growth factor receptor mutation detection for lung cancer: a pilot study. Thorac Cancer. 2016;7(4):428–36.

63. Wei F, Strom CM, Cheng J, Lin CC, Hsu CY, Soo Hoo GW, Chia D, Kim Y, Li F, Elashoff D, Grognan T, Tu M, Liao W, Xian R, Grody WW, Su WC, Wong DTW. Electric field-induced release and measurement liquid biopsy for noninvasive early lung Cancer assessment. J Mol Diagn. 2018;20(6):738–42.

64. Issa IA, Noureddine M. Colorectal cancer screening: an updated review of the available options. World J Gastroenterol. 2017;23(28):5086–96.

65. Wright CL, Pan Q, Knopp MV, Tweedle MF. Advancing theranostics with tumor-targeting peptides for precision otolaryngology. World J Otorhinolaryngol Head Neck Surg. 2016;2(2):98–108.
66. Mayerhoefer ME, Prosch H, Beer L, et al. PET/MRI versus PET/CT in oncology: a prospective single-center study of 330 examinations focusing on implications for patient management and cost considerations. Eur J Nucl Med Mol Imaging. 2020;47:51–60.
67. Frangioni JV. New technologies for human cancer imaging. J Clin Oncol. 2008;26(24):4012–21.
68. Economopoulou P, de Bree R, Kotsantis I, Psyrri A. Diagnostic tumor markers in head and neck squamous cell carcinoma (HNSCC) in the clinical setting. Front Oncol. 2019;9:827.
69. Higgins LJ, Pomper MG. The evolution of imaging in cancer: current state and future challenges. Semin Oncol. 2011;38(1):3–15.
70. Warram JM, de Boer E, Sorace AG, Chung TK, Kim H, Pleijhuis RG, van Dam GM, Rosenthal EL. Antibody-based imaging strategies for cancer. Cancer Metastasis Rev. 2014;33(2–3):809–22.
71. Spiegelberg D, Nilvebrant J. CD44v6 targeted imaging of head and Neck squamous cell carcinoma: antibody-based approaches. Contrast Media Mol Imaging. 2017;2017:2709547.
72. Huizing FJ, Garousi J, Lok J, Franssen G, Hoeben BAW, Frejd FY, Boerman OC, Bussink J, Tolmachev V, Heskamp S. CAIX targeting radiotracers for hypoxia imaging in head and neck cancer models. Sci Rep. 2019;9(1):18898. https://doi.org/10.1038/s41598-019-54824-5. PMID: 31827111; PMCID: PMC6906415.
73. Lu M, Kang N, Chen C, Yang L, Li Y, Hong M, Luo X, Ren L, Wang X. Plasmonic enhancement of cyanine dyes for near-infrared light-triggered photodynamic/photothermal therapy and fluorescent imaging. Nanotechnology. 2017;28(44):445710.
74. Madamsetty VS, Mukherjee A, Mukherjee S. Recent trends of the bio-inspired nanoparticles in cancer theranostics. Front Pharmacol. 2019;10:1264.
75. Kooijmans SAA, Schiffelers RM, Zarovni N, Vago R. Modulation of tissue tropism and biological activity of exosomes and other extracellular vesicles: new nanotools for cancer treatment. Pharmacol Res. 2016;111:487–500.
76. Moor J. The Dartmouth College artificial intelligence conference: the next fifty years. AI Mag. 2006;27(4):87–91.
77. Jiang F, Jiang Y, Li H, et al. Artificial intelligence in healthcare: past, present and future. Stroke Vasc Neurol. 2017;2(4):230–43.
78. Borkowski AA, Wilson CP, Borkowski SA, Thomas LB, Deland LA, Grewe SJ, Mastorides SM. Comparing artificial intelligence platforms for histopathologic Cancer diagnosis. Fed Pract. 2019;36(10):456–63.
79. Chishti S, Jaggi KR, Saini A, Agarwal G, Ranjan A. Artificial intelligence-based differential diagnosis: development and validation of a probabilistic model to address lack of large-scale clinical datasets. J Med Internet Res. 2020;22(4):e17550.
80. Samuel AL. Some studies in machine learning using the game of checkers. IBM J Res Dev. 1959;3(3):210–29.
81. Schmidhuber J. Deep learning in neural networks: an overview. Neural Netw. 2015;61:85–117.
82. LeCun Y, Bengio Y, Hinton G. Deep learning. Nature. 2015;521(7553):436–44.
83. Deo RC. Machine learning in medicine. Circulation. 2015;132(20):1920–30.
84. Bi WL, Hosny A, Schabath MB, Giger ML, Birkbak NJ, Mehrtash A, Allison T, Arnaout O, Abbosh C, Dunn IF, Mak RH, Tamimi RM, Tempany CM, Swanton C, Hoffmann U, Schwartz LH, Gillies RJ, Huang RY, Aerts HJWL. Artificial intelligence in cancer imaging: clinical challenges and applications. CA Cancer J Clin. 2019;69(2):127–57.
85. Summerton N, Cansdale M. Artificial intelligence and diagnosis in general practice. Br J Gen Pract. 2019;69(684):324–5.
86. Seeburg DP, Baer AH, Aygun N. Imaging of patients with head and neck cancer: from staging to surveillance. Oral Maxillofac Surg Clin North Am. 2018;30(4):421–33.
87. Mehanna H, Wong WL, McConkey CC, Rahman JK, Robinson M, Hartley AG, Nutting C, Powell N, Al-Booz H, Robinson M, Junor E, Rizwanullah M, von Zeidler SV, Wieshmann

H, Hulme C, Smith AF, Hall P. Dunn J; PET-NECK trial management group. PET-CT surveillance versus neck dissection in advanced head and neck cancer. N Engl J Med. 2016;374(15):1444–54.

88. Siegel RL, Miller KD, Jemal A. Cancer statistics, 2016. CA Cancer J Clin. 2016;66:7–30.

89. Goel R, Moore W, Sumer B, Khan S, Sher D, Subramaniam RM. Clinical practice in PET/CT for the management of head and neck squamous cell cancer. AJR Am J Roentgenol. 2017;209(2):289–303.

90. Forghani R. An update on advanced dual-energy CT for head and neck cancer imaging. Expert Rev Anticancer Ther. 2019;19(7):633–44.

91. Lee B, Choi YJ, Kim SO, Lee YS, Hong JY, Baek JH, Lee JH. Prognostic value of radiologic extranodal extension in human papillomavirus-related oropharyngeal squamous cell carcinoma. Korean J Radiol. 2019;20(8):1266–74.

92. Maxwell JH, Rath TJ, Byrd JK, Albergotti WG, Wang H, Duvvuri U, Kim S, Johnson JT, Branstetter BF 4th, Ferris RL. Accuracy of computed tomography to predict extracapsular spread in p16-positive squamous cell carcinoma. Laryngoscope. 2015;125:1613–8.

93. Carlton JA, Maxwell AW, Bauer LB, McElroy SM, Layfield LJ, Ahsan H, Agarwal A. Computed tomography detection of extracapsular spread of squamous cell carcinoma of the head and neck in metastatic cervical lymph nodes. Neuroradiol J. 2017;30:222–9.

94. Ando T, Kato H, Kawaguchi M, Tanahashi Y, Aoki M, Kuze B, Matsuo M. Diagnostic ability of contrast-enhanced computed tomography for metastatic cervical nodes in head and neck squamous cell carcinomas: significance of additional coronal reconstruction images. Pol J Radiol. 2020;85:e1–7.

95. Kann BH, Aneja S, Loganadane GV, Kelly JR, Smith SM, Decker RH, Yu JB, Park HS, Yarbrough WG, Malhotra A, Burtness BA, Husain ZA. Pretreatment identification of head and neck cancer nodal metastasis and extranodal extension using deep learning neural networks. Sci Rep. 2018;8(1):14036.

96. Balachandar N, Chang K, Kalpathy-Cramer J, Rubin DL. Accounting for data variability in multi-institutional distributed deep learning for medical imaging. J Am Med Inform Assoc. 2020;pii:ocaa017.

97. Kar A, Wreesmann VB, Shwetha V, Thakur S, Rao VUS, Arakeri G, Brennan PA. Improvement of oral cancer screening quality and reach: the promise of artificial intelligence. J Oral Pathol Med 2020. https://doi.org/10.1111/jop.13013.

98. Tax CL, Haslam SK, Brillant M, Doucette HJ, Cameron JE, Wade SE. Oral cancer screening: knowledge is not enough. Int J Dent Hyg. 2017;15(3):179–86.

99. Sharma G. Diagnostic aids in detection of oral cancer: an update. World J Stomatol. 2015;4(3):115–20.

100. Ilhan B, Lin K, Guneri P, Wilder-Smith P. Improving Oral Cancer outcomes with imaging and artificial intelligence. J Dent Res. 2020;99(3):241–8.

101. Jeyaraj PR, Samuel Nadar ER. Computer-assisted medical image classification for early diagnosis of oral cancer employing deep learning algorithm. J Cancer Res Clin Oncol. 2019;145(4):829–37.

102. Fei B, Lu G, Wang X, Zhang H, Little JV, Patel MR, Griffith CC, El-Diery MW, Chen AY. Label-free reflectance hyperspectral imaging for tumor margin assessment: a pilot study on surgical specimens of cancer patients. J Biomed Opt. 2017;22(8):1–7.

103. Aubreville M, Knipfer C, Oetter N, Jaremenko C, Rodner E, Denzler J, Bohr C, Neumann H, Stelzle F, Maier A. Automatic classification of cancerous tissue in laserendomicroscopy images of the oral cavity using deep learning. Sci Rep. 2017;7(1):11979.

104. Song S, Sunny S, Uthoff RD, Patrick S, Suresh A, Kolur T, Keerthi G, Anbarani A, Wilder-Smith P, Kuriakose MA, et al. Automatic classification of dual-modality, smartphone-based oral dysplasia and malignancy images using deep learning. Biomed Opt Express. 2018;9(11):5318–29.

105. Coppola F, Faggioni L, Regge D, Giovagnoni A, Golfieri R, Bibbolino C, Miele V, Neri E, Grassi R. Artificial intelligence: radiologists' expectations and opinions gleaned from a nationwide online survey. Radiol Med. 2020. https://doi.org/10.1007/s11547-020-01205-y.

Chapter 3
Microfluidic Technologies for Head and Neck Cancer: From Single-Cell Analysis to Tumor-on-a-Chip

Yamin Yang and Hongjun Wang

Introduction

Head and neck squamous cell carcinoma (HNSCC) is the sixth most common malignancy worldwide, with approximately 550,000 new cases diagnosed every year [1]. HNSCC accounts for approximately 6% of all cancer cases and is responsible for an estimated 1–2% of cancer deaths [2, 3]. Oral squamous cell carcinoma (OSCC) is the most common oral cancer, representing up to 80–90% of all malignant neoplasms of the oral cavity [4]. OSCC constitutes 90% of all cases of head and neck cancer, with a rising incidence in young adults [5]. Currently, oral cancers are typically diagnosed through a combination of surgical biopsy, radiology, and pathological assessment of tissue specimens [6]. However, due to the lack of reliable tumor-associated biomarkers and indistinct morphological characteristics of early-stage cancer, most OSCC cases are not detected until their late stages [7]. OSCC is usually treated surgically, with or without radiation and chemotherapy. The cure rate for advanced HNSCC and OSCC remains poor, mainly due to late diagnosis and the resistance of tumor cells to treatments at advanced stages [8, 9]. Therefore, there is an urgent need for new biomarkers and methodologies for early detection of HNSCC and OSCC. In addition, better understanding of the specific molecular mechanisms involved in HNSCC and OSCC carcinogenesis and progression can improve the survival and prognosis. Meanwhile, it is essential to establish model systems recapitulating the key pathophysiological features of HNSCC and

Y. Yang
Department of Biomedical Engineering, Nanjing University of Aeronautics and Astronautics, Nanjing, Jiangsu, China
e-mail: yaminyang@nuaa.edu.cn

H. Wang (✉)
Department of Biomedical Engineering, Stevens Institute of Technology, Hoboken, NJ, USA
e-mail: hongjun.wang@stevens.edu

© Springer Nature Switzerland AG 2021
R. El Assal et al. (eds.), *Early Detection and Treatment of Head & Neck Cancers*, https://doi.org/10.1007/978-3-030-69859-1_3

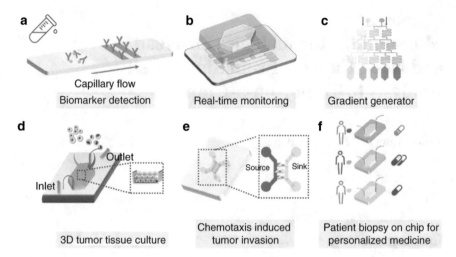

Fig. 3.1 Schematic illustration of representative applications of microfluidics-based platforms for early detection and therapeutic evaluation of head and neck cancers. (**a**) Microfluidics-based multiplexed biomarker detection via antibody binding through capillary flow for early screening of oral cancer in a highly sensitive and efficient manner. (**b**) Embedded electrodes in microfluidic devices enable real-time multiparametric electrical measurements for oral cancer diagnosis. (**c**) A typical microchannel network allows serial dilution of a single concentration into a gradient range of five concentration doses. (**d**) Tumor-on-chip platform for in vitro resembling 3D multicellular tumor constructs by co-culturing heterogeneous cells. (**e**) Representative microfluidic design for inducing in vivo emulating chemotactic heterogeneity for motility analysis or tumor cell invasion study. (**f**) Personalized patient-tumor-biopsy-on-chip for customizing the treatment regimens

OSCC in studying their progression and evaluating their response to various therapeutic modalities. The emerging microfluidic technologies that involve miniaturization, yield high-throughput capability, and integrate with various detection modalities hold intriguing advantages for cancer diagnosis, on-chip single-cell analysis, tumor microenvironment recapitulation, and drug evaluation [10, 11]. In this chapter, we summarize recent advances in microfluidic technologies for diagnostic and therapeutic applications in head and neck cancer. As shown in Fig. 3.1, the most significant advances in the biomarker development for early detection and tumor microenvironment reconstruction for drug evaluation are particularly highlighted.

General Background of Microfluidic Technologies

Microfluidics deals with the precise control and manipulation of fluids, usually in the range of microliters (10^{-6} liter) to picoliters (10^{-12} liter), which are geometrically constrained to networks of channels with dimensions from tens to hundreds of micrometers. The network of microchannels can be incorporated into the microfluidic chip, in which fluids are processed to transport, mix, separate, or attain multiplexing [12]. Microfluidic applications operate on the integrated microfabrication and specific physicochemical properties of designed microstructures. To precisely manipulate the fluids inside the microchannels, the microfluidic systems need to be designed specifically. Typically, the microfluidic systems include an on-chip fluid control using capillary forces, embedded elements such as Quake valves, or microsystems (e.g., liquid pumps, gas valves, pressure controllers) for handling off-chip fluids. Materials used to fabricate the microfluidic chips have rapidly evolved from rigid glass and silicon chips to biodegradable hydrogel materials. Most microfluidic chips are made of polydimethylsiloxane (PDMS), owning to its good biocompatibility, gas permeability, and low cost [13]. Fabrication techniques for the microfluidic chips are also dependent on the materials and geometries. The basis for most microfluidic fabrication processes by far was introduced by Whitesides in 1998 using soft lithography [14]. During the microfabrication process of a typical PDMS-based microfluidic device, a master mold is often fabricated using SU-8 photolithography. That is, photomask microchannels are transferred onto a silicon wafer spin-coated with SU-8 photoresist, and the unpolymerized regions of SU-8 are washed away to form a SU8 master mold with desired microfeatures. Premixed, degassed PDMS is poured over the mold master. A cured PDMS layer is then peeled off and chemically bonded to another layer or glass slide upon oxygen plasma treatment. As an alternative to lithography, rapid prototyping and 3D printing, such as stereolithography, have recently emerged for the direct production of complex 3D structures in microfluidic devices [15].

With the capability of multi-functionality in modern microfluidics, an environment closer to in vivo can be recapitulated in vitro by replicating various physiologically relevant parameters, such as cell-matrix, flow rate, and chemical gradients [16]. First, as the dimensions of microfluidic channels are well-suited to the physical scale of eukaryotic cells, microfluidic techniques hold immense promise as a platform to study cell behavior from single- to multicellular organism levels that are not possible using conventional macroscale petri-dish or well-plate techniques [17]. Second, compared to the conventional 2D static petri-dish culture, the dynamic culture conditions provided by microfluidics not only enable sufficient nutrient supply via perfusion, along with timely removal of wastes for long-term cell culture, but also simulate the in vivo dynamic cell processes by providing complex interactions between cells and their residing microenvironments [18]. Third, the laminar flow of microfluidics at the micron scale also enables the creation of stable chemical gradients with spatial control for understanding the chemotactic effects on cells or investigating the cellular responses to drugs in a series of concentration gradients [19, 20]. Last but not least, the ease of integration of microfluidics with other sensing or diagnostic techniques allows real-time detection and simultaneous analysis of different analytes in a single device, with a significant reduction in sample processing time and with simplified procedures [21].

Lab-on-a-Chip Approaches for Early Diagnosis of Head and Neck Cancer

Biomarkers Associated with HNSCC and OSCC

HNSCC and OSCC comprise a wide spectrum of heterogeneous neoplasms for which biomarkers are needed for earlier diagnosis and targeted therapy response. With the identification of human papillomavirus (HPV) as an etiologic agent in a subset of HNSCC, p16 overexpression is employed as a surrogate biomarker in HPV-associated HNSCC in clinical practice [22]. Plasma Epstein-Barr virus (EBV) DNA also plays a role as a predictive and prognostic biomarker specifically in patients with nasopharyngeal carcinoma [23]. Some membrane-associated cell proteins singularly expressed in dysplastic and cancer cells of the oral cavity, such as heat shock protein 47 (Hsp-47), epithelial cell adhesion molecule (EpCAM) [24], and the unique gene transcription profiles of cancer cells, such as p53, cyclin D1, and epidermal growth factor receptor (EGFR) gene, have also been utilized as HNSCC and OSCC biomarkers [25].

Microfluidic-Based Techniques for Detection of HNSCC and OSCC Biomarkers

Conventional methods for HNSCC and OSCC biomarker detection, such as immunohistochemistry (IHC) assays and antibody-based immunoassays, can be expensive and time-consuming [26]. Lab-on-a-chip approaches integrate sample processing steps including concentration, reaction, and detection into chip-scale devices with fluidic microchannels. Diverse technologies, such as electrochemical, optical biosensing, and nanoparticle amplification, have been incorporated into the microfluidic platform for on-chip diagnosis and real-time monitoring [27]. In an earlier review, Ziober et al. discussed the applications of the lab-on-a-chip technology for biomarker detection in the early screening of oral cancer [28]. Compared to the conventional methods, microfluidics-based devices can analyze diverse clinical samples from patients in small amounts and allow for straightforward measurement of multiplexed biomarkers of HNSCC and OSCC in a highly sensitive and efficient manner. In one study, Soares et al. developed a microfluidics-based genosensor for detecting HPV16 in solution as well as HPV16-infected HNSCC cell lines with high sensitivity and specificity [29]. Microfluidic interdigitated electrodes were functionalized with a layer-by-layer film of chitosan and chondroitin sulfate and modified with a DNA probe for anchoring HPV16. The strong specific interaction between the immobilized DNA probe and complementary chain enables the detection of HPV16 at hybridization temperatures with the impedance spectroscopy measurements [29]. Weigum et al. developed a nano-bio-chip (NBC) sensor technique targeting biochemical and morphological changes in exfoliative cytology specimens of oral lesions from 41 dental patients and 11 healthy volunteers [30]. A total of 51 measurement parameters were extracted using the custom image analysis macros, among which four key parameters were significantly elevated in both dysplastic and malignant lesions relative to the healthy oral epithelium, including EGFR labeling intensity, cell and nuclear size, and the nuclear-to-cytoplasmic ratio. Because of the heterogeneity of head and neck tumors, the integration of multiplexed biomarker detection is necessary to provide more reliable diagnoses of oral cancer. Malhotra et al. developed a multiplexed biomarker detection approach using an ultrasensitive electrochemical microfluidic array for accurate oral cancer diagnostics [31]. (Fig. 3.2a) A four-protein panel of biomarkers (8-sensor immunoarray), including interleukin (IL)-6, IL-8, VEGF, and VEGF-C, in serum samples of 78 patients with oral cancer and 49 controls was first captured off-line by massively labeled paramagnetic beads (MB) bioconjugates with ~400,000 horseradish peroxidase (HRP) enzyme and 120,000 Ab2 (Ab2-MB-HRP). After the capture of analyte proteins, Ab2-MB-HRP beads were magnetically separated and injected into the microfluidic array modified with specific antibodies. Changes of amperometric signals in eight nanostructured sensors in the microfluidic device were recorded upon specific protein adsorption and demonstrated a sensitive response to the presence of corresponding analytes. Their nanostructured microfluidic immunoarray provides a rapid serum test for oral cancer detection with a clinical diagnostic sensitivity of 89% and specificity of 98%.

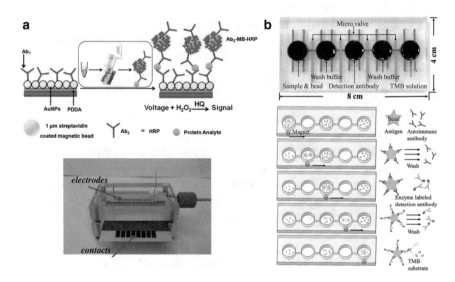

Fig. 3.2 (**a**) A gold nanoparticle (AuNP) immunoarray in a microfluidic channel pumped with massively labeled paramagnetic beads (MB) for ultrasensitive, multiplexed detection of biomarkers in serum samples of patients with oral cancer (Ab1: primary antibodies; Ab2: secondary antibody, PDDA: poly[diallyldimethylammonium chloride]; HRP: horseradish peroxidase; HQ: hydroquinone). (Adapted with permission from Ref. [31]. Copyright (2012) *American Chemical Society*) (**b**) Multiple reaction microwells separated by microvalves to mix antibody-labeled magnetic beads with testing saliva samples to quantify the concentration of anti-p53 in saliva. (Adapted from Ref. [40], CC BY-NC 3.0)

Microfluidic Chip-Based Biosensors for Saliva Analysis

Saliva is an easily obtained bodily fluid containing early-stage diagnostic analytes, including exfoliated normal and potentially abnormal cells, making it an ideal liquid biopsy in the detection and management of HNSCC and OSCC. Saliva could also be used to detect promoter region hypermethylation of cancer-related genes, a process that occurs early in carcinogenesis. More than 100 different salivary constituents have been suggested as potential OSCC markers [32–37]. With the ease of manipulation of liquid at the microscale, target protein biomarkers, DNA, mRNA, electrolytes, and small molecules in saliva can be detected by the combination of microfluidics with electrochemical sensing or immunoassay. In a pilot study, Gau et al. have developed a sensor array chip for direct electrochemical detection of the biomarkers from saliva [38]. Two salivary proteomic biomarkers (thioredoxin and IL-8) and four salivary mRNA biomarkers (salivary transcriptome (SAT), Oz/ten-m homolog (ODZ), IL-8, and IL-1b) associated with oral cancer can be detected with high specificity and sensitivity relying on the efficient binding of target RNA molecules or proteins onto the sensor surface. Wang et al. developed a microfluidic chip-based fluorescent DNA biosensor for the detection of oral cancer-related, single-base mismatch DNA in saliva and serum samples [39]. The target DNA can effectively hybridize with fluorescently labeled signals and capture probes to form a stable "sandwich" structure on the surface of magnetic beads. The magnetic beads in the microfluidic chip are then electrokinetically driven to the detection area by magnets, and the corresponding fluorescence signal is detected by sensitive laser-induced fluorescence (LIF) detection with a high discrimination ability and sensitivity. To achieve higher efficiency than traditional immunoassay and to prevent cross-contamination, an automated microfluidic system was developed by Lin et al. to quantify the concentration of anti-p53 in saliva [40]. As illustrated in Fig. 3.2b, instead of manipulating fluid, a magnet was used to move the p53-antigen-labeled magnetic beads between reaction wells. After antibody capture and series of mixing and washing steps, magnetic beads were reacted with an enzyme substrate (TMB), and the color intensity was related to the concentration of antibodies captured. In addition, automation software and hardware were integrated into the system to control the movement of magnetic beads, the actuation of micromixers, and the opening and closing of microvalves between reaction wells, which further decreased the immunoassay detection time to approximately 60 min.

Microfluidic-Assisted Single-Cell Analysis in HNSCC and OSCC

HNSCC is characterized by significant genomic instability that could lead to intratumor clonal heterogeneity and resistance to chemotherapy and radiation. Detailed analysis of HNSCC ecosystems with single-cell resolution, including the biological behavior and molecular profiling, will greatly improve our understanding of initiation, invasion, metastasis, and therapy resistance during HNSCC progression [41–43]. Comprehensive single-cell research relies heavily on the use of high-throughput and efficient tools for manipulating and analyzing cells. Accompanying the tremendous progress of experimental single-cell sequencing technologies, microfluidic sorting has also provided many technical advantages of single-cell analysis with high specificity and temporal resolution. Microscale devices have been fabricated for trapping single cells with an array of precisely designed microscale structures. Moreover, various approaches, including hydrodynamic, electrical, optical, acoustic, magnetic, and micro-robotic methods, were involved for diverse microfluidic single-cell manipulations. In one example, He et al. fabricated a microfluidic device with a hydrodynamic shuttle to capture individual OSCC cells and to pair them with lymphatic endothelial cells for an in vitro co-culture study [44]. Different types of single cells can repeatedly transport to the culture chamber in the microfluidic device, and cell-cell interactions were monitored with time-lapse microscopy. The authors found that the migration behavior of individual OSCCs was affected by the coexistence of lymphatic endothelial cells in a triple-culture setting, highlighting the importance of the cellular heterogeneity for OSCC biology and medical research. In another study, the deformability properties of single cells in response to mechanical stress was determined as an inherent cell marker to distinguish the malignant transformation of oral cancer cells in a microfluidic device [45]. Individual OSCC cells and cells collected from brush biopsy flew through a microfluidic channel were trapped and stretched out along the laser beam axis. Due to their unique cytoskeleton composition, malignant cells showed significant viscoelastic extension behavior in comparison to benign cells. The relative deformation of cells with the increase in laser power was calculated based on the phase-contrast images. This microfluidic-based optical stretching approach owns its potential as a sensitive tool for quantitative and automated cytological sample screening of oral carcinoma. To develop robust classification models and to evaluate a Multivariate Analytical Risk Index for Oral Cancer (MARIO), Abram et al. developed a "cytology-on-a-chip" approach capable of executing high-content analysis at the single-cell level over 200 cellular features related to biomarker expression, nuclear parameters, and cellular morphology [30, 46–48]. As shown in Fig. 3.3a [48], sample cells were processed through a microfluidic cartridge containing an embedded nanoporous membrane, which captured and isolated single cells for fluorescent biomarker labeling. Single-cell data with approximately 300 cytomorphometric parameters extracted from multispectral fluorescence images were analyzed with machine-learning-assisted methods. Key parameters, including cell circularity, Ki67 and EGFR expression, nuclear-cytoplasmic ratio, nuclear area, and cell area, were identified. Their model yielded an overall diagnostic accuracy of 72.8% with the potential to provide a quantitative risk assessment for monitoring the lesion progression in oral cancer.

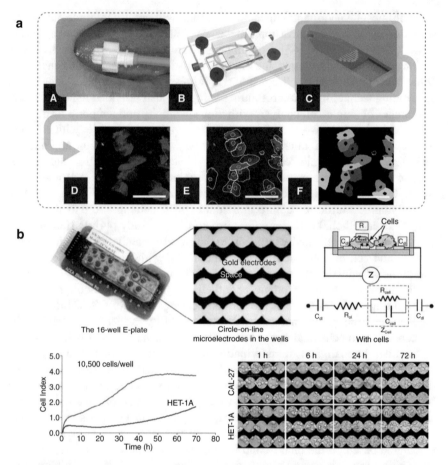

Fig. 3.3 (**a**) A "cytology-on-a-chip" approach including brush cytology sample collection, sample loading, cell capture, multispectral fluorescence image recording, image analysis for single cell identification and region extraction. (Adapted with permission from Ref. [48]. Copyright (2016) *Elsevier Ltd*) (**b**) A real-time impedance measurement system to distinguish oral cancer cells (CAL27 cells) from non-cancer oral epithelial cells (Het-1A cells) based on the impedance-based cell index. (Adapted with permission from Ref. [53]. Copyright (2010) *Springer Nature*)

On-Chip Monitoring of HNSCC and OSCC Characteristics

Another feature of the microfluidics platform is its ease of integration with other electrical and biochemical sensing approaches and in-field measurement tools. For instance, dielectrophoresis (DEP) can be readily incorporated with microfluidic chips to obtain multiparametric measurements of cell electrical properties. Mulhall et al. reported their study distinguishing primary normal oral keratinocytes from precancerous and cancerous oral keratinocyte cell lines in a DEP-microwell electrode system [49]. As cell electric properties were associated with different cell types and transition stages, increasing effective membrane capacitance and decreasing cytoplasmic conductivity were found to correlate with disease progression. Thus, this DEP-on-chip showed its potential for label-free detection of oral cancer and oral precancer. In a similar study, Broche et al. utilized a DEP-based approach to characterize the dielectric differences in the cytoplasm and membrane between a human OSCC cell line H357 and a human HPV-16 transformed keratinocyte cell line [50]. They demonstrated that DEP could be used to isolate cancer cells from normal epithelial cells relying on the size difference between two cell lines by applying a signal of frequency between 5 and 10 kHz, highlighting the utility of DEP in oral cancer detection [51].

Aside from DEP, electrical impedance spectroscopy (EIS) is another label-free method for characterizing biological samples based on cellular dielectric properties, such as the absolute impedance, phase, conductance, and capacitance. Embedded electrodes in microfluidic devices have enabled long-term, real-time EIS for multiparametric measurements for oral cancer diagnosis [52]. Yang et al. designed a real-time impedance measurement system to distinguish oral cancer cells and non-cancer oral epithelial cells based on the kinetics of cell spreading and the static impedance-based cell index [53]. This impedance-based method could be a rapid label-free and noninvasive approach to distinguish a spreading OSCC cell line CAL 27 from a non-cancer-derived oral epithelial cell line Het-1A (Fig. 3.3b).

Cancer cell electrotaxis, which refers to the directional migration towards either cathode or anode under a direct current electric field, is closely related to their metastatic potentials. Microfluidic-based electrotaxis measurement can overcome the disadvantages of conventional dish-based methods by miniaturizing the experimental setup and increasing the throughput. Tsai et al. utilized a microfluidic device to study the electrotaxis of an OSCC cell line HSC-3 [54]. Three different electric field strengths were achieved in the microdevice based on an interconnecting network of microfluidic segments while simultaneously providing a uniform flow field. According to their results, OSCC cells showed weaker electrotaxis response as compared to lung adenocarcinoma cell lines.

Microfluidic Technology for Isolation and Detection of Circulating Tumor Cells in HNSCC

Circulating tumor cells (CTCs) have been identified as a potential marker for early metastatic disease, response to treatment, and surveillance in HNSCC. Taking advantage of the physical and biological differences between CTCs and normal cells, microfluidic technologies enable precise isolation of CTCs from the blood. Some epithelial-specific surface markers (e.g., EpCAM, EGFR, human epidermal growth factor receptor 2 (HER2), and Mucin 1, cell surface associated (MUC1)) expressed on CTCs can be employed for CTC isolation in HNSCC patients. As CTCs can undergo epithelial-to-mesenchymal-transition (EMT),

EMT-related markers such as neurotrophin receptor B and inflammatory cyto-kines (IL-1β) are also considered as potential targets for isolating CTCs [55]. Maremanda et al. designed a flat channel PDMS microfluidic device functional-ized with locked nucleic acid (LNA)-modified aptamers that targeted EpCAM and nucleolin expression to capture CTCs [56]. An average capture of 5 ± 3 CTCs per mL were obtained from 22 of 25 blood samples from patients with head and neck cancer by using the EpCAM LNA aptamer-functionalized chip. These chips were demonstrated to be reusable, increasing their sustainability. As CTCs are usually larger than normal blood cells, size-based CTC isolation methods have also been adapted to the design of microfluidic devices. As a result of laminar flow, the low shear stress acting on CTCs within microchannels allows for accu-rate isolation of intact CTCs for subsequent assays and culture. Kulasinghe et al. designed a straight microfluidic chip for efficient sorting and preservation of single CTCs, CTC clusters, and circulating tumor microemboli from 10 of 21, 9 of 21, and 2 of 21 patient samples, respectively [57]. According to the two-stage migration model of inertial microfluidics, cells flowing inside the straight low-aspect-ratio microchannels are dominated by the inertial force, which depends on the size of cells. That is, larger individual CTCs, CTC clusters, or CTMs migrate much faster into their equilibrium positions at the centerline near the top and bot-tom walls, while smaller normal blood cells distribute throughout the cross-sec-tion of channels. Such differential diameter-dependent cell migration offers unparalleled convenience for label-free cell separation. As shown in Fig. 3.4a, the same group recently evaluated the use of spiral microfluidic chips for CTC

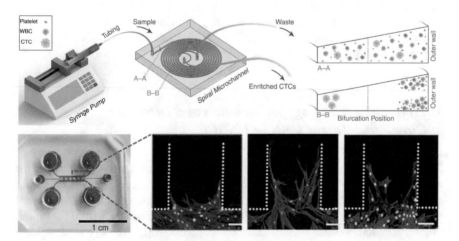

Fig. 3.4 (**a**) A spiral microfluidic chip setup for the enrichment of circulating head and neck tumor cells. Adapted from Ref. [58], CC BY 4.0. (**b**) Microfluidic-based cell invasion assay showing the invasion areas of primary CAFs from patients with ACC were significantly greater than that of the fibroblasts isolated from normal gingival tissues. (Adapted from Ref. [61], CC BY 4.0)

enrichment with a detection rate of 54% for patients with head and neck cancer [58]. The curvilinear microchannels in the spiral chip provide hydrodynamic forces for size-based cell sorting, which help separate and enrich CTCs from the lysed whole blood.

Tumor-on-Chip Platforms for Cancer Biology Investigation in HNSCC and OSCC

Tumor Invasion and Metastasis

It is well recognized that cancer invasion and metastasis are the most important prognostic factor in OSCC. The invasion front of OSCC harbors the most aggressive cells of cancer progression. Compared to traditional transwell chamber-based methods, microfluidic devices offer a promising avenue to generate artificial chemokine gradients to induce cell migration and enable real-time observation of cell invasion processes. Liu et al. designed a microfluidic device with two parallel perfusion channels for characterizing the invasion of oral cancer cells [59]. Later, they modeled the OSCC invasion front in the microfluidic chip by confining UM-SCC6 cells to the culture channel and collecting migrated cells through a matrix channel filled with Matrigel. The miRNA profiles of the isolated invasion front cells were compared with those of the cells in the tumor mass by small RNA sequencing. Key miRNA and pathways involved in OSCC invasiveness were determined, which may serve as useful targets for oral cancer therapy [60]. In a similar study (Fig. 3.4b), they evaluated the invasive potential of carcinoma-associated fibroblasts (CAFs) in salivary gland adenoid cystic carcinoma (ACC) [61]. Primary CAFs from two patients with ACC were isolated and co-cultured with ACC cells in the microfluidic invasive model. ACC-derived CAFs showed increased migration and invasion activity by secreting more soluble factors and forming an invasive track in the extracellular matrix (ECM).

Recent evidence suggests that the metastatic spread of HNSCC requires the function of cancer stem cells endowed with multipotency, self-renewal, and high tumorigenic potential. Chen et al. designed a single-cell migration chip that generated a chemoattractant gradient in the narrow migration channels [62]. Utilizing this microfluidic migration platform, they assessed the migration ability of cancer stem cells with the presence of the endothelial cell-conditioned medium [63]. In comparison to the conventional static transwell system, microfluidic platforms can better recapitulate the in vivo emulating chemotactic heterogeneity while allowing for motility analysis of single cells in real time. Their results showed that endothelial cell-secreted IL-6 enhanced the survival of highly tumorigenic cancer stem cells and induced the progression of carcinoma cells towards blood vessels by creating a chemotactic gradient. To study the chemotactic response of multicellular OSCC spheroids, Ayuso et al. designed a microfluidic device comprising a central microchamber and two lateral channels through which different reagents can be introduced to generate gradients across the central chamber [64]. Chemotactic behavior of tumor spheroids towards the direction of fetal bovine serum gradient was identified with a greater invaded area under the gradient conditions.

Tumor-Associated Angiogenesis

The microenvironmental conditions of a tumor impact the surrounding vasculature formation, also known as tumor angiogenesis, which is a critical hallmark in tumor development. To investigate the role of cell-cell interactions in modulating the angiogenic capability of oral cancer cells, Tan et al. developed a peel-off cell-culture array chip to control interactions between tumor cells spatiotemporally and to analyze angiogenic factor secretion [65]. An array of rectangular cavities were etched into parylene substrate and filled with fibronectin for cell adhesion. Human OSCC3 and human prostate carcinoma (DU145) were cultured in such micropatterning chips at the single-cell level in comparison with cell clusters dependent on the size of fibronectin features. The key functions of cell-cell interaction in regulating tumor angiogenesis were determined by quantitatively profiling the angiogenic factor proteins (i.e., VEGF and IL-8) secreted from tumor cell clusters.

High microvessel density has been found in both salivary gland ACC and OSCC and correlates with poor prognosis. Inhibition of blood vessel growth has, therefore, become a new strategy in anti-oral cancer therapy. Microfluidic technology has proved to be an ideal platform for elucidating the mechanism of angiogenesis and validating antiangiogenic drugs. Liu et al. developed a biomimetic microfluidic model for assessing the angiogenic capabilities of salivary gland ACC cells and OSCC cells [66]. In the angiogenesis-mimicking unit, tumor cells were seeded into the cell culture chamber, and HUVEC were seeded into the parallel vessel channels with basement membrane extract loaded in between. The biomimetic model reproduced the typical features of pathophysiological angiogenesis, including tumor-induced tip cell differentiation, ECM invasion, and capillary-like formation. The microfluidic model was subsequently used to evaluate the effect of antiangiogenic drugs on ACC- and SCC-induced angiogenesis and demonstrated good similarity with therapeutic response in vivo.

Microfluidic Technologies for Drug Evaluation in HNSCC and OSCC

Compared to the conventional cell-based drug screening performed in well plates, microfluidic technology provides new experimental possibilities of assessing the therapeutic efficacy in treating HNSCC and OSCC. Typical advantages of a microfluidic platform for anticancer therapeutic evaluation include (1) offering heterogeneous tumor tissue recapitulation with higher biological relevance, (2) real-time monitoring of in vivo mimicking dynamic cell-drug interactions, (3) delivery of drugs in gradients with microscale manipulations, and (4) high-throughput screening.

Multicellular Tumor Spheroid Formation and Tumor Microenvironment Reconstruction in Microdevice

Resistance to chemotherapy is a major obstacle to the successful treatment of HNSCC and OSCC. While chemoresistance is dependent on the heterogeneity of cancer cells with a variety of genetic and epigenetic alterations at cellular levels, the tumor microenvironment has emerged as a key player in malignant progression and the development of chemoresistance. Multiple in vitro tumor models are being developed for recapitulating the in vivo tumor microenvironment, among which multicellular tumor spheroids can represent a spectrum of physiologically relevant growth phenotypes closely aligned with solid tumors. Compared to traditional sedimentation or hanging drop methods, uniform spheroid can be created in the confined microfluidic device with precise control of the spheroid size. Microdevices have been fabricated to trap tumor spheroids or to generate uniform spheroids of HNSCC and OSCC, on which chemotherapeutic efficacy has been determined. Kochanek et al. characterized the morphologies, viability, and growth behaviors of multicellular tumor spheroids produced by 11 different HNSCC cell lines in 384-well ultra-low attachment plates [67]. Anticancer drug uptake, penetration, and distribution gradients in the HNSCC monocarboxylate transporters (MCTS) as well as doxorubicin-induced cytotoxicity were investigated by high-content imaging analysis. Tanaka et al. established in vitro HNSCC cancer organoids from 43 patients' samples with a success rate of 30.2% [68]. Responses to cisplatin and docetaxel treatment in vivo were found to be similar to the IC50 calculated from organoid-based drug sensitivity assays in vitro, suggesting these cancer tissue-originated spheroids may represent useful tools to predict in vivo drug sensitivity. These microwell array and micropatterning approaches are highly effective in the massive formation of tumor spheroids, but they have limitations in fully predicting the drug response, due to the lack of microcirculation-like fluidic channels. As compared to static microwell arrays for tumor spheroid construction, microfluidic spheroid perfusion culture devices could sustain long-term survival and proliferation of 3D tumor aggregates by promoting biochemical mass transport and nutrient delivery. Ong et al. reported their study about the fabrication of a microfluidic device using 3D printing technologies for multicellular spheroid cultures [69]. As illustrated in Fig. 3.5a, tumor cells were immobilized within fluidic channels in a microfluidic device fabricated with stereolithography (SLA) printing techniques. Patient-derived parental and metastatic OSCC tumor spheroids can be maintained in this

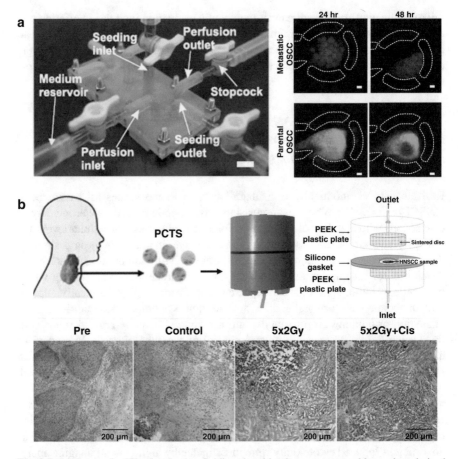

Fig. 3.5 (**a**) Setup of a 3D printed microfluidic spheroid culture system enables patient-derived parental and metastatic OSCC tumor spheroids growth with good viability and functionality. (Adapted with permission from Ref. [69]. Copyright (2017) *IOP Publishing Ltd*). (**b**) Tissue from surgical resection was sliced (precision cut tumor slices, PCTS), and loaded into tumor-on-chip devices. Tumor tissues from laryngeal squamous cell carcinoma in the tumor-on-chip device before and following radiation treatment in the addition of concurrent cisplatin were assessed by H&E staining. (Adapted from Ref. [76], CC BY 4.0)

microfluidic culture device via gravity-driven flow perfusion for up to 72 h with good viability and functionality. Considering the important role that immune cells play in altering tumor microenvironment and cancer immunotherapy, Al-Samadi et al. developed an in vitro microfluidic chip assay to test immunotherapeutic drugs against HNSCC patient samples [70]. Cancer cells isolated from patient-derived tumor tissue biopsy were embedded in human tumor-based ECM "myogel/fibrin." The microfluidic device contains a central chamber for immune cells, which is connected to the neighboring cancer cell-containing chambers via microchannels. Isolated cancer cells and patients' serum and immune cells were loaded into the microfluidic chip, with or without immunomodulators to test both the immune cell migration towards cancer cells and their cytotoxic activity. Although no in vivo evidence was obtained for validation, the efficacy variability of immunotherapeutic drugs was found between two patients with HNSCC in the humanized in vitro microfluidic chip assay.

Microfluidics Enables Dynamic Cell-Drug Interactions

The unique physical behavior of fluids within a microfluidic network can give insights into new ways to resolve the current challenges of evaluating the cellular responses to therapeutics on the basis of dynamic interactions. To mimic the intravenous administration of anticancer drugs in vivo, Jin et al. developed a microfluidic-based perivascular SCC tumor model to assess drug sensitivity in 3D cultured tumor spheroids and toxicity in endothelium in parallel [71]. The microfluidic device was composed of a glass substrate and two layers of PDMS membrane separated by a porous membrane, where HUVECs were seeded in the top chamber, while 3D SCC or ACC spheroids were loaded in the bottom chamber. It was found that the combination of low concentrations of therapeutic drugs presented less toxicity to the HUVEC layer than monotherapy and effectively induced apoptosis of head and neck cancer cells. This model was also applied to test the effects of combinations of drugs on primary cells isolated from patient tissues, demonstrating its clinical potential to facilitate cancer therapy for individuals.

Microfluidic Devices Enable High-Throughput Drug Screening and Online Monitoring

Microfluidic technologies not only have the potential to enhance the biological relevance of cell models in response to different drugs but also can also maintain or increase the throughput of current drug screening methods. For example, with the design of the concentration gradient generator, different concentrations of therapeutics can be generated in the diffusive gradient mixers and sequentially perfused to cells cultured in downstream microchambers. In the example discussed above [71], six concentrations of candidate drugs were created with a concentration gradient generator integrated into the device design, enabling possible evaluation of the therapeutic effects of drugs in various combinations.

With the ease of integration with on-line detection, as introduced in the previous section, cellular response to different treatments can be examined in a real-time manner aside from the end-point analysis of cell viability to draw a more comprehensive conclusion about drug chemosensitivity. Hsieh et al. developed a microfluidic cell culture platform with embedded microheaters, temperature sensors, and micropumps for investigating the interactions between oral cancer cells and anticancer drugs [72]. They emphasized that the choice of cell culture formats (i.e., 2D, 3D, or spheroid culture models) might play an important role in the physiology (i.e., metabolic activity or cell proliferation) of cultured cells and lead to overestimate or underestimate the chemosensitivity outcomes.

Personalized Tumor-Biopsy-on-Chip for Customizing the Treatment Regimens

The use of patient biopsy or patient-derived xenograft models can provide definitive evidence of HNSCC and OSCC metastatic status and offer a more predictable therapeutic response for customizing the treatment formula. Microfluidic platforms exhibit the potential to overcome many technical challenges in biopsy processing as well as to provide an in vivo *pseudo*-microenvironment for maintaining the patient-derived tumor tissue for a relatively long term. Greenman et al. have published a series of studies regarding the culture of ex vivo tissue specimens of head and neck tumors in the microfluidic environment with various biomimetic flow attributes [73–80]. As demonstrated in Fig. 3.5c, the tissue chamber loaded with a patient biopsy was sealed with a threaded adaptor filled with PDMS during perfusion. The microchannel network around the tumor tissue biopsy provides continuous medium flow over the tissue to support its growth by pumping the syringe linked to the inlet via flexible tubing. After confirming the viability of cultured tissues, this ex vivo tissue-on-chip platform was used to investigate the response of fresh and cryogenically frozen primary HNSCC or metastatic lymph node samples to X-irradiation [74, 76] and various chemotherapy drugs (e.g., cisplatin, 5-fluorouracil, and docetaxel) [75, 78, 79]. Upon treatment, a clear inter- and intra-patient variability was observed, as demonstrated with a variety of apoptotic biomarkers and the characteristics of tissue architecture, offering potential approaches to provide clinically valuable information and to create personalized treatment regimens.

Conclusion

HNSCC and OSCC are characterized by high morbidity and poor survival rate. The emergence of microfluidic culture technologies hold promises in single-cell analysis and the possibility of replicating the in vivo tumor environment for HNSCC and OSCC, which offers a potential avenue for both early diagnosis and therapeutic evaluation. Here, we reviewed the recent advances of microfluidic platforms in HNSCC and OSCC for biomarker analysis, single cancer cell detection, and a tumor-on-chip model reconstruction for drug evaluation. Microfluidic technology has proven to reflect the physiological tumor complexities by offering precise control of physical and chemical cues in microarchitecture. With the ease of integration with various sensing and detection modalities, microfluidics is suitable for early cancer detection, high-throughput screening, and mechanistic study of anti-cancer therapeutics. All these attractive features make microfluidics a powerful platform for enhancing in-depth understanding of the molecular pathogenesis and cell-drug interaction involved in HNSCC and OSCC development and intervention. However, the state-of-the-art microfluidic technologies are still in their infancy; more validations by comparing with in vivo results are required prior to the adoption for clinical utilization. Theoretical simulation should be carried out to optimize the microstructure design for minimizing the need for complex fluidic actuation networks and external pumps. Simplified micromanufacturing processes of microfluidic devices with the assistance of automated handling systems are also of particular interest in bringing this platform closer to point-of-care use.

References

1. Vigneswaran N, Williams MD. Epidemiological trends in head and neck cancer and aids in diagnosis. Oral Maxillofac Surg Clin North Am. 2014;26:123–41.
2. Jemal A, et al. Global cancer statistics. CA Cancer J Clin. 2011;61:69–90.
3. Sabaila A, Fauconnier A, Huchon C. Cancer incidence and mortality worldwide: sources, methods and major patterns in GLOBOCAN 2012. Int J Cancer. 2015;43:66–7.
4. Pires FR, et al. Oral squamous cell carcinoma: clinicopathological features from 346 cases from a single Oral pathology service during an 8-year period. J Appl Oral Sci. 2017;21:460–7.
5. Noguti J, et al. Metastasis from oral cancer: an overview. Cancer Genomics Proteomics. 2012;9:329–36.
6. Akbulut N, Altan A. Early detection and multidisciplinary approach to oral cancer patients. Prevention, detection and management of oral cancer (ed. Sundaresan, S.) 13 (IntechOpen, 2018).
7. Yakob M, Fuentes L, Wang MB, Abemayor E, Wong DTW. Salivary biomarkers for detection of oral squamous cell carcinoma: current state and recent advances. Curr Oral Heal Rep. 2014;1:133–41.
8. Rivera C. Essentials of oral cancer. Int J Clin Exp Pathol. 2015;8:11884–94.
9. Cognetti DM, Weber RS, Lai SY. Head and neck cancer: an evolving treatment paradigm. Cancer. 2008;113:1911–32.
10. Sackmann EK, Fulton AL, Beebe DJ. The present and future role of microfluidics in biomedical research. Nature. 2014;507:181–9.
11. Ahn J, Sei Y, Jeon N, Kim Y. Tumor microenvironment on a chip: the progress and future perspective. Bioengineering. 2017;4:64.
12. Mark D, Haeberle S, Roth G, Von Stetten F, Zengerle R. Microfluidic lab-on-a-chip platforms: requirements, characteristics and applications. Chem Soc Rev. 2010;39:1153–82. https://doi.org/10.1039/b820557b.
13. Ren K, Zhou J, Wu H. Materials for microfluidic chip fabrication. Acc Chem Res. 2013;46:2396–406.
14. Ashley JF, Cramer NB, Davis RH, Bowman CN. Soft-lithography fabrication of microfluidic features using thiol-ene formulations. Lab Chip. 2011;11:2772–8.
15. Zips S, et al. Direct stereolithographic 3D printing of microfluidic structures on polymer substrates for printed electronics. Adv Mater Technol. 2019;4:1–5.

16. Coluccio ML, et al. Microfluidic platforms for cell cultures and investigations. Microelectron Eng. 2019;208:14–28.
17. Duncombe TA, Tentori AM, Herr AE. Microfluidics: reframing biological enquiry. Nat Rev Mol Cell Biol. 2015;16:554–67.
18. Tehranirokh M, Kouzani AZ, Francis PS, Kanwar JR. Microfluidic devices for cell cultivation and proliferation. Biomicrofluidics. 2013;7:1–32.
19. Wang X, Liu Z, Pang Y. Concentration gradient generation methods based on microfluidic systems. RSC Adv. 2017;7:29966–84.
20. Kim SH, Lee GH, Park JY, Lee SH. Microplatforms for gradient field generation of various properties and biological applications. J Lab Autom. 2015;20:82–95.
21. Luka G, et al. Microfluidics integrated biosensors: a leading technology towards lab-on-A-chip and sensing applications. Sensors (Switzerland). 2015;15:30011–31.
22. Eze N, Lo Y-C, Burtness B. Biomarker driven treatment of head and neck squamous cell cancer. Cancers Head Neck. 2017;2:1–12.
23. Ferrari D, et al. Role of plasma EBV DNA levels in predicting recurrence of nasopharyngeal carcinoma in a western population. BMC Cancer. 2012;12:208.
24. Pandya D, Nagarajappa AK, Reddy S, Bhasin M. Lab-on-a-Chip-oral cancer diagnosis at your door step. J Int Oral Heal. 2015;7:122–8.
25. Thomas GR, Nadiminti H, Regalado J. Molecular predictors of clinical outcome in patients with head and neck squamous cell carcinoma. Int J Exp Pathol. 2005;86:347–63.
26. Hayes B, Murphy C, Crawley A, O'Kennedy R. Developments in point-of-care diagnostic technology for cancer detection. Diagnostics. 2018;8:39.
27. Rackus DG, Shamsi MH, Wheeler AR. Electrochemistry, biosensors and microfluidics: a convergence of fields. Chem Soc Rev. 2015;44:5320–40.
28. Mauk MG, Ziober BL, Chen Z, Thompson JA, Bau HH. Lab-on-a-chip technologies for oral-based cancer screening and diagnostics: capabilities, issues, and prospects. Ann N Y Acad Sci. 2007;1098:467–75.
29. Soares AC, et al. Microfluidic-based genosensor to detect human papillomavirus (HPV16) for head and neck cancer. ACS Appl Mater Interfaces. 2018;10:36757–63.
30. Weigum SE, et al. Nano-Bio-Chip sensor platform for examination of oral exfoliative cytology. Cancer Prev Res. 2010;3:518–28.
31. Malhotra R, et al. Ultrasensitive detection of cancer biomarkers in the clinic using a nanostructured microfluidic array. Anal Chem. 2012;84:6249–55.
32. Wang A, Wang CP, Tu M, Wong DTW. Oral biofluid biomarker research: current status and emerging frontiers. Diagnostics. 2016;6:PMC5192520.
33. Herr AE, et al. Microfluidic immunoassays as rapid saliva-based clinical diagnostics. Proc Natl Acad Sci. 2007;104:5268–73.
34. Kaczor-Urbanowicz KE, et al. Emerging technologies for salivaomics in cancer detection. J Cell Mol Med. 2017;21:640–7.
35. Khan R, Khurshid Z, Yahya Ibrahim Asiri F. Advancing Point-of-Care (PoC) testing using human saliva as liquid biopsy. Diagnostics. 2017;7:39.
36. Zilberman Y, Sonkusale SR. Biosensors and bioelectronics microfluidic optoelectronic sensor for salivary diagnostics of stomach cancer. Biosens Bioelectron. 2015;67:465–71.
37. Herr AE, et al. Integrated microfluidic platform for oral diagnostics. Ann N Y Acad Sci. 2007;1098:362–74.
38. Gau V, Wong D. Oral Fluid Nanosensor Test (OFNASET) with advanced electrochemical-based molecular analysis platform. Ann N Y Acad Sci. 2007;1098:401–10.
39. Wang Z, et al. A microfluidic chip-based fluorescent biosensor for the sensitive and specific detection of label-free single-base mismatch via magnetic beads-based 'sandwich' hybridization strategy. Electrophoresis. 2013;34:2177–84.
40. Lin YH, et al. Detection of anti-p53 autoantibodies in saliva using microfluidic chips for the rapid screening of oral cancer. RSC Adv. 2018;8:15513–21.

41. López-Verdín S, et al. Molecular markers of anticancer drug resistance in head and neck squamous cell carcinoma: a literature review. Cancers (Basel). 2018;10:1–15.
42. Canning M, et al. Heterogeneity of the head and neck squamous cell carcinoma immune landscape and its impact on immunotherapy. Front Cell Dev Biol. 2019;7:1–19.
43. Reese JB, et al. Single-cell transcriptomic analysis of primary and metastatic tumor ecosystems in head and neck cancer. Cell. 2018;123:4757–63.
44. He CK, Chen YW, Wang SH, Hsu CH. Hydrodynamic shuttling for deterministic high-efficiency multiple single-cell capture in a microfluidic chip. Lab Chip. 2019;19:1370–7.
45. Runge J, et al. Evaluation of single-cell biomechanics as potential marker for oral squamous cell carcinomas: a pilot study. Oral Dis. 2014;20:120–7.
46. Weigum SE, Floriano PN, Christodoulides N, McDevitt JT. Cell-based sensor for analysis of EGFR biomarker expression in oral cancer. Lab Chip. 2007;7:995–1003.
47. Abram TJ, et al. Development of a cytology-based multivariate analytical risk index for oral cancer. Oral Oncol. 2019;92:6–11.
48. Abram TJ, et al. Cytology-on-a-chip' based sensors for monitoring of potentially malignant oral lesions. Oral Oncol. 2016;60:103–11.
49. Mulhall HJ, et al. Cancer, pre-cancer and normal oral cells distinguished by dielectrophoresis. Anal Bioanal Chem. 2011;401:2455–63.
50. Broche LM, et al. Early detection of oral cancer – is dielectrophoresis the answer? Oral Oncol. 2007;43:199–203.
51. Adekanmbi EO, Srivastava SK. Dielectrophoretic applications for disease diagnostics using lab-on-a-chip platforms. Lab Chip. 2016;16:2148–67.
52. Cheung KC, et al. Microfluidic impedance-based flow cytometry. Cytom Part A. 2010;77:648–66.
53. Yang L, Arias LR, Lane TS, Yancey MD, Mamouni J. Real-time electrical impedance-based measurement to distinguish oral cancer cells and non-cancer oral epithelial cells. Anal Bioanal Chem. 2011;399:1823–33.
54. Tsai HF, Peng SW, Wu CY, Chang HF, Cheng JY. Electrotaxis of oral squamous cell carcinoma cells in a multiple-electric-field chip with uniform flow field. Biomicrofluidics. 2012;6:34116.
55. Perumal V, et al. Circulating tumour cells (CTC), head and neck cancer and radiotherapy; future perspectives. Cancers (Basel). 2019;11:1–25.
56. Maremanda NG, et al. Quick chip assay using locked nucleic acid modified epithelial cell adhesion molecule and nucleolin aptamers for the capture of circulating tumor cells. Biomicrofluidics. 2015;9:1–20.
57. Kulasinghe A, Zhou J, Kenny L, Papautsky I, Punyadeera C. Capture of circulating tumour cell clusters using straight microfluidic chips. Cancers (Basel). 2019;11:1–11.
58. Kulasinghe A, et al. Enrichment of circulating head and neck tumour cells using spiral microfluidic technology. Sci Rep. 2017;7:1–10.
59. Liu T, et al. A microfluidic device for characterizing the invasion of cancer cells in a 3-D matrix. Electrophoresis. 2009;30:4285–91.
60. Li X, et al. Downregulation of miR-218-5p promotes invasion of oral squamous cell carcinoma cells via activation of CD44-ROCK signaling. Biomed Pharmacother. 2018;106:646–54.
61. Li J, et al. Carcinoma-associated fibroblasts lead the invasion of salivary gland adenoid cystic carcinoma cells by creating an invasive track. PLoS One. 2016;11:1–15.
62. Chen YC, et al. Single-cell migration chip for chemotaxis-based microfluidic selection of heterogeneous cell populations. Sci Rep. 2015;5:1–13.
63. Kim HS, et al. Endothelial-derived interleukin-6 induces cancer stem cell motility by generating a chemotactic gradient towards blood vessels. Oncotarget. 2017;8:100339–52.
64. Ayuso JM, et al. Study of the chemotactic response of multicellular spheroids in a microfluidic device. PLoS One. 2015;10:1–16.
65. Tan CP, et al. Parylene peel-off arrays to probe the role of cell-cell interactions in tumour angiogenesis. Integr Biol. 2009;1:587–94.

66. Liu L, et al. Biomimetic tumor-induced angiogenesis and anti-angiogenic therapy in a microfluidic model. RSC Adv. 2016;6:35248–56.
67. Kochanek SJ, Close DA, Johnston PA. High content screening characterization of head and neck squamous cell carcinoma multicellular tumor spheroid cultures generated in 384-well ultra-low attachment plates to screen for better cancer drug leads. Assay Drug Dev Technol. 2019;17:17–36.
68. Tanaka N, et al. Head and neck cancer organoids established by modification of the CTOS method can be used to predict in vivo drug sensitivity. Oral Oncol. 2018;87:49–57.
69. Ong LJY, et al. A 3D printed microfluidic perfusion device for multicellular spheroid cultures. Biofabrication. 2017;9:45005.
70. Al-samadi A, et al. In vitro humanized 3D microfluidic chip for testing personalized immunotherapeutics for head and neck cancer patients. Exp Cell Res. 2019;383:111508.
71. Jin D, et al. Application of a microfluidic-based perivascular tumor model for testing drug sensitivity in head and neck cancers and toxicity in endothelium. RSC Adv. 2016;6:29598–607.
72. Hsieh CC, Huang S, Bin W, C P, Shieh DB, Lee GB. A microfluidic cell culture platform for real-time cellular imaging. Biomed Microdevices. 2009;11:903–13.
73. Bower R, et al. Maintenance of head and neck tumor on-chip: gateway to personalized treatment? Futur. Sci. OA. 2017;3:FSO174.
74. Cheah R, et al. Measuring the response of human head and neck squamous cell carcinoma to irradiation in a microfluidic model allowing customized therapy. Int J Oncol. 2017;51:1227–38.
75. Hattersley SM, et al. A microfluidic system for testing the responses of head and neck squamous cell carcinoma tissue biopsies to treatment with chemotherapy drugs. Ann Biomed Eng. 2012;40:1277–88.
76. Kennedy R, et al. A patient tumour-on-a-chip system for personalised investigation of radiotherapy based treatment regimens. Sci Rep. 2019;9:1–10.
77. Tanweer F, Green VL, Stafford ND, Greenman J. Application of microfluidic systems in management of head and neck squamous cell carcinoma. Head Neck. 2014;36:1391.
78. Riley A, et al. A novel microfluidic device capable of maintaining functional thyroid carcinoma specimens ex vivo provides a new drug screening platform. BMC Cancer. 2019;19:1–13.
79. Sylvester D, Hattersley SM, Stafford ND, Haswell SJ. Development of microfluidic-based analytical methodology for studying the effects of chemotherapy agents on cancer tissue. Curr Anal Chem. 2012;9:2–8.
80. Sylvester D, Hattersley S, Haswell S. Development of microfluidic based devices for studying tumour biology and evaluating treatment response in head and neck cancer biopsies. 14th Int Conf Miniaturized Syst Chem Life Sci. 2010:1472–4.

Chapter 4
Nanotechnology for Diagnosis, Imaging, and Treatment of Head and Neck Cancer

Mehdi Ebrahimi

Introduction

According to the World Health Organization's (WHO's) International Agency for Research on Cancer (IARC) and the National Cancer Institute (NCI), cancer is one of the leading causes of death in the twenty-first century, and the number of people with cancer is going to increase significantly within the next two decades. The number of new cancer cases per year is expected to rise to 23.6 million by 2030 [1, 2]. Therefore, the main global strategies are based on the following topics: (i) monitoring the incidence and prevalence of cancer, (ii) identifying the etiology and mechanism of carcinogenesis, and (iii) developing scientific strategies for cancer control.

Classical treatment modalities for head and neck cancer (HNC) are limited to surgery, radiotherapy, and chemotherapy, which are associated with disadvantages, such as low specificity, systemic toxicity, and inadequate or unfavorable results (e.g., remnant tumor cells or tissue after surgery, tumor recurrence, and functional and esthetic impairments). The low survival rate of HNC is mainly associated with the lack of proper drug delivery systems (DDS) that could specifically target the tumor cells with high sensitivity and low systemic toxicity. Considering all of these aspects, there is a high demand for the introduction of novel techniques in the diagnosis, treatment, and follow-up of patients with HNC. Early screening and diagnosis of HNC is of particular interest to prevent complications associated with local invasion and metastasis of cancer [3, 4].

M. Ebrahimi (✉)
Prince Philip Dental Hospital, The University of Hong Kong, Sai Ying Pun, Hong Kong
e-mail: ebrahimi@connect.hku.hk

© Springer Nature Switzerland AG 2021   63
R. El Assal et al. (eds.), *Early Detection and Treatment of Head & Neck Cancers*, https://doi.org/10.1007/978-3-030-69859-1_4

For the past few decades, the emergence of nanotechnology and its application in medicine offered a new insight into the diagnosis and management of many diseases. The first attempted application of nanotechnology in medicine in the late 1960s at ETH Zurich initiated substantial interest in research in this field [5]. The first significant breakthrough in nanomedicine for cancer was in 1995 when the Food and Drug Administration (FDA) approved Doxil, known outside the US as "Caelyx," for the treatment of Kaposi's sarcoma and ovarian cancer [6–8]. Later on, in 2004, FDA approved Cetuximab (Erbitux®) as a nanoscale epidermal growth factor receptor (EGFR) antagonist for locally/regionally advanced, recurrent, or metastatic head and neck squamous cell carcinoma (HNSCC) [9, 10].

Coupling nanotechnology with biology necessitates the engineering of functional systems at the molecular or nanoscale level. The term "nano" has been defined as the size range less than 100 nm; however, there are controversies in the application of this term in the literature [11, 12]. As such the size of nanomaterials or nanoparticles (NP) would be in the range of fundamental macromolecules and cells; DNA double-helix (2 nm diameter), carbon-carbon bond (0.12–0.15 nm), enzymes, and receptors. Nanoscale materials smaller than 50 nm can enter human cells and those less than 20 nm can exit blood vessels. In this context, the importance of nanotechnology is related to the fact that the unusual biological processes at the nanoscale level lead to initiation, multiplication, and metastasis of cancer cells.

Thus, nanotechnology can offer great opportunities for researchers to study and target cancer cells at an early stage. Nanotechnology can also provide rapid and sensitive detection of cancer biomarkers and can cross biological barriers such as the blood-brain barrier. NP and nanomaterials have the potential to be functionalized and tuned for diagnostic and therapeutic applications through passive and active tumor targeting. These systems offer reduced cytotoxicity, controllable distribution pattern, and predefined interaction with desired ligands.

The literature applies different terminologies related to nanotechnology in medicine or nanomedicine including NP, nanomaterials, nanodevices, nanoprobes, nanosensors, and nanocarriers. Disclosure of these terminologies and their applications are beyond the scope of this chapter; therefore, the interested readers are referred to the related literature in each particular field. This chapter provides a general overview of the application of nanotechnology in medicine and the mechanism of interaction of NP at the molecular level. A particular focus is made to cover the current application of nanomedicine in the treatment of HNC including ongoing clinical trials for the treatment of refractory and metastatic cancers.

Classification of NP

In general, the NP are classified into two broad groups: organic and inorganic (Table 4.1). Organic NP could be of polymeric or lipid-based types.

Table 4.1 Classification of currently applied NP in nanotechnology-based management of diseases

Nanoparticles	Group	Examples
	Inorganic	Metallic; Au, Ag
		Magnetic; Fe
		Fullerenes
		Ceramic; Ca-P
		Quantum dot
		Silica
	Organic	Micelle
		Nanocapsule
		Hydrogel
		Dendrimer
		Carbone
		Cyclodextrin
		Solid lipid
		Liposome
		Exosome

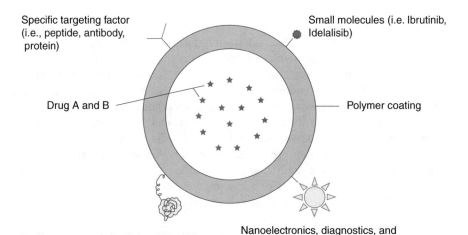

Specific targeting factor (i.e., peptide, antibody, protein)

Small molecules (i.e. Ibrutinib, Idelalisib)

Drug A and B

Polymer coating

Genetic contents (i.e., DNA, siRNA, miRNA)

Nanoelectronics, diagnostics, and molecular imaging agent (i.e., AuNP, AgNP)

Fig. 4.1 NP with multifunctional properties

The Impact of NP Size on Biological Behaviors

Nanocarriers are NP platforms (i.e., liposome, lipid, dendrimer, micelle, gold NP, silver NP, and copper NP) with significantly high surface area (>1000 m^2/g) and unique physicochemical properties. They can be used to carry countless molecules and drugs for selective delivery to cancer tissue and to overcome bioavailability- and instability-associated problems [13]. There is a possibility of cofunctionalizing the NP with different moieties, imaging agents, and drugs for the simultaneous diagnosis, imaging, treatment, and follow-up. "Theranostics" are referred to the field of personalized medicine using multifunctional NP (Fig. 4.1) [14, 15].

Although the size range of "nano" is strictly defined as being less than 100 nm, many forms of nanoparticulate anticancer products are larger than 100 nm such as liposomal/albumin-bound NP (100–1000 nm), paclitaxel-albumin (130 nm), Lipoplatin (110 nm), non-pegylated doxorubicin liposome (180 nm), and cationic liposome containing paclitaxel (230 nm) [16, 17]. Therefore, the size range may not be critical to adversely affect the improved bioavailability and reduced toxicity of drug formulations. However, the increased size can affect the drug half-life in the circulation (i.e., rapid detection and clearance of large particles by phagocytic cells and liver), optical (photonic) properties or emitted color of particles, quantum effects, and available surface area that would impact the in vivo behavior [18]. In general, the characteristics of the nanoparticle-based delivery system, such as size, charge, shape, type of surface modification, and biocompatibility, have a significant impact on the distribution and clearance of nanomedicine [19].

Mechanism of Interaction of NP at the Tumor Site

A tumor is defined as uncontrolled rapid cell growth that results in a mass with defective and irregular vasculature, improper lymphatic drainage, and reduced flow of interstitial fluid. The tumor microenvironment is a dynamic system of extracellular matrix with unique properties. NP encounter both functional (i.e., high interstitial fluid pressure, hypoxic condition, and acidic environment) and biological barriers (i.e., cell density such as the blood-brain barrier) that limit the drug distribution and bioavailability in the tumor microenvironment [20]. Another main challenge is the lack of the desired selectivity of available treatment modalities for cancer (i.e., surgery, radiation, chemotherapy, immunotherapy, hormone therapy, or combination of these) that result in detrimental side effects on healthy tissues [21, 22]. Furthermore, the emergence of multidrug resistance (MDR) becomes a major concern in the therapeutic protocol of cancer and is the main reason for treatment failure [23].

To address these limitations, researchers are studying alternative approaches to enhance tumor penetration of therapeutic agents by directly targeting the tumor cells through targeted DDSs. The advent of nanotechnology in medicine would allow the therapeutic agents to be encapsulated within the NP, adsorbed or conjugated onto the surface of the NP followed by tissue-specific delivery of therapeutic agents and tumor cell-targeting while sparing the healthy cells [24]. This is expected to increase the drug concentration in the tumor site by active and passive internalization with an improved pharmacokinetic and pharmacodynamic profile. Additional desirable features include improved stability, solubility, biocompatibility, biodistribution, bioavailability, and efficacy with reduced systemic toxicity [22, 25]. In fact, the dimensional similarity of NP to biomolecules and their unique physicochemical properties (i.e., high surface-to-volume ratio, possible surface engineering) have made them a promising tool in the management of cancer [26, 27].

Passive Tumor Targeting

An ideal cancer-targeting device should target tumor cells selectively while sparing the healthy surrounding cells. Passive targeting and NP accumulation in the tumor site is a size-dependent process that was first defined as the "enhanced permeability and retention (EPR) effect" [28, 29]. However, healthy tissues are resistant to the passage of NP due to the presence of tight junctions.

Traditionally, the EPR is based on the defective vasculature of tumor tissue as a result of fast angiogenesis, thus the vessel walls containing many pores of 40 nm to 1 μm. Furthermore, tumor mass lacks a functional organized lymphatic system with a very limited clearance rate. This favors extravasation and accumulation of NP (8–100 nm) at the tumor site, which forms the base for the treatment of solid tumor [30, 31].

However, the NP are easily recognized as foreign bodies and soon opsonized by the mononuclear phagocyte of the reticuloendothelial system. The NP should be available in the circulation long enough for the EPR to take place. For this purpose, the hydrophobic nanomaterials or drugs can be masked with hydrophilic polymers of varying molecular weight and chain length such as polyethylene glycol (PEG), a process that is known as "stealth" delivery system [32]. Another challenge for the EPR would be the inaccessibility to the central region of large or solid tumors. This is addressed by additional steps that would enhance EPR such as (i) infusion of angiotensin II to increase systolic blood pressure, (ii) application of NO-releasing agent for vasodilation, and (iii) photodynamic therapy (PDT) or photothermal therapy (PTT). Different factors impacting the EPR efficacy should be considered beforehand during designing nanomedicine, including the size and molecular weight of NP, surface charge, and biocompatibility [33].

Active Tumor Targeting

It is clear that the EPR effect of drug accumulation at the tumor tissue does not assure the delivery of NP into the cells for the desired action. Furthermore, EPR is heterogeneous with variable effectiveness depending on the tumor type and the patient. As such when the drug activation within the cell is required, treatment objectives cannot be achieved solely through EPR. The entry of drugs into the tumor cell is a membrane-specific process that should be achieved through attachment of the designed nanoscale ligand to the specific receptors on the surface of tumor cells followed by phagocytosis/endocytosis mechanism that results in internalization of the drug [34]. For this reason, tumor-targeting can be achieved through NP surface modifications (i.e., with molecules, antibodies, peptides, and aptamers) to target the tumor cells, uncontrolled cell proliferation, or tumor angiogenesis. Therefore, active drug targeting can be applied for tumor-specific drug delivery using overexpressed receptors or biomarkers at the cancer sites. Examples include, (i) transferrin receptor: a cell membrane-associated glycoprotein [35, 36], (ii) folate receptors: a cell membrane-associated glycoprotein [37], (iii) endothelial growth factor receptor (EGFR): endothelial-specific receptor tyrosine kinases (Cetuximab is a clinically approved anti-EGFR as a receptor-blocking monoclonal antibody) [38], (iv) endothelial growth factor (EGF): a potent angiogenic signaling protein (nanocarrier can be conjugated with EGF to enhance tumor cell-specific delivery and internalization) [39, 40], and (v) $\alpha v\beta 3$ integrins (vitronectin receptor) and matrix metalloproteinase receptors: zinc-dependent endopeptidases for targeting uncontrolled cell proliferation [41–43].

New Insight of NP Pathway into the Tumor

Originally, the principle of NP delivery into tumors was defined in 1986 when two independent research groups demonstrated accumulation of dyes and proteins in carcinoma and sarcoma models [28, 44]. In 1998, Hobbs et al. [45] associated this phenomenon with the existence of large permeable inter-endothelial gaps (with a size range of up to 2000 nm) that occur in tumor vasculature during angiogenesis [44–46]. Later, it was proposed that the permeability of blood vessels includes a dynamic vent that forms transient openings and closings at the leaky vascular burst with the vigorous outward flow of fluid (named "eruptions") into the tumor interstitial space [47].

For three decades, this rationale was the base for engineers and scientists to design NP with tunable size and shape to penetrate these inter-endothelial gaps into the tumor. However, the traditional concept of EPR as a passive mechanism of accumulation of NP at the tumor site has been challenged recently [48–52]. This is due to the heterogeneity of tumor vasculature across different species and tumors, the variability of tumor microenvironments, and the infrequent occurrence of inter-endothelial gaps that do not correspond to the presence of NP at the tumor site [53, 54]. Furthermore, there is a lack of original data about active or passive transportation of NP into the tumor [50, 55]. This is because of the inability to directly analyze this mechanism as there is no suitable technique for visualization of NP entry into the tumor. For example, TEM cannot provide dynamic nanoscale resolutions and intravital confocal laser scanning microscopy has a limited resolution despite its real-time analysis ability [47].

As such, the new pieces of evidence suggest endothelial transcytosis as a dominant mechanism of extravasation of NP [50, 56]. This is an active vesicle-mediated transport mechanism to assist macromolecules' crossing of biological barriers and it acts as a trans-endothelial nutritional pathway for some tumors. Figure 4.2 demonstrates the potential mechanisms of entry of NP into the tumor tissue and cells.

Sindhwani group [53] reported that the tumor vasculature is mostly continuous and endothelial gaps occur rarely, thus the NP tumor accumulation cannot be merely explained by the frequency of these endothelial gaps. In fact, the measured tumor accumulation of NP was 60-fold higher than the observed number of these gaps. It

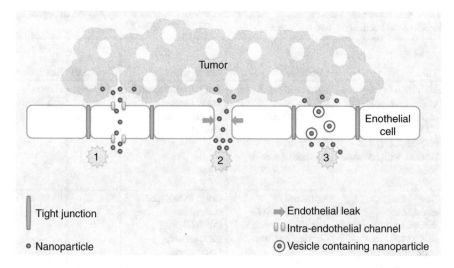

Fig. 4.2 Potential mechanisms of NP' entry into the tumor

was concluded that passive extravasation plays only a minor role, and the dominant mechanism of NP extravasation is the active trans-endothelial pathways. Indeed, 97% of NP enter the tumor using an active process. This could be through intra-endothelial channels or vesicles or other active mechanisms that need to be discovered (Fig. 4.1). Of particular importance during this active intracellular transportation mechanism is the physicochemical properties of NP (i.e., composition, geometry, dimension, surface topography, charge, and mechanical properties) that have a significant impact on the nature of interactions between NP and biological barriers as well as the mechanism of transcytosis [57].

Nanotechnology for the Management of Cancer

Currently, the application of nanotechnology for the diagnosis, imaging, and treatment of tumors is in the early developmental stage. However, several clinical trials are running and there are a few FDA-approved nanomedicines and nanocarriers for cancer (Table 4.2).

Nanotechnology for Early Detection of Cancer

Early detection and diagnosis of cancer is the key factor that significantly reduces the mortality rate by allowing management of cancer before metastasis. Currently, varieties of imaging techniques (i.e., X-ray, MRI, computed tomography (CT),

Table 4.2 Example of current and ongoing clinical trials on nanotechnology-based strategies for targeting the head, neck, and oral cancer

Title	Conditions	Interventions	Enrolment	Study phase / References
Metronomic oral vinorelbine plus anti-PD-L1/anti-CTLA4 immunotherapy in patients with advanced solid tumors (*2018–2023*)	Advanced solid tumors Breast cancer HNC Cervix cancer Prostate cancer	Drug: Durvalumab + Tremelimumab +metronomic vinorelbine	150	Phase 1 and 2 [58]
Basket study to evaluate the therapeutic activity of RO6874281 as a combination therapy in participants with advanced and/or metastatic solid tumors (*2017–2020*)	Advanced or metastatic HNC esophageal cancers Cervical cancers	Drug: RO6874281, atezolizumab (MPDL3280A), gemcitabine, vinorelbine	322	Phase 2 [59]
Ferumoxytol - iron oxide nanoparticle magnetic resonance dynamic contrast-enhanced MRI (*2013–2022*)	HNC	Procedure: MRI Drug: Ferumoxytol	7	Early phase 1 [60]
Paclitaxel albumin-stabilized nanoparticle formulation and carboplatin followed by chemoradiation in treating patients with recurrent head and neck cancer (*2013–2022*)	Tongue cancer Salivary gland SCC Recurrent salivary gland cancer Recurrent HNSCC Recurrent verrucous Carcinoma of the larynx and oral cavity	Drug: carboplatin, paclitaxel albumin-stabilized nanoparticle formulation, fluorouracil, hydroxyurea Procedure: conventional surgery Radiation: radiation therapy, HFRT, Other: LBA	61	Phase 1 [61]
Dose escalation study of mRNA-2752 for intratumoral injection to patients with advanced malignancies (*2018–2021*)	Dose escalation: Relapsed/refractory Solid tumor malignancies or lymphoma Dose expansion: Triple negative breast cancer, HNSCC, non-Hodgkin lymphoma, and urothelial cancer	Biological: mRNA-2752 + durvalumab	126	Phase 1 [62]

Table 4.2 (continued)

Title	Conditions	Interventions	Enrolment	Study phase / References
Induction chemotherapy with ACF followed by chemoradiation therapy for adv. Head and neck cancer (*2012–2023*)	Head and neck neoplasms	Drug: paclitaxel albumin-stabilized nanoparticle formulation, cisplatin, fluorouracil, cetuximab Radiation: IMRT Procedure: Quality-of-life assessment	30	Phase 2 [63–65]
Chemotherapy and locoregional therapy trial (surgery or radiation) for patients with head and neck cancer (*2017–2020*)	HPV-Related HNSCC	Drug: nab-paclitaxel, carboplatin, nivolumab, cisplatin, hydroxyurea, 5-FU, dexamethasone, famotidine, paclitaxel diphenhydramine	56	Phase 2 [66]
Recombinant EphB4-HSA fusion protein with standard chemotherapy regimens in treating patients with advanced or metastatic solid tumors (*2015–2020*)	HNSCC Non-resectable cholangiocarcinoma Pancreatic adenocarcinoma Recurrent gallbladder carcinoma	Drug: Cisplatin, docetaxel, gemcitabine hydrochloride, paclitaxel albumin-stabilized nanoparticle formulation Other: LBA and pharmacological study Biological: Recombinant EphB4-HAS fusion protein	61	Phase 1 [67]
Targeted silica NP for real-time image-guided intraoperative mapping of nodal metastases (*2014–2021*)	Head and neck melanoma Breast cancer Colorectal cancer	Drug: fluorescent cRGDY-PEG-Cy5.5-C dots	105	Phase 1 and 2 [68]
Ficlatuzumab w/wo cetuximab in patients w/cetuximab-resistant, recurrent, or metastatic head/neck squamous cell carcinoma (*2017–2020*)	Head and neck basaloid carcinoma Recurrent and stage IV HNSCC Recurrent oropharyngeal SCC	Biological: Cetuximab Drug: Ficlatuzumab	74	Phase 2 [69]

(continued)

Table 4.2 (continued)

Title	Conditions	Interventions	Enrolment	Study phase / References
Panitumumab IRDye800 optical imaging study (*2016–2022*)	HNC	Drug: Panitumumab IRDye 800 Device: da Vinci Firefly Device: IMAGE1 + ICG Hopkins telescope and/or VITOM	23	Phase 1 [70, 71]
Panitumumab-IRDye800 and 89Zr-panitumumab in identifying metastatic lymph nodes in patients with squamous cell head and neck cancer (*2019–2022*)	HNSCC Carcinoma of the head and neck	Drug: Panitumumab-IRDye800 Drug: Zirconium Zr-89 panitumumab Device: fluorescence imaging system Device: camera (Explorer Air, PDE-NEO II) Device: da Vinci Firefly imaging system Device: IGP-ELVIS-v4 macroscopic specimen imager	14	Phase 1 [72]
Panitumumab-IRDye800 compared to sentinel node biopsy and (Selective) neck dissection in identifying metastatic lymph nodes in patients with head and neck cancer (*2019–2021*)	HNSCC	Drug: Panitumumab-IRDye800, Lymphoseek	20	Phase 2 [73]
Carboplatin, nab-paclitaxel, durvalumab before surgery and adjuvant therapy in head and neck squamous cell carcinoma (*2017–2026*)	SCC Oral cancer Oropharynx cancer Larynx cancer Lip cancer Esophageal cancer	Drug: Durvalumab, carboplatin, nab-paclitaxel, cisplatin Procedure: Ssurgical resection Radiation: IMRT	39	Phase 2 [74]

Abbreviations: *MRI* magnetic resonance imaging, *IMRT* intensity-modulated radiation therapy, *NP* nanoparticles, *HNC* head and neck cancer, *SCC* squamous cell carcinoma, *HNSCC* head and neck squamous cell carcinoma, *HFRT* hyper-fractionated radiation therapy, *LBA* laboratory biomarker analysis endoscopy, and ultrasound) and morphological cell/tissue analysis (i.e., histopathology and cytology) are applied for the diagnosis of cancer. Unfortunately, these methods are not molecular-based therefore they are limited to detection of cancer only after visible and remarkable tissue change with possible metastasis. Furthermore, they are not effectively and independently applicable and they lack the required sensitivity and specificity to diagnose cancer at the early stage [75]. Similarly, surgical removal of the cancer is not a precise cellular-based method and the uncertainty about the exact tumor margin necessitates resection of a safety margin of healthy tissue along with the tumor. Therefore, to limit the serious complications and negative life impacts, the development of new technologies is essential for the early detection of cancer.

Currently, three main approaches can implement the nanotechnology for cancer detection in the early stage (Fig. 4.3);

1. Tumor imaging: passive targeting and active targeting.

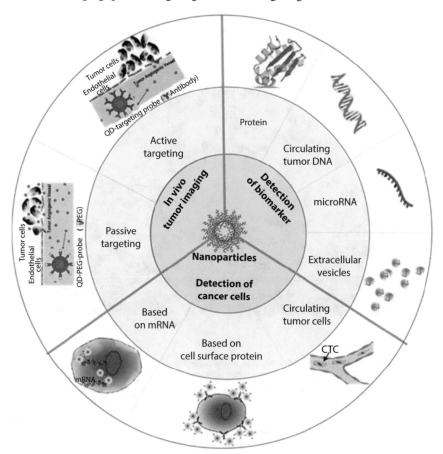

Fig. 4.3 Nanotechnology-supported cancer diagnosis and imaging. NP can be applied for the detection of cancer cells or biomarkers as well as tumor imaging. (Reprinted with permission from reference [4])

2. Detection of biomarkers: protein, circulating tumor DNA, microRNA, mRNA, extracellular vesicles, and exosomes.
3. Detection of cancer cells: circulating tumor cells (CTC) and CTC-clusters.

In the field of cancer imaging, nanotechnology can provide molecular materials or contrast agents that enable early and more precise detection and monitoring of cancer. Nanotechnology-based imaging can greatly enhance in vivo tumor detection using conventional scan devices such as MRI, PET (positron emission tomography), and CT scans. Figure 4.4 demonstrates the principle of a triple-modality MRI-photoacoustic-Raman NP for clinical use. Moreover, modern nanotechnology imaging allowed imaging modalities including photoacoustic tomography, Raman spectroscopic imaging, and multimodal imaging with the capacity of real-time imaging of cancer [76–81] (Fig. 4.5).

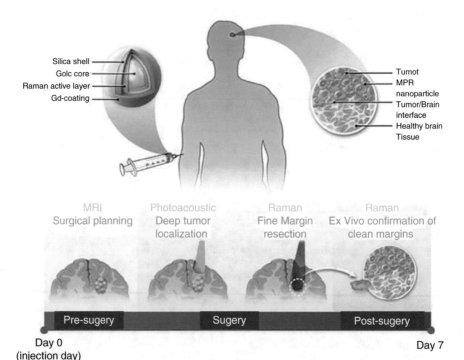

Fig. 4.4 Graphic showing the "Principle of a triple-modality MRI-photoacoustic-Raman NP for clinical use." After intravenous injection of NP, contrast agents are stably internalized within the brain tumor cells, allowing the whole spectrum from preoperative MRI for surgical planning to intraoperative imaging to be performed with a single injection. During the surgery, photoacoustic imaging with its greater depth penetration and 3D imaging capabilities can be used to guide the gross resection steps, while Raman imaging can guide the resection of the microscopic tumor at the resection margins. (*Used with permission of the U.S. National Cancer Institute (NCI). Source: Dr. Moritz Kircher, Dana Farber Cancer Institute*)

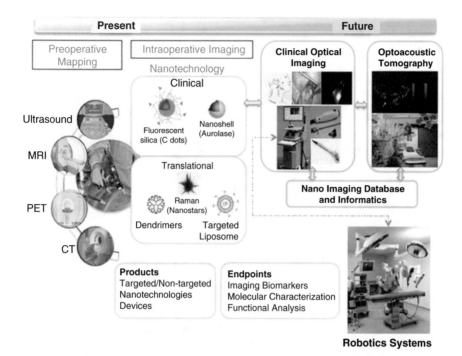

Fig. 4.5 Graphic showing "Present and future of NanoOncology Image-guided Surgical Suite." Preoperative conventional imaging tools are used to screen for disease and inform optically driven minimally invasive and open surgical procedures. Clinically available particle platforms can be monitored in real time using portable multichannel camera systems. Representative translational probes and devices for future clinical use are also shown. In the future, the operating surgeon will select suitable probe-device combinations for specific indications, and be provided with structural, functional, and/or molecular-level data for further treatment management. (*Used with permission of the U.S. National Cancer Institute (NCI). Source: Dr. Michelle Bradbury, Memorial Sloan Kettering Cancer Center*)

Furthermore, nanotechnology may aid in the early detection of cancer through the capture of cancer biomarkers. Cancer biomarkers are detectable and measurable biological molecules in body fluids that are secreted by the body or cancer cells including; (i) proteins, (ii) carbohydrates, and (iii) nucleic acids [82, 83]. Examples include cancer-associated proteins, cell surface proteins (i.e., vimentin, glycan, EpCAM), circulating tumor DNA, DNA methylation, microRNA, CTC, extracellular vesicles, and exosomes [84–87]. Due to significantly high surface-to-volume ratio [88], NP surface can be equipped and modified with varieties of moieties and binding ligands (i.e., peptides, aptamers, nucleic acid molecules, and antibodies) with multivalent effects to recognize cancer biomarkers and molecules with high specificity and sensitivity (Fig. 4.6) [4]. However, the application of NP as a real-time and cost-effective cancer diagnosis method is in the early developmental phase [89].

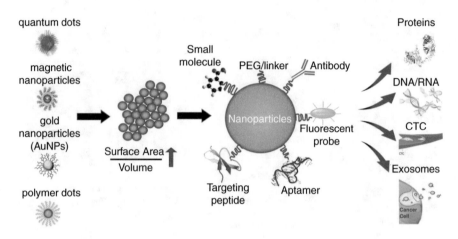

Fig. 4.6 Various agents can be coupled or conjugated with NP due to their high surface-to-volume ratio for cancer management (Reprinted with permission from Ref. [4])

There are several limiting factors in the use of biomarkers such as (i) low concentration of biomarkers, (ii) heterogeneity in the presentation of biomarkers within patients, and (iii) problems for conduction of prospective studies [90]. Biosensors could be coupled with nanotechnology to offer specific targeting and simultaneous multiple measurements with improved selectivity and sensitivity for the detection and monitoring of cancer [91, 92]. Examples include NP probes such as magnetic NP (MNPs), quantum dots (QDs), gold NPs, polymer dots (PDs), nanowires, nanopillars, silicon nanopillars, carbon nanotubes, dendrimers, and polymers [93, 94]. These NP biosensors or probes could be designed for the early detection of cancer biomarkers and metastatic cancer cells [4]. As such, since the majority of death is attributed to metastasis [95, 96], early and accurate detection of cancer and metastasis using nanotechnology could significantly improve the survival rate among cancer patients.

Recent innovations involving nanomaterials-based microfluidic systems offer high detection sensitivity, capture purity, and downstream functional characterization of circulating tumor cells, tumor DNA, and other tumor biomarkers [97, 98]. For example, "NanoVelcro" chips were applied as cell-affinity substrates where CTC capture agent-coated nanostructured substrates were utilized to immobilize CTCs with remarkable efficiency. The fourth-generation NanoVelcro chip can purify CTCs with the preservation of RNA transcripts for downstream analysis of several cancer-specific RNA biomarkers [99].

Nanotechnology-Based Treatment Modalities in the Treatment of Cancer

Nanotechnology as an Adjuvant to Cancer Chemoradiotherapy

Systemic toxicity is the major challenge in chemotherapy and radiotherapy that results in a significant impact on patient lifestyle [100, 101]. Selective targeting of tumor cells by chemical anticancer agents is a critical issue that can decrease the systemic toxicity of chemotherapy. NP through their unique physicochemical properties can improve chemotherapy by an increase in the overall therapeutic index of conjugated or encapsulated drugs to their surface. This is achieved through the accumulation of drugs in the tumor microenvironment followed by controllable site and timing of drug release [102]. Furthermore, nanotechnology could support radiotherapy through enhancement or augmentation of its effect during the application of PDT and PTT [103, 104]. NP through their inherent atomic features can interact with X-ray photons and increase the efficacy of traditional radiation therapy without the need for a higher dosage. Furthermore, nanocarriers could deliver sensitizing agents locally at the tumor site that enhance radiotherapy efficacy while reducing systemic toxicity [105, 106].

Nanotechnology to Support Cancer Immunotherapy

Immunotherapy is a new promising field in the management of cancer; however, a better understanding of the nature of the interaction between tumor and host immune system is required. Analysis of functional immune system responses to therapy at the cellular and molecular levels using nanodevices and nanomaterials is under process. NP and nanodevices are also being investigated to sort, image, and characterize T cells and to deliver immunomodulatory molecules and antigens along with chemotherapy and radiotherapy. This is aimed to raise T cell response, stimulate multiple dendritic cell targets, or suppress immune responses [105, 107–109].

Nanotechnology as a Promising Pathway in Cancer Genetic Therapeutics

Nucleic acid-based drugs (i.e., aptamers, siRNA, and anti-sense DNA/RNA) have shown promising results in cancer therapy. One of the main challenges in gene therapy is the issue of sensitivity and high instability of the nucleic acid since they are targeted and eliminated from circulation through opsonization, serum nuclease, macrophage, and renal system. The ultimate goal of drug delivery is to maintain the desired drug concentration at the target site for an optimal time. Therefore, the application of the nanocarrier-based DDS is intended to overcome this limitation. Genetic therapeutics involving siRNA, miRNA, and DNA encapsulated or conjugated onto the surface of NP have been reported to increase the stability and half-life of the nucleic acid in the systemic circulation [110].

DNA Nanotechnology for Cancer Therapy

DNA is a biocompatible molecule with low cytotoxicity. Nanotechnology-based DNA can be useful in various applications including (i) scaffolds to arrange organic, inorganic, and biomolecules into defined morphology as molecular transporters, (ii) highly sensitive nucleic acid detection as bio-sensor, (iii) single-molecule spectroscopy, (iv) protein structure determination, and (v) drug delivery [111, 112].

Nanotechnology for Small Interfering RNA (siRNA) Delivery

siRNA is a small double-stranded molecule that can regulate or suppress the gene expression in the target cells following a process known as RNA interference (RNAi). RNAi is a posttranscriptional process involving suppression of gene expression through cleavage on a specified area of target messenger RNA (mRNA). This technology has shown promising results in the treatment of a variety of diseases including cancer [113].

   Current studies in the development of effective nanotechnology-based siRNA delivery systems are to address therapeutic drawbacks such as lack of stability due to fast biodegradation in cellular cytoplasm and plasma, poor cellular uptake of unmodified siRNAs, and low bioavailability issue. To overcome these limitations, siRNA molecules need to be conjugated or encapsulated with appropriate carrier systems to secure safe and efficient in vivo delivery to the target site [114]. Various nanoparticle-based delivery systems have been investigated or are under clinical trials including biodegradable polymeric NP (i.e., liposomes, chitosan, polyethyleneimine, PEG, cyclodextrin, polylactic acid-co-glycolic acid (PLGA), poly amidoamine dendrimers), and nonbiodegradable inorganic NP (i.e., magnetic iron oxide, gold, silica NP, semiconductor quantum dots) [113, 114].

Nanotechnology for Tumor microRNA (miRNA) Profiling and Delivery

The miRNA is an endogenous single noncoding RNA that acts by repressing protein production through mRNA destabilization or by blocking translation of target mRNA thus regulating the development, proliferation, differentiation, and apoptosis. The miRNA profile is altered in disease conditions, as such restoration of downregulated or overexpressed miRNA to its normal state is the premise of miRNA-based therapy. For this reason, miRNA is suggested and investigated as a promising valuable biomarker and therapeutics for various disease conditions such as cancer, diabetes, and cardiovascular disease [115]. Precise and sensitive assessment of altered miRNA levels can lead to early and correct disease diagnosis [116].

Real-time quantitative polymerase chain reaction (qRT-PCR) and microarrays are the conventional detection methods of miRNA. These methods lack high accuracy and need legitimate and valid internal control that challenges the designing of probes and primers [115, 117]. Additional challenges in miRNA-based therapy are related to the successful delivery of miRNA due to biological instability and short circulation half-life, reduced intracellular delivery, and off-target effects with associated toxicity [115]. Aiming to overcome these limitations, nanotechnology seems to be a strong alternative to conventional methods in miRNA sensing and as a potential carrier system for effective miRNA delivery [116]. Oligonucleotides (i.e., siRNA, anti-miRNA, and miRNA) can be linked with nanocarriers to improve their resistance to nuclease degradation, to reduce the chance of immune rejection, and to enhance cellular uptake. Nanotechnology-assisted miRNA delivery involves a variety of inorganic (e.g., gold, silver, calcium phosphate, graphene, quantum dots, iron oxide, and silica), organic (e.g., chitosan, liposomes, proteins/peptides, and aptamers), and polymers-based NP and nanomaterials.

NP to Overcome the Problem of MDR in Cancer Therapy

The next challenging phenotype in the treatment of cancer is MDR, which is mainly associated with inadequate drug delivery to tumor cells and overexpression of P-glycoprotein (P-gp), which is a member of ATP-dependent multidrug efflux membrane transporters. Their action results in the intracellular sublethal concentration of drugs due to cellular evasion of cytotoxicity that leads to treatment failure [118]. Nanotechnology can be applied to overcome MDR by designing NP to simultaneously deliver the drug and block the MDR proteins thus rendering the tumor sensitive to cytotoxic agents. NP can also overcome the P-glycoprotein-mediated resistance by partial bypassing of the efflux pump [119, 120] or through siRNA for downregulating the expression of P-glycoprotein [121, 122].

Intra-tumoral heterogeneity is another contributing factor to drug resistance that is usually managed by chemo-modulators using combination therapy. However, this approach is limited by dose-dependent toxicity and altered drug disposition pattern [123]. The application of NP is a promising approach due to their ability to encapsulate or conjugate multiple agents and drugs simultaneously [124]. For example, solid polymer lipid NP were suggested as a combination approach (diffusion and phagocytosis) to overcome P-glycoprotein overexpression and increase the cellular accumulation and retention of doxorubicin [125]. Other approaches to overcome MDR and improve cellular uptake of doxorubicin included doxorubicin-loaded magnetic silk fibroin-based NP [126], doxorubicin-loaded PEGylated gold NP

[127, 128], nanocrystalline silver with a TAT-enhanced cell-penetrating peptide [129], as well as co-delivery of doxorubicin and therapeutic siRNA using cationic/anionic liposome-polycation-DNA combined with vascular endothelial growth factor siRNA [130–132].

Nanotechnology-Based Therapeutics for Head, Neck, and Oral Cancer

The majority of the head and neck cancers that originate in the lip, oral cavity, oropharynx, nasopharynx, hypopharynx, and larynx are of the squamous cell histopathology nature [133]. HNSCC passes through many phases originating from normal histology and transforming into hyperplasia, dysplasia, carcinoma in situ, and invasive carcinoma [134]. HNSCC remains the most challenging condition because about 60% of the cases are diagnosed with the locally advanced disease upon initial examinations with a high risk of recurrence [135]. Moreover, approximately 10% of diagnosed cases are metastatic diseases [136]. Besides, the treatment has a significant impact on the patient's quality of life by impairing the vital functions and patient appearance [137, 138].

The management of the HNSCC requires a complex well-planned multidisciplinary approach based on tumor staging [139]. Early diagnosed cases of stage I and II usually undergo surgical resection of the primary tumor and draining lymph nodes followed by adjuvant radiotherapy. For patients with locoregionally advanced or unresectable disease, a combined approach is recommended involving platinum-based chemotherapy or primary definitive concurrent chemo-radiation [140, 141]. This approach is also indicated postoperatively in patients with high-risk pathological findings at surgical resection. A major drawback to this approach is the development of recurrence or distant metastasis in the majority of cases.

The standard multimodal approach includes surgical resection with adjuvant chemotherapy and radiotherapy. This approach is suggested in advanced cases with positive surgical margin and lymphovascular or neural invasion. New treatment modalities involve IMRT with 3D planned resection and reconstruction.

There has not been a remarkable improvement in the prognosis of HNSCC despite the advancement in treatment modalities over the last few decades. As such modification of the current approach and development of novel techniques for early diagnosis and better management remain the main priority and challenges [135]. Cancer nanotechnology is a multidisciplinary field (i.e., medicine, biology, chemistry, engineering, and physics) that promises new insights for the management of head and neck cancer [142, 143]. In particular, nanotechnology-based approaches for the treatment of oral cavity carcinoma include NP (i.e., polysaccharides, proteins, and polymers), liposomes (i.e., phospholipids and cholesterol), hydrogels, and liquid crystals as carriers for drug delivery [144–147].

Therapeutic Strategies in the Head, Neck, and Oral Cancer

Immunotherapy

Ideally, the immune system recognizes and eliminates premalignant tumor cells. However, head, neck, and oral cancers are categorized as immune-suppressive diseases that interfere with the patient normal immune responses. This is because of the lower absolute lymphocyte count and altered antigen presentation that inhibit tumor cell detection and immune-mediated clearance [148].

Therefore, immunotherapy based on nanotechnology could offer new promising modalities in the management of head and neck cancers by enhancing the immune system activity to eradicate the tumor cells in particular the refractory solid tumor [149, 150]. The first evidence to treat cancer by targeting the immune system was reported in 1891 [151]. Immunotherapy aims to boost the patient immune reaction or to block the tumor pathways in resisting the immune responses [152]. Due to altered antigen-presenting function, the head and neck carcinoma tumors poorly present tumor antigen (TA) on their cell surface. Nowadays, the use of humanized monoclonal antibodies has been approved as an effective protocol for cancer therapy, metastatic cancer, and those with failed chemotherapy. Monotherapeutic monoclonal antibodies are one avenue for targeted therapy that improves TA presentation (Table 4.3). [209].

Immunotherapy targeting cancer may involve systemic therapy (i.e., systemic cytokines), locally targeted therapy (i.e., molecular inhibitors or immune checkpoints for immune-modulation of tumor microenvironment), or recent combinatorial approaches under study [210, 211]. The monoclonal antibodies such as immune checkpoint inhibitors are agents that reactivate the antitumor immune responses through targeting and blocking the inhibitory immune checkpoint receptors expressed on T cell and NK cells (i.e., cytotoxic T lymphocyte antigen 4 (CTLA4) and its ligands CD80 and CD86, and program death 1 (PD1) and its ligands PD-L1 and PD-L2) [212]. Expression and activation of these inhibitory receptors result in a dysfunctional state with reduced proliferative and cytolytic activities of lymphocytes, which can be reversed with inhibitory checkpoint receptor blockade [213]. Examples of approved agents include anti-PD-1 (i.e., nivolumab and pembrolizumab), anti- CTLA4 (i.e., ipilimumab), and EGFR inhibitors (i.e, cetuximab, bevacizumab, erlotinib) [148, 214–218].

These immunotherapy strategies can improve the cancer survival rate by effective immune control of the tumor [219]. However, the application of immunotherapy faces challenges such as autoimmune adverse effects, inability to target slowly growing cold tumors, high cost, and variable and unsatisfactory patient response rate [210, 220]. To address these limitations, there is a growing interest to investigate combinational approaches (i.e., combination immunotherapy and immunotherapy with chemoradiotherapy) aiming to improve the response rate and duration with minimum toxicity [148, 221].

Table 4.3 Monoclonal antibodies-based therapies for the treatment of head and neck cancer

Drugs	Mechanism of Action	Reference
Cetuximab, Panitumumab, Zalutumumab and Nimotuzumab	EGFR inhibitors	[153–162]
Gefitinib, Erlotinib, Lapatinib, Afatinib and Dacomitinib	EGFR tyrosine kinase inhibitors	[163–172]
Bevacizumab	VEGF inhibitors	[162]
Sorafenib, Sunitinib and Vandetanib	VEGFR inhibitors	[162]
Rapamycin, Temsirolimus, Everolimus, torin1, PP242 and PP30, BYL719	PI3K/AKT/mTOR pathway inhibitors	[162, 173]
Pembrolizumab, Nivolumab, Atezolizumab, Durvalumab, Avelumab)	Anti-PD1/PD-L1 antibody	[154, 162, 174–181]
Motolimod (VTX-2337)	TLR8 agonist	[182–187]
AZD1775 (Adavosertib)	Elective small molecule inhibitor of WEE1 G2 checkpoint serin/threoin/protein kinase	[188, 189]
Abemaciclib (LY2835219)	Cyclin-dependent kinase inhibitor	[190, 191]
TPST-1120	Selective antagonist of PPARα	[192]
Sitravatinib (MGCD516)	RTK inhibitor	[193]
Nintedanib (BIBF1120)	Triple receptor tyrosine kinase inhibitor (PDGFR/FGFR and VEGFR)	[194, 195]
Tremelimumab and Ipilimumab,	Anti-CTLA4 antibody	[179, 196–198]
Relatlimab (BMS-986016)	LAG-3 inhibitor	[199–201]
Danvatirsen (AZD9150)	STAT3 inhibitor	[202–204]
AZD5069	CXCR2 Inhibitor	[203, 205, 206]
Epacadostat and Navoximod	IDO1 Inhibitor	[207, 208]

Abbreviations: *EGFR* epidermal growth factor receptor, *VEGF* vascular endothelial growth factor, *VEGFR* VEGF receptor, *PI3K* phosphatidylinositol 3-kinase, *AKT* serine/threonine-specific protein kinase, *mTOR* mammalian target of rapamycin, *PD-1* program death receptor 1, *TLR8* a selective toll-like receptor 8, *PPARα* peroxisome proliferator-activated receptor-alpha, *RTK* receptor tyrosine kinase, *PDGF-R* platelet-derived growth factor receptor, *CTLA4* cytotoxic T-lymphocyte associated antigen-4, *IgG1κ* human immunoglobulin G1 kappa, *WEE1* wee1-like protein kinase, *IDO1* indoleamine 2,3-dioxygenase 1, *LAG-3* lymphocyte activation gene 3, *STAT3* signal transducers, and activators of transcription 3, *CXCR2* C-X-C motif chemokine receptor 2

Clinical trials are underway for evaluation of anti-PD1 + anti-CTLA4 combination immunotherapy (i.e., Durvalumab (MEDI4736) + tremelimumab, Nivolumab + ipilimumab) [222–226]. Other ongoing clinical trials are evaluating immunotherapy (i.e., anti-PD-1 and anti-PD-L1) in conjunction with radiotherapy for treatment of locally advanced, refractory recurrent, or metastatic HNSCC [227]. Ionizing radiotherapy would trigger immunogenic cell death (ICD) that may be synergistic with immunotherapy [228]. ICD can potentially promote systemic responses through an "abscopal effect" where a systemic response is initiated after local therapy that continues to be active after radiotherapy [229]. This could alter the tumor microenvironment rendering it more sensitive to PD-1 and CTLA4 pathway inhibitors [230, 231].

Additionally, radiotherapy would induce direct DNA damage or upregulation of PD-L1 on tumor cells [230, 232, 233]. Current clinical trials are exploring the proper techniques and dosing fractionation for optimum response to synergistic radiotherapy and immunotherapy [234–239]. The addition of immunotherapy to traditional chemotherapy is another alternative option under investigation. The interim analysis result showed that pembrolizumab in combination with weekly cisplatin-based chemoradiotherapy was safe and did not impair the safety of standard chemoradiotherapy [240]. However, the complete results from randomized trials are required to confirm the exact impact of this approach [241, 242]. Other alternative approaches include small molecule immunotherapy and nano-based DDS that facilitate intracellular penetration by direct targeting of tumor cells. Combined immunotherapy with nano-based DDS would enhance the benefits of current anticancer therapy while minimizing the undesirable toxic effects [243, 244].

Small Molecule Immunotherapeutics

Small molecule-based immunotherapy can be designed to target the immune-suppressive mechanism or to promote activation of cytotoxic lymphocyte responses to the tumor. This novel strategy in immunotherapy offers inherent advantages over biologic immunotherapies since they can access a wider spectrum of intra-tumoral or intra-cellular molecular targets with reduced immune-related adverse effects. Additional advantages of small molecules over biologics include precise formulations and dosing options, proper oral bioavailability, and greater ability to penetrate the physiological barriers, tumor milieu, and cell membranes [245, 246]. Another key advantage of small molecules is their affordable lower cost that would allow greater patient access to advanced immunotherapy [247, 248].

The diversity of immune cells, receptors, and molecular pathways involved in tumor pathogenesis offer great potential for the molecular targeting approach in cancer therapy (Table 4.4). Such novel treatment strategies might be used as monotherapy or in combination modalities with other anticancer therapies (i.e., biologics, chemo- and radiotherapy) to improve their quality and efficacy [220, 245].

DDS Formulated Agents for Targeting the Head, Neck, and Oral Cancer

Anti-cancer agents are usually administered intravenously; however, several recent formulations have been approved by the FDA for intraoral administration. This can improve patient compliance in particular when prolonged exposure is required [297]. Due to the physicochemical nature of anticancer drugs and their poor

Table 4.4 Examples of small molecule immunotherapeutics (compiled from reference [220])

Small Molecule	Molecular Target	Study phase/References
BMS-1001	PD-L1 antagonist	Preclinical [245, 249]
BMS-1116	PD-L1 antagonist	Preclinical [245, 249]
CA-170	PD-L1/VISTA antagonist	Phase I [250]
CA-327	PD-L1/TIM-3 antagonist	Preclinical [251]
Imiquimod	TLR7/8 agonist	Approved [252–255]
Resiquimod	TLR7/8 agonist	Phase I/ II [256]
852A	TLR7 agonist	Phase II [257]
VTX-2337	TLR8 agonist	Phase II [258]
ADU-S100	STING agonist	Phase I [259–261]
MK-1454	STING agonist	Phase I [260–262]
Ibrutinib	Btk/Itk inhibitor	Approved [263–266]
3 AC	SHIP1 inhibitor	Preclinical [267, 268]
Idelalisib	PI3K-δ inhibitor	Approved [269–271]
IPI-549	PI3K-γ inhibitor	Phase I [272]
CPI-444	A2A receptor antagonist	Phase I/ II [273]
Vipadenant	A2A receptor antagonist	Preclinical [274, 275]
Preladenant	A2A receptor antagonist	Phase I [276]
PBF 509	A2A receptor antagonist	Phase II [277]
AZD4635	A2A receptor antagonist	Phase I/ II [278]
Galuniseritib	TGF-βR1 kinase/Alk5 inhibitor	Preclinical [279]
OTX015/MK-8628	Bromodomain inhibitor	Phase II [280]
CPI-0610	Bromodomain inhibitor	Phase II [281]

Table 4.4 (continued)

Small Molecule	Molecular Target	Study phase/References
D1MT	IDO1 inhibitor	Phase I/ II [282–287]
INCB024360	IDO1 inhibitor	Phase II/III [288–290]
GDC-0901 (navoximod)	IDO1 inhibitor	Phase I [291–293]
PF-0684003 (EOS-200271) BMS-986205 (ONO-7701)	IDO1 inhibitor	Phase I/ II [294–296]

hydrophilicity, the formulation of oral administration faces major challenges [298]. This can be addressed by the incorporation of a carefully designed nanocarrier for controlled and/or targeted DDS to improve both local and intravenous administrations of anticancer drugs [299]. Common examples of anticancer agents formulated with this technology for the treatment of head, neck, and oral cavity cancer include; Paclitaxel, Cisplatin, Doxorubicin, Docetaxel, Methotrexate, and Fluoropyrimidine 5-Fluorouracil.

The most commonly applied regimen for the management of oral cavity carcinoma is the intravenous administration of cisplatin every 3 weeks (100 mg/m^2) in combination with standard fractionated radiotherapy [300, 301]. Cisplatin (cis-diamino-dichloro platinum, CDDP) is an alkylating agent forming intra-strand (95%) or inter-strand (5%) DNA cross-links [302] that interferes with DNA repair mechanisms resulting in apoptosis [303]. Cisplatin suffers from poor systemic stability, limited hydrophilicity, and systemic toxicity (e.g., bone marrow depression, nephrotoxicity, ototoxicity). To address these limitations, cisplatin can be prepared using NP formulations such as PLGA-PEG (poly (lacticco-glycolic acid)-poly(ethylene)glycol) [304].

Overexpression of epidermal growth factor and its ligand transforming growth factors alpha is early independent prognostic biomarkers in HNSCC. Cetuximab is a monoclonal antibody of the immunoglobulin G1 class with a high affinity to the extracellular domain of EGFR. It acts by blocking the endogenous ligands with inhibition of receptor function as well as by downregulation of EGFR [305, 306]. These nanoformulations can facilitate targeted drug accumulation and intracellular uptake at the tumor site. In addition, they can improve the synergistic actions of chemotherapy with intensified radiotherapy that inhibit intra-fraction tumor growth [307].

There are several alternative strategies for DDS to overcome current challenges with parenteral administration of chemotherapeutic agents including; (i) intratumoral injection, (ii) local drug delivery, (iii) phototherapy approaches (i.e., PDT and PTT), and (iv) micro-bubbles mediated ultrasound delivery [103].

NP as Nanocarriers for Controlled/Targeted DDS

Different carrier systems have been designed for controlled release and targeted drug delivery. This can improve the selectivity and efficacy, while enhancing the prolonged release of drug at the target site that subsequently reduce the cytotoxicity and other adverse effects of traditional therapeutic approaches [308]. Nanocarriers for delivery of chemotherapeutic agents in the head, neck, and oral cancer include polymeric NP, inorganic NP, lipid-based NP, hydrogels, and exosomes (Table 4.5) [103].

The Nanotechnology-Based Approach in the Management of Cancer and Other Diseases

Safety

The nature of physiological responses to NP and nanocarriers are not clearly understood, a fact that delayed their clinical translation. For example, cytotoxicity of silver NP and the accumulation of NP in the skin have been reported [358]. Other studies reported systemic toxicities such as pneumonia, colitis, and autoimmune endocrinopathies associated with nanotechnology-based immunotherapeutic agents ipilimumab (anti-CTLA4 agent) and nivolumab (anti-PD1 agents), respectively [359, 360]. As such, this should be kept in mind that the great advantageous potential of NP in medicine may be also associated with critical unexplored risks and complications.

Nanoparticles occur naturally and are not inherently unsafe, but as a standard protocol, the safety and potential risks associated with the use and application of new technologies need to be carefully evaluated. For this purpose, NCI's Alliance for Nanotechnology in Cancer ensures responsible development of nanotechnology for cancer applications by offering its service of Nanotechnology Characterization

Table 4.5 Carriers for drug delivery in the head, neck, and oral cancer

Carriers for Drug Delivery	Examples of application	Properties
Polymeric NP	Polysaccharides, PLA, PGA, and their copolymers. PEG-PGA copolymer for cisplatin delivery [309–311]. PCL NP coated with the polysaccharide chitosan for curcumin delivery [312–314]. Ellagic acid loaded chitosan NP [311, 315].	Biodegradable and biocompatible Suitable for controlled DDS Difficult handling due to particle aggregation Not suitable for the release of proteins including antibodies Local toxicity upon degradation [316–319]

Table 4.5 (continued)

Carriers for Drug Delivery	Examples of application	Properties
Inorganic NP	Silver NP as highly sensitive NP probes and nanoelectronics for targeting, diagnosis, and imaging of small molecules, DNA, proteins, and cells including cancer [320–322]. Silver NP as antibacterial and anticancer agents [323–325] Silver NP as anti-angiogenic and anti-proliferative agents [326, 327] PLGA/quinacrine/silver NP with improved ability to inhibit proliferation and neo-angiogenesis of head and neck carcinoma [311, 328] Gold NP for tumor diagnosis and imaging, photothermal therapy, radiofrequency therapy, drug delivery, and angiogenesis modulation [329, 330] Anti-EGFR antibody-conjugated gold NP for photothermal destruction of EGFR-overexpressing malignant cells using NIR laser light [331]. Anti-EGFR-antibody conjugated with PEGylated titanium dioxide (TiO_2) Up-conversion NP for increased tissue penetration of NIR laser light and enhanced apoptosis and tumor growth inhibition [332, 333]. μ-oxo N,N′-bis (salicylidene) ethylenediamine iron (Fe(Salen)) magnetic NP for targeted delivery of anticancer agents activated using an AMF combining chemotherapy and hyperthermia [334, 335]. Silica mesoporous NP copolymer with high porosity and carrying capacity [336, 337].	Higher photostability and optical properties compared to organic dyes The target can be site-specific by attaching the ligand to the nanoparticle (e.g., magnetic NP) Toxicity Limited effective delivery due to limited penetration depth for photothermal therapy Cannot deliver biomacromolecules (e.g., proteins) [338, 339]
Nanolipids	SLN carriers [340, 341]. NLC consisting of both solid and lipids in the core matrix can overcome the limited loading capacity of SLN [342–344].	Higher stability against chemical degradation Suitable for controlled release and local delivery of anticancer drugs Improve solubility and bioavailability Able to penetrate deeply into tumors The crystalline structure provides limited drug loading capacity Aggregation of NLC during storage Associated with immune response [145, 314, 319, 345, 346].

(continued)

Table 4.5 (continued)

Carriers for Drug Delivery	Examples of application	Properties
Hydrogels	Delivery of hydrophilic and hydrophobic drugs, protein, and other macromolecules [347, 348]. Coadministration of multiple drugs with synergistic anti-cancer effects and decreased drug resistance [297, 349].	Injectable to a specific site Do not dissolve in water at physiological temperature and pH Stable structural integrity and elasticity High drug loading capacity Poor mechanical properties Difficult handling Expensive [350, 351]
Exosomes	As a vehicle for chemotherapeutic agents such as curcumin, doxorubicin, and paclitaxel [351–353].	Ability to deliver different types of biomolecules and play an essential role in intercellular communication [354] Ability to act as targeted DDS due to their binding to the cell membrane through adhesion proteins and ligands [353, 355] Limited loading capacity difficult purification, analysis, and administration [356] May induce adverse immune reactions [357]

Abbreviations: *PLA* polylactic acid, *PGA* polyglycolic acid, *PEG* polyethylene glycol, *PGA* polyglutamic acid, *PCL* polycaprolactone, *DDS* drug delivery system, *PLGA* poly lactic-co-glycolic acid, *EGFR* epithelial growth factor receptor, *NIR* near-infrared, *AMF* alternating magnetic field, *SLN* solid lipid nanoparticle, *NLC* nanostructured lipid carrier

Laboratory (NCL) available to the nanotech and cancer research communities. To date, NCL tests have evaluated the physicochemical properties, biocompatibility, and efficacy of over 125 different NP for medical applications. NCL also works closely with the FDA and National Institutes of Standards and Technology (NIST) to set, validate, and disseminate relevant experimental protocols to the nanotech and cancer research communities.

Advantages

Due to their high surface-to-volume ratio, the NP have relatively higher intracellular uptake and efficacy and can be administered via various routes: oral, nasal, intra-ocular, parenteral [361]. Furthermore, the strong link between NP and drug facilitates on-demand site-specific drug release and altered organ distribution and clearance of the drug [362]. NP can allow the incorporation of a large number of drugs without the need for a chemical reaction. Drug chemical stability can also be increased by a nanocarrier that prevents biodegradation of encapsulated contents particularly in dry solid forms [363]. The possibility of the application of polymeric NP as biosensors for imaging and targeted therapy is due to the ease of surface engineering and modification [364]. Further potential applications of NP are under investigation in basic, preclinical, and clinical studies.

Limitations

Synthesis of NP is a technique-sensitive procedure that requires strict control over manufacturing parameters (i.e., temperature, pressure) for precise control over particle properties such as size, shape, crystallinity, and surface properties. Compared to conventional procedures, the production of NP is costly due to difficulty in the control of the manufacturing parameters, physicochemical properties, and reproducibility [365]. Due to the relative instability of NP, uncontrolled manufacturing or prolonged storage may change their crystallinity and result in particle agglomeration and sedimentation [363]. This may affect their physicochemical properties and in turn biological behaviors.

Challenges in Clinical Translations

Nanomedicines are a highly diverse group of drug products including polymer–protein conjugates, polymeric micelles, inorganic NP, protein-based NP, and lipid-based NP [366]. Despite three decades of active research in the field of cancer nanomedicine, the actual clinical impact on patient life at the bedside has been disappointing. Since the development of liposomal doxorubicin in 1995 and despite a large number of nanomaterials under investigation, the overall efficacy and survival rate have been very limited [56]. Only a few nanomedicines are in phase III or IV clinical trials and just some passed the regulatory approval in the US and Europe [55, 367], while there are hundreds of published papers and ongoing clinical trials [368]. This mismatch is due to several obstacles that involve the development of nanomedicine. The majority of nanomedical products are the reformulations of available active clinically approved pharmaceutical drugs. This is because developing an entirely new formulation with unknown biocompatibility behaviors in humans is more challenging and requires a longer time for clinical approval [365]. However, the reformulated nanomedicine drugs and carriers encounter similar difficulties in passing through the approval process compared to the parent formulation. This is because of the minimal improvement in clinical performances that may not be worth the expense, effort, and time of developing and commercializing the new formulations [369].

There are several developmental challenges before clinical translations that involve investors, commercial parties, insurance agencies, and patients. The first challenge is the formulation of cost-effective drugs with clear benefits to patients that would promote patient compliance (i.e., improved clinical administration with lower dosing, increased therapeutic efficacy, and higher safety with lower adverse effects) [365]. This involves proper manufacturing methods to precisely control the physicochemical properties of nanomedicine according to the standards of quality control (CMC), good manufacturing practice (GMP), and quality-by-design (QbD). Other factors to be considered before successful clinical translation include scalability of the manufacturing process, sterility and manufacturing-related impurities, and storage feasibility [4, 370–372]. The second challenge is related to the design of proper clinical trials with potentially more relevant clinical outcomes and patient benefits so that all relevant bodies (i.e., government and insurance party) are willing to invest in [57, 373]. The third challenge is the lack of predictability in translating the preclinical efficacy of nanomedicine to real clinical outcomes when considering the variability in response rates and therapeutic effects among the patients. The inter- and intra-tumor differences in vascularization, stroma, and macrophage population among different patients are already reported. These factors would potentially impact the NP targeted drug release [373, 374]. This poses another challenge in shifting from preclinical toxicology studies to safety assurance in the patients. Due to the unique nature of NP, the delivery and biodistribution of molecules are unpredictable with the possible overexpression in certain tissues and organs. This may result in unexpected nanomedicine-related toxicity and immunological responses, since the results of the animal studies are not necessarily applicable to human studies [375].

Future Direction

3D Optical Imaging of Cancer Tissue

A better understanding of the disease mechanism of head and neck cancer may be possible with the advances in chemical probe design and microscopy. Recently, there has been a focus on the designing of chemical probes for 3D tissue bioimaging, which allow labeling-specific biomolecules in cells and tissues, thus providing optical contrast for biological molecular visualization [376, 377]. The ability to image deep into tissue is necessary to accurately reconstruct the 3D microstructure within whole organs. The 3D optical imaging of NP distribution within cells and tissues can also provide insights into barriers to NP transport in vivo [378]. For this purpose, small organic fluorescent molecules conjugated to antibodies and fluorescent proteins have been chemically designed to target specific receptors on cell surface followed by optical microscopy imaging to visualize the spatial context of disease mechanisms [379] However, these molecules suffer from autofluorescence, photobleaching, and weak signal. Similarly, other imaging approaches based on photoacoustic tomography and Raman scattering either cannot provide cellular resolution or suffer from low acquisition speed [27].

Nanoparticle-based probes can overcome several limitations of both small organic molecules and fluorescent proteins because they have been demonstrated to produce large extinction coefficients [380]. It has been shown that metal NP scattering can provide ideal optical properties for 3D ultrasensitive imaging of intact and transparent tissues. The NP can also act as a template for the chemical growth of a metal layer to further amplify the scattering signal. The use of chemically grown NP (i.e., gold or silver ions) in whole tissues can amplify the optical scattering to produce a significantly higher optical signal than with common fluorophores. These probes are nonphotobleaching and can be used alongside fluorophores without interference. The three distinct potential biomedical applications of these probes are (i) molecular imaging of blood vessels, (ii) tracking of nanodrug carriers in tumors, and (iii) mapping of lesions and immune cells. In addition to these applications, molecular labeling of cleared tissues can be achieved by conjugating proteins to the NP surface. This could be combined to obtain correlative live and ex vivo imaging data by photoacoustic tomography and surface-enhanced Raman scattering using a single set of metallic probes [381]. Currently, the main challenge is the lack of proper tools for capturing the 3D distribution of NP with respect to biological structures at subcellular resolution [382]. Researchers are now investigating new approaches to allow deep and good quality imaging into the tissue to fully resolve complex biological structures and luminescent NP labeled with fluorescent tags such as gold and silica NP [383].

There is good literature supporting the application of NP (i.e., in particular, gold NP and silver NP) as nanoprobes and radiosensitizers for molecular imaging and cellular targeting (Table 4.5). Their co-application in IMRT has shown great promises in clinical trials. This is due to their unique optical properties and proven impact in radiobiology (e.g., radiosensitivity, repair, reoxygenation, redistribution, and repopulation) [320–322, 329, 330]. Further basic studies and clinical trials are necessary to disclose the full potential of NP in the diagnosis, imaging, and treatment of cancers, autoimmune diseases, and other human diseases.

Lymphotropic NP for Diagnosis of Metastasis

Treatment strategy of the head, neck, and oral cavity carcinoma and necessity of neck dissection is dependent on the accurate nodal staging. Current diagnostic recommendations for the detection of suspicious metastatic lymph nodes using standard MRI contrast imaging are prone to error due to relatively high false-negative reports (15–25%) [384, 385]. Although a spherical lymph node >10 mm with central necrosis and/or extra-capsular spread is categorized as metastatic, a small lymph node of 5–10 mm without necrosis and/or extra-capsular spread is questionable [386].

The development of lymphotropic NP as a new class of MRI contrast agents is expected to improve the sensitivity of diagnostic procedures, in particular in head and neck cancer [387]. A potential example includes Ferumoxtran-10 (Combidex), which is a biodegradable ultra-small super-paramagnetic iron oxide (USPIO) particle covered with low-molecular-weight dextran with a diameter of 17–21 nm. It enters the physiologic iron metabolic pathway and can be used for lymph node evaluation later during its distribution phase [388]. It can easily cross the capillary wall and localize within the lymph nodes to allow robust characterization of normal-sized metastatic nodes from reactive nodes independent of the size criterion [389]. Compared to traditional imaging, Ferumoxtran-10 is more sensitive in detecting minimal metastatic nodal disease particularly in normal-sized lymph nodes; however, the main limit is the need for additional time (1–2 days after injection to get the maximum iron peak in lymph nodes) to perform post-contrast MRI.

The sentinel lymph node is the first lymph node that receives drainage from the primary tumor. Localization of this lymph node is important to identify the possible cervical metastasis in patients with early-stage cancer. Classically, in the case of a positive biopsy of the sentinel lymph node, the patient must undergo complete prophylactic lymphadenectomy [390]. NP structures can be used to incorporate tracing agents such as Methylene blue dye and indocyanine green-loaded NP (< 50 nm in diameter) to map sentinel lymph node [391, 392]. These NP can improve the accumulation of tracing agents in the sentinel lymph node, protract tracer circulation, and improve its stability to facilitate near-infrared fluorescence imaging (NIRF). NIRF imaging is an attractive modality for sentinel lymph node mapping with the ability to bypass the blue dye's radioactive issues, low spatial resolution, and allergic reactions [393, 394]. Further research is essential to disclose the full potential of NP in the early detection of cancer metastasis.

Multifunctional Smart Nanomaterials

Multifunctional smart nanomaterials would be a promising future breakthrough in head and neck cancer with the potential to be programmed to target and act at different levels. The advent of these nanomaterials would offer several advantages including minimized systemic toxicity and adverse reactions, lower chance of drug interactions, reduced cost of therapy associated with multiple traditional medicines, and higher patient compliance. A potential example includes D-α-tocopheryl polyethylene glycol 1000 succinate or TPGS which is a water-soluble derivative of natural lipid-soluble vitamin E. It is a safe FDA-approved chemical agent that has been utilized for numerous purposes in pharmaceutical and nutraceutical applications. In the future, the potential applications of TPGS in management of cancer in particular the head and neck cancer would be based on four main properties of TPGS: (i) emulsifier property by acting as coating molecules to increase the encapsulation efficiency and cellular uptake of drug-loaded NP (i.e., microemulsion vehicle and carrier of drugs and imaging agents) which enhance permeation and reduce drug sensitivity in the tissue [395–399], (ii) anti-tumor and antioxidant property by inducing apoptosis, acting as a prodrug to enhance chemotherapy, and exhibiting synergistic effects with other anticancer drugs [400, 401], (iii) solubilizer and permeability enhancer to increase the oral bioavailability of anticancer and poorly water-soluble drugs in the TPGS-based DDS, where it can extend the half-life of the drug in plasma by increasing their cellular uptake [402, 403], and (iv) P-glycoprotein (P-gp) inhibitory activity of TPGS, which can function as a means to overcome MDR cancer cells (i.e., a paclitaxel-encapsulated nanocrystal formulation using TPGS [404]). These properties along with its apoptotic potential render the TPGS-based nanoparticulate application a promising approach to improve the therapeutic efficacy of cancer chemotherapeutic agents by better internalization and sustained release kinetics of the NP [405].

Unlocking the Power of Nanotechnology in Cancer Management

Nanotechnology in cancer management has proved to be a valuable adjuvant to traditional chemotherapy, radiotherapy, and immunotherapy that altogether would reduce the impact of surgical resection in patients. Nanotechnology could offer highly sensitive nanoprobes for accurate imaging and diagnosis of cancer and for tracing lymphadenopathy. Furthermore, nanotechnology offers variable treatment strategies by directly targeting the small molecules, DNA, proteins, and cells including cancer. Nanotechnology aids in the application of controlled and targeted DDSs through nanocarriers that increase the efficiency and bioavailability of drugs. It is also a powerful means for cases with MDR to conventional therapies. However, there are several challenges in the clinical translation of a nanotechnology-based management of cancer. First of all, further investigations are necessary to fill our knowledge gap about the mechanism of NP entry into the tumor. This would include the studies to identify (i) the molecular mechanisms that play major roles in modulating the NP entry into tumor cells, (ii) the impact of surface-adsorbed proteins on NP interactions, (iii) the role of different tumor vasculature in extravasation of NP with varying physicochemical properties, and (iv) the impact of other cells (i.e., immune cells) in the generation of transient permeability. Sound knowledge of these factors would help to overcome the poor clinical translation of nanomedicines in cancer management [53, 406, 407].

Furthermore, it is critical to obtain the reliability of the detection results, to maintain the high sensitivity and reproducibility during large-scale production, to secure the long-term storage stability, to minimize the possible systemic toxicity, and to consider cost-efficiency for realistic clinical translation. Continued interdisciplinary collaborative strategies involving basic research, preclinical, and clinical studies are essential to utilize the full potential of nanotechnology for different applications in medicine, in particular, for patients suffering from head and neck cancer and autoimmune diseases. The ultimate goal would be the development of personalized or customized nanomedicine tailored to the unique genetic and molecular characteristics of diseases.

References

1. NCI. Understanding cancer. p. https://www.cancer.gov/about-cancer/understanding/.
2. IARC. The International Agency for Research on Cancer. p. https://www.iarc.fr/.
3. Choi Y-E, Kwak J-W, Park JW. Nanotechnology for early cancer detection. Sensors (Basel) [Internet]. 2010;10(1):428–55. Available from: http://www.ncbi.nlm.nih.gov/pubmed/22315549.
4. Zhang Y, Li M, Gao X, Chen Y, Liu T. Nanotechnology in cancer diagnosis: progress, challenges and opportunities. J Hematol Oncol [Internet]. 2019;12(1):137. Available from: https://jhoonline.biomedcentral.com/articles/10.1186/s13045-019-0833-3.
5. Kreuter J. Nanoparticles--a historical perspective. Int J Pharm [Internet]. 2007;331(1):1–10. Available from: http://www.ncbi.nlm.nih.gov/pubmed/17110063.
6. FDA approves KS drug. Food and Drug Administration. Florida Department of Health and rehabilitation services. AIDS Alert [Internet]. 1996;11(1):11–2. Available from: http://www.ncbi.nlm.nih.gov/pubmed/11363227.
7. Doxil receives FDA market clearance. AIDS Patient Care STDS [Internet]. 1996;10(2):135. Available from: http://www.ncbi.nlm.nih.gov/pubmed/11361702.
8. DOXIL approved by FDA. AIDS Patient Care [Internet]. 1995;9(6):306. Available from: http://www.ncbi.nlm.nih.gov/pubmed/11361446.
9. Bonner JA, Harari PM, Giralt J, Azarnia N, Shin DM, Cohen RB, et al. Radiotherapy plus cetuximab for squamous-cell carcinoma of the head and neck. N Engl J Med [Internet]. 2006;354(6):567–78. Available from: http://www.ncbi.nlm.nih.gov/pubmed/16467544.
10. Bonner JA, Harari PM, Giralt J, Cohen RB, Jones CU, Sur RK, et al. Radiotherapy plus cetuximab for locoregionally advanced head and neck cancer: 5-year survival data from a phase 3 randomised trial, and relation between cetuximab-induced rash and survival. Lancet Oncol [Internet]. 2010;11(1):21–8. Available from: http://www.ncbi.nlm.nih.gov/pubmed/19897418.
11. Directorate-General for Health and Food Safety (European Commission). Scientific basis for the definition of the term "nanomaterial." 2012 [cited 2020 May 8]; Available from: https://op.europa.eu/en/publication-detail/-/publication/fddead88-e1a6-4b40-8e22-8a7089ee47c3/language-en.
12. Ebrahimi M, Botelho MG, Dorozhkin SV. Biphasic calcium phosphates bioceramics (HA/TCP): concept, physicochemical properties and the impact of standardization of study protocols in biomaterials research. Mater Sci Eng C Mater Biol Appl [Internet]. 2017;71:1293–312. Available from: https://linkinghub.elsevier.com/retrieve/pii/S0928493116316721.
13. Peer D, Karp JM, Hong S, Farokhzad OC, Margalit R, Langer R. Nanocarriers as an emerging platform for cancer therapy. Nat Nanotechnol [Internet]. 2007;2(12):751–60. Available from: http://www.nature.com/articles/nnano.2007.387.
14. Omidi Y. Smart multifunctional theranostics: simultaneous diagnosis and therapy of cancer. Bioimpacts [Internet]. 2011;1(3):145–7. Available from: http://www.ncbi.nlm.nih.gov/pubmed/23678419.
15. Jain KK. Role of nanodiagnostics in personalized cancer therapy. Clin Lab Med [Internet]. 2012;32(1):15–31. Available from: http://www.ncbi.nlm.nih.gov/pubmed/22340841.
16. Bawa R. Patents and nanomedicine. Nanomedicine (Lond) [Internet]. 2007;2(3):351–74. Available from: http://www.ncbi.nlm.nih.gov/pubmed/17716180.

17. Mattheolabakis G, Rigas B, Constantinides PP. Nanodelivery strategies in cancer chemotherapy: biological rationale and pharmaceutical perspectives. Nanomedicine (Lond) [Internet]. 2012;7(10):1577–90. Available from: http://www.ncbi.nlm.nih.gov/pubmed/23148540.
18. Woodle MC, Matthay KK, Newman MS, Hidayat JE, Collins LR, Redemann C, et al. Versatility in lipid compositions showing prolonged circulation with sterically stabilized liposomes. Biochim Biophys Acta [Internet]. 1992;1105(2):193–200. Available from: http://www.ncbi.nlm.nih.gov/pubmed/1586658.
19. Moghimi SM, Hunter AC, Andresen TL. Factors controlling nanoparticle pharmacokinetics: an integrated analysis and perspective. Annu Rev Pharmacol Toxicol [Internet]. 2012;52:481–503. Available from: http://www.ncbi.nlm.nih.gov/pubmed/22035254.
20. Nguyen KT. Targeted nanoparticles for cancer therapy: promises and challenges. J Nanomed Nanotechnol [Internet]. 2011;02(05). Available from: https://www.omicsonline.org/targeted-nanoparticles-for-cancer-therapy-promises-and-challenges-2157-7439.1000103e.php?aid=2090.
21. Jabir NR, Anwar K, Firoz CK, Oves M, Kamal MA, Tabrez S. An overview on the current status of cancer nanomedicines. Curr Med Res Opin [Internet]. 2018;34(5):911–21. Available from: http://www.ncbi.nlm.nih.gov/pubmed/29278015.
22. Awasthi R, Roseblade A, Hansbro PM, Rathbone MJ, Dua K, Bebawy M. Nanoparticles in cancer treatment: opportunities and obstacles. Curr Drug Targets [Internet]. 2018;19(14):1696–709. Available from: http://www.ncbi.nlm.nih.gov/pubmed/29577855.
23. Callaghan R, Luk F, Bebawy M. Inhibition of the multidrug resistance P-glycoprotein: time for a change of strategy? Drug Metab Dispos [Internet]. 2014;42(4):623–31. Available from: http://www.ncbi.nlm.nih.gov/pubmed/24492893.
24. Dua K, Shukla SD, de Jesus Andreoli Pinto T, Hansbro PM. Nanotechnology: advancing the translational respiratory research. Interv Med Appl Sci [Internet]. 2017;9(1):39–41. Available from: http://www.ncbi.nlm.nih.gov/pubmed/28932494.
25. Pillai G. Nanotechnology toward treating cancer. In: Applications of targeted nano drugs and delivery systems [Internet]. Elsevier; 2019. p. 221–56. Available from: https://linkinghub.elsevier.com/retrieve/pii/B9780128140291000090.
26. Sanvicens N, Marco MP. Multifunctional nanoparticles--properties and prospects for their use in human medicine. Trends Biotechnol [Internet]. 2008;26(8):425–33. Available from: http://www.ncbi.nlm.nih.gov/pubmed/18514941.
27. Lee D-E, Koo H, Sun I-C, Ryu JH, Kim K, Kwon IC. Multifunctional nanoparticles for multimodal imaging and theragnosis. Chem Soc Rev [Internet]. 2012;41(7):2656–72. Available from: http://www.ncbi.nlm.nih.gov/pubmed/22189429.
28. Matsumura Y, Maeda H. A new concept for macromolecular therapeutics in cancer chemotherapy: mechanism of tumoritropic accumulation of proteins and the antitumor agent smancs. Cancer Res [Internet]. 1986;46(12 Pt 1):6387–92. Available from: http://www.ncbi.nlm.nih.gov/pubmed/2946403.
29. Sinha R, Kim GJ, Nie S, Shin DM. Nanotechnology in cancer therapeutics: bioconjugated nanoparticles for drug delivery. Mol Cancer Ther [Internet]. 2006;5(8):1909–17. Available from: http://www.ncbi.nlm.nih.gov/pubmed/16928810.
30. Bertrand N, Wu J, Xu X, Kamaly N, Farokhzad OC. Cancer nanotechnology: the impact of passive and active targeting in the era of modern cancer biology. Adv Drug Deliv Rev [Internet]. 2014;66:2–25. Available from: http://www.ncbi.nlm.nih.gov/pubmed/24270007.
31. Li H, Jin H, Wan W, Wu C, Wei L. Cancer nanomedicine: mechanisms, obstacles and strategies. Nanomedicine (Lond) [Internet]. 2018;13(13):1639–56. Available from: http://www.ncbi.nlm.nih.gov/pubmed/30035660.
32. Danhier F, Feron O, Préat V. To exploit the tumor microenvironment: passive and active tumor targeting of nanocarriers for anti-cancer drug delivery. J Control Release [Internet]. 2010;148(2):135–46. Available from: http://www.ncbi.nlm.nih.gov/pubmed/20797419.
33. Bazak R, Houri M, El Achy S, Hussein W, Refaat T. Passive targeting of nanoparticles to cancer: a comprehensive review of the literature. Mol Clin Oncol [Internet]. 2014;2(6):904–8. Available from: http://www.ncbi.nlm.nih.gov/pubmed/25279172.

34. Torchilin VP. Targeted pharmaceutical nanocarriers for cancer therapy and imaging. AAPS J [Internet]. 2007;9(2):E128–47. Available from: http://www.ncbi.nlm.nih.gov/pubmed/17614355.

35. Gaspar MM, Radomska A, Gobbo OL, Bakowsky U, Radomski MW, Ehrhardt C. Targeted delivery of transferrin-conjugated liposomes to an orthotopic model of lung cancer in nude rats. J Aerosol Med Pulm Drug Deliv [Internet]. 2012;25(6):310–8. Available from: http://www.ncbi.nlm.nih.gov/pubmed/22857016.

36. Daniels TR, Bernabeu E, Rodríguez JA, Patel S, Kozman M, Chiappetta DA, et al. The transferrin receptor and the targeted delivery of therapeutic agents against cancer. Biochim Biophys Acta [Internet]. 2012;1820(3):291–317. Available from: http://www.ncbi.nlm.nih.gov/pubmed/21851850.

37. Lu Y, Low PS. Folate-mediated delivery of macromolecular anticancer therapeutic agents. Adv Drug Deliv Rev [Internet]. 2012;64:342–52. Available from: https://linkinghub.elsevier.com/retrieve/pii/S0169409X12002803.

38. Harding J, Burtness B. Cetuximab: an epidermal growth factor receptor chemeric human-murine monoclonal antibody. Drugs Today (Barc) [Internet]. 2005;41(2):107–27. Available from: http://www.ncbi.nlm.nih.gov/pubmed/15821783.

39. Le UM, Hartman A, Pillai G. Enhanced selective cellular uptake and cytotoxicity of epidermal growth factor-conjugated liposomes containing curcumin on EGFR-overexpressed pancreatic cancer cells. J Drug Target [Internet]. 2018;26(8):676–83. Available from: http://www.ncbi.nlm.nih.gov/pubmed/29157028.

40. Master AM, Sen Gupta A. EGF receptor-targeted nanocarriers for enhanced cancer treatment. Nanomedicine (Lond) [Internet]. 2012;7(12):1895–906. Available from: http://www.ncbi.nlm.nih.gov/pubmed/23249333.

41. Quintero-Fabián S, Arreola R, Becerril-Villanueva E, Torres-Romero JC, Arana-Argáez V, Lara-Riegos J, et al. Role of matrix metalloproteinases in angiogenesis and cancer. Front Oncol [Internet]. 2019;9:1370. Available from: http://www.ncbi.nlm.nih.gov/pubmed/31921634.

42. Eck SM, Blackburn JS, Schmucker AC, Burrage PS, Brinckerhoff CE. Matrix metalloproteinase and G protein coupled receptors: co-conspirators in the pathogenesis of autoimmune disease and cancer. J Autoimmun [Internet]. 33(3–4):214–21. Available from: http://www.ncbi.nlm.nih.gov/pubmed/19800199.

43. Awasthi R, Pant I, Kulkarni GT, Satiko Kikuchi I, de Jesus Andreoli Pinto T, Dua K, et al. Opportunities and challenges in nano-structure mediated drug delivery: where do we stand? Curr Nanomedicine [Internet]. 2016;6(2):78–104. Available from: http://www.eurekaselect.com/openurl/content.php?genre=article&issn=2468-1873&volume=6&issue=2&spage=78.

44. Gerlowski LE, Jain RK. Microvascular permeability of normal and neoplastic tissues. Microvasc Res [Internet]. 1986;31(3):288–305. Available from: https://linkinghub.elsevier.com/retrieve/pii/002628628690018X.

45. Hobbs SK, Monsky WL, Yuan F, Roberts WG, Griffith L, Torchilin VP, et al. Regulation of transport pathways in tumor vessels: role of tumor type and microenvironment. Proc Natl Acad Sci [Internet]. 1998;95(8):4607–12. Available from: http://www.pnas.org/cgi/doi/10.1073/pnas.95.8.4607.

46. Hashizume H, Baluk P, Morikawa S, McLean JW, Thurston G, Roberge S, et al. Openings between defective endothelial cells explain tumor vessel leakiness. Am J Pathol [Internet]. 2000;156(4):1363–80. Available from: https://linkinghub.elsevier.com/retrieve/pii/S0002944010650067.

47. Matsumoto Y, Nichols JW, Toh K, Nomoto T, Cabral H, Miura Y, et al. Vascular bursts enhance permeability of tumour blood vessels and improve nanoparticle delivery. Nat Nanotechnol [Internet]. 2016;11(6):533–8. Available from: http://www.nature.com/articles/nnano.2015.342.

48. WCW C. Nanomedicine 2.0. Acc Chem Res [Internet]. 2017;50(3):627–32. Available from: https://pubs.acs.org/doi/10.1021/acs.accounts.6b00629.

49. Rosenblum D, Joshi N, Tao W, Karp JM, Peer D. Progress and challenges towards targeted delivery of cancer therapeutics. Nat Commun [Internet]. 2018;9(1):1410. Available from: http://www.nature.com/articles/s41467-018-03705-y.

50. Nel A, Ruoslahti E, Meng H. New insights into "permeability" as in the enhanced permeability and retention effect of cancer nanotherapeutics. ACS Nano [Internet]. 2017;11(10):9567–9. Available from: https://pubs.acs.org/doi/10.1021/acsnano.7b07214.

51. Nakamura Y, Mochida A, Choyke PL, Kobayashi H. Nanodrug delivery: is the enhanced permeability and retention effect sufficient for curing cancer? Bioconjug Chem [Internet]. 2016;27(10):2225–38. Available from: https://pubs.acs.org/doi/10.1021/acs.bioconjchem.6b00437.

52. Danhier F. To exploit the tumor microenvironment: since the EPR effect fails in the clinic, what is the future of nanomedicine? J Control Release [Internet]. 2016;244:108–21. Available from: https://linkinghub.elsevier.com/retrieve/pii/S0168365916307799.

53. Sindhwani S, Syed AM, Ngai J, Kingston BR, Maiorino L, Rothschild J, et al. The entry of nanoparticles into solid tumours. Nat Mater [Internet]. 2020;19(5):566–75. Available from: http://www.nature.com/articles/s41563-019-0566-2.

54. de Lázaro I, Mooney DJ. A nanoparticle's pathway into tumours. Nat Mater [Internet]. 2020;19(5):486–7. Available from: http://www.nature.com/articles/s41563-020-0669-9.

55. Wilhelm S, Tavares AJ, Dai Q, Ohta S, Audet J, Dvorak HF, et al. Analysis of nanoparticle delivery to tumours. Nat Rev Mater [Internet]. 2016;1(5):16014. Available from: http://www.nature.com/articles/natrevmats201614.

56. Petersen GH, Alzghari SK, Chee W, Sankari SS, La-Beck NM. Meta-analysis of clinical and preclinical studies comparing the anticancer efficacy of liposomal versus conventional non-liposomal doxorubicin. J Control Release [Internet]. 2016;232:255–64. Available from: https://linkinghub.elsevier.com/retrieve/pii/S0168365916302413.

57. Shi J, Kantoff PW, Wooster R, Farokhzad OC. Cancer nanomedicine: progress, challenges and opportunities. Nat Rev Cancer [Internet]. 2017;17(1):20–37. Available from: http://www.nature.com/articles/nrc.2016.108.

58. ClinicalTrials.gov U.S. National Library of Medicine. Metronomic oral vinorelbine plus anti-PD-L1/anti-CTLA4 immunotherapy in patients with advanced solid tumours (MOVIE) [Internet]. Available from: https://clinicaltrials.gov/ct2/show/NCT03518606.

59. ClinicalTrials.gov U.S. National Library of Medicine. Basket study to evaluate the therapeutic activity of RO6874281 as a combination therapy in participants with advanced and/or metastatic solid tumors [Internet]. Available from: https://clinicaltrials.gov/ct2/show/NCT03386721.

60. ClinicalTrials.gov U.S. National Library of Medicine. Ferumoxytol - iron oxide nanoparticle magnetic resonance dynamic contrast enhanced MRI [Internet]. Available from: https://clinicaltrials.gov/ct2/show/NCT01895829.

61. ClinicalTrials.gov U.S. National Library of Medicine. Paclitaxel albumin-stabilized nanoparticle formulation and carboplatin followed by chemoradiation in treating patients with recurrent head and neck cancer [Internet]. Available from: https://clinicaltrials.gov/ct2/show/NCT01847326.

62. ClinicalTrials.gov U.S. National Library of Medicine. Dose escalation study of mRNA-2752 for intratumoral injection to patients with advanced malignancies [Internet]. Available from: https://clinicaltrials.gov/ct2/show/NCT03739931.

63. Adkins D, Ley J, Oppelt P, Gay HA, Daly M, Paniello RC, et al. Impact on health-related quality of life of induction chemotherapy compared with concurrent cisplatin and radiation therapy in patients with head and neck cancer. Clin Oncol (R Coll Radiol) [Internet]. 2019;31(9):e123–31. Available from: http://www.ncbi.nlm.nih.gov/pubmed/31147146.

64. Adkins D, Ley J, Oppelt P, Wildes TM, Gay HA, Daly M, et al. Nab-Paclitaxel-based induction chemotherapy with or without cetuximab for locally advanced head and neck squamous cell carcinoma. Oral Oncol [Internet]. 2017;72:26–31. Available from: http://www.ncbi.nlm.nih.gov/pubmed/28797458.

65. ClinicalTrials.gov U.S. National Library of Medicine. Induction chemotherapy with ACF followed by chemoradiation therapy for Adv Head & Neck Cancer [Internet]. Available from: https://clinicaltrials.gov/ct2/show/NCT01566435.

66. ClinicalTrials.gov U.S. National Library of Medicine. Chemotherapy and locoregional therapy trial (surgery or radiation) for patients with head and neck cancer (OPTIMA-II) [Internet]. Available from: https://clinicaltrials.gov/ct2/show/NCT03107182.

67. ClinicalTrials.gov U.S. National Library of Medicine. Recombinant EphB4-HSA fusion protein with standard chemotherapy regimens in treating patients with advanced or metastatic solid tumors [Internet]. Available from: https://clinicaltrials.gov/ct2/show/NCT02495896.

68. ClinicalTrials.gov U.S. National Library of Medicine. Targeted silica nanoparticles for real-time image-guided intraoperative mapping of nodal metastases [Internet]. Available from: https://clinicaltrials.gov/ct2/show/NCT02106598.

69. ClinicalTrials.gov U.S. National Library of Medicine. Ficlatuzumab w/wo cetuximab in patients w/cetuximab-resistant, recurrent or metastatic head/neck squamous cell carcinoma [Internet]. Available from: https://clinicaltrials.gov/ct2/show/NCT03422536.

70. Fakurnejad S, van Keulen S, Nishio N, Engelen M, van den Berg NS, Lu G, et al. Fluorescence molecular imaging for identification of high-grade dysplasia in patients with head and neck cancer. Oral Oncol [Internet]. 2019;97:50–5. Available from: http://www.ncbi.nlm.nih.gov/pubmed/31421471.

71. ClinicalTrials.gov U.S. National Library of Medicine. Panitumumab IRDye800 optical imaging study [Internet]. Available from: https://clinicaltrials.gov/ct2/show/NCT02415881.

72. ClinicalTrials.gov U.S. National Library of Medicine. Panitumumab-IRDye800 and 89Zr-panitumumab in identifying metastatic lymph nodes in patients with squamous cell head and neck cancer [Internet]. Available from: https://clinicaltrials.gov/ct2/show/NCT03733210.

73. ClinicalTrials.gov U.S. National Library of Medicine. Panitumumab-IRDye800 compared to sentinel node biopsy and (selective) neck dissection in identifying metastatic lymph nodes in patients with head & neck cancer [Internet]. Available from: https://clinicaltrials.gov/ct2/show/NCT03405142.

74. ClinicalTrials.gov U.S. National Library of Medicine. Carboplatin, nab-paclitaxel, durvalumab before surgery and adjuvant therapy in head and neck squamous cell carcinoma [Internet]. Available from: https://clinicaltrials.gov/ct2/show/NCT03174275.

75. Chinen AB, Guan CM, Ferrer JR, Barnaby SN, Merkel TJ, Mirkin CA. Nanoparticle probes for the detection of cancer biomarkers, cells, and tissues by fluorescence. Chem Rev [Internet]. 2015;115(19):10530–74. Available from: http://www.ncbi.nlm.nih.gov/pubmed/26313138.

76. Chakravarty R, Goel S, Dash A, Cai W. Radiolabeled inorganic nanoparticles for positron emission tomography imaging of cancer: an overview. Q J Nucl Med Mol Imaging [Internet]. 2017;61(2):181–204. Available from: http://www.ncbi.nlm.nih.gov/pubmed/28124549.

77. Chen F, Ma K, Benezra M, Zhang L, Cheal SM, Phillips E, et al. Cancer-targeting ultrasmall silica nanoparticles for clinical translation: physicochemical structure and biological property correlations. Chem Mater [Internet]. 2017;29(20):8766–79. Available from: http://www.ncbi.nlm.nih.gov/pubmed/29129959.

78. D'Hollander A, Mathieu E, Jans H, Vande Velde G, Stakenborg T, Van Dorpe P, et al. Development of nanostars as a biocompatible tumor contrast agent: toward in vivo SERS imaging. Int J Nanomedicine [Internet]. 2016;11:3703–14. Available from: http://www.ncbi.nlm.nih.gov/pubmed/27536107.

79. Han L, Duan W, Li X, Wang C, Jin Z, Zhai Y, et al. Surface-enhanced resonance raman scattering-guided brain tumor surgery showing prognostic benefit in rat models. ACS Appl Mater Interfaces [Internet]. 2019;11(17):15241–50. Available from: http://www.ncbi.nlm.nih.gov/pubmed/30896915.

80. Neuschmelting V, Harmsen S, Beziere N, Lockau H, Hsu H-T, Huang R, et al. Dual-modality surface-enhanced resonance raman scattering and multispectral optoacoustic tomography

nanoparticle approach for brain tumor delineation. Small [Internet]. 2018;14(23):e1800740. Available from: http://www.ncbi.nlm.nih.gov/pubmed/29726109.

81. Kircher MF, de la Zerda A, Jokerst JV, Zavaleta CL, Kempen PJ, Mittra E, et al. A brain tumor molecular imaging strategy using a new triple-modality MRI-photoacoustic-Raman nanoparticle. Nat Med [Internet]. 2012;18(5):829–34. Available from: http://www.ncbi.nlm. nih.gov/pubmed/22504484.

82. Borrebaeck CAK. Precision diagnostics: moving towards protein biomarker signatures of clinical utility in cancer. Nat Rev Cancer [Internet]. 2017;17(3):199–204. Available from: http://www.ncbi.nlm.nih.gov/pubmed/28154374.

83. Chevillet JR, Lee I, Briggs HA, He Y, Wang K. Issues and prospects of microRNA-based biomarkers in blood and other body fluids. Molecules [Internet]. 2014;19(5):6080–105. Available from: http://www.ncbi.nlm.nih.gov/pubmed/24830712.

84. Li H, Meng QH, Noh H, Somaiah N, Torres KE, Xia X, et al. Cell-surface vimentin-positive macrophage-like circulating tumor cells as a novel biomarker of metastatic gastrointestinal stromal tumors. Oncoimmunology [Internet]. 2018;7(5):e1420450. Available from: http:// www.ncbi.nlm.nih.gov/pubmed/29721368.

85. Wang D, Wu L, Liu X. Glycan markers as potential immunological targets in circulating tumor cells. Adv Exp Med Biol [Internet]. 2017;994:275–84. Available from: http://www. ncbi.nlm.nih.gov/pubmed/28560680.

86. Schneck H, Gierke B, Uppenkamp F, Behrens B, Niederacher D, Stoecklein NH, et al. EpCAM-independent enrichment of circulating tumor cells in metastatic breast cancer. PLoS One [Internet]. 2015;10(12):e0144535. Available from: http://www.ncbi.nlm.nih.gov/ pubmed/26695635.

87. Jia S, Zhang R, Li Z, Li J. Clinical and biological significance of circulating tumor cells, circulating tumor DNA, and exosomes as biomarkers in colorectal cancer. Oncotarget [Internet]. 2017;8(33):55632–45. Available from: http://www.ncbi.nlm.nih.gov/pubmed/28903450.

88. Song S, Qin Y, He Y, Huang Q, Fan C, Chen H-Y. Functional nanoprobes for ultrasensitive detection of biomolecules. Chem Soc Rev [Internet]. 2010;39(11):4234–43. Available from: http://www.ncbi.nlm.nih.gov/pubmed/20871878.

89. Chen X-J, Zhang X-Q, Liu Q, Zhang J, Zhou G. Nanotechnology: a promising method for oral cancer detection and diagnosis. J Nanobiotechnology [Internet]. 2018;16(1):52. Available from: https://jnanobiotechnology.biomedcentral.com/articles/10.1186/s12951-018-0378-6.

90. Hull LC, Farrell D, Grodzinski P. Highlights of recent developments and trends in cancer nanotechnology research--view from NCI Alliance for Nanotechnology in Cancer. Biotechnol Adv [Internet]. 32(4):666–78. Available from: http://www.ncbi.nlm.nih.gov/ pubmed/23948249.

91. Doria G, Conde J, Veigas B, Giestas L, Almeida C, Assunção M, et al. Noble metal nanoparticles for biosensing applications. Sensors (Basel) [Internet]. 2012;12(2):1657–87. Available from: http://www.ncbi.nlm.nih.gov/pubmed/22438731.

92. Sharifi M, Avadi MR, Attar F, Dashtestani F, Ghorchian H, Rezayat SM, et al. Cancer diagnosis using nanomaterials based electrochemical nanobiosensors. Biosens Bioelectron [Internet]. 2019;126:773–84. Available from: http://www.ncbi.nlm.nih.gov/pubmed/30554099.

93. Harun NA, Benning MJ, Horrocks BR, Fulton DA. Gold nanoparticle-enhanced luminescence of silicon quantum dots co-encapsulated in polymer nanoparticles. Nanoscale [Internet]. 2013;5(9):3817–27. Available from: http://www.ncbi.nlm.nih.gov/pubmed/23519376.

94. Zhang H, Lv J, Jia Z. Efficient fluorescence resonance energy transfer between quantum dots and gold nanoparticles based on porous silicon photonic crystal for dna detection. Sensors [Internet]. 2017;17(5):1078. Available from: http://www.mdpi.com/1424-8220/17/5/1078.

95. Chaffer CL, Weinberg RA. A perspective on cancer cell metastasis. Forensic Sci Int. 2011;331(6024):1559–64. Available from: http://www.ncbi.nlm.nih.gov/pubmed/21436443.

96. Gupta GP, Massagué J. Cancer metastasis: building a framework. Cell [Internet]. 2006;127(4):679–95. Available from: http://www.ncbi.nlm.nih.gov/pubmed/17110329.

97. Lin M, Chen J-F, Lu Y-T, Zhang Y, Song J, Hou S, et al. Nanostructure embedded micro-chips for detection, isolation, and characterization of circulating tumor cells. Acc Chem Res [Internet]. 2014;47(10):2941–50. Available from: http://www.ncbi.nlm.nih.gov/pubmed/25111636.

98. Park S-M, Wong DJ, Ooi CC, Kurtz DM, Vermesh O, Aalipour A, et al. Molecular profiling of single circulating tumor cells from lung cancer patients. Proc Natl Acad Sci U S A [Internet]. 2016;113(52):E8379–86. Available from: http://www.ncbi.nlm.nih.gov/pubmed/27956614.

99. Jan YJ, Chen J-F, Zhu Y, Lu Y-T, Chen SH, Chung H, et al. NanoVelcro rare-cell assays for detection and characterization of circulating tumor cells. Adv Drug Deliv Rev [Internet]. 2018;125:78–93. Available from: http://www.ncbi.nlm.nih.gov/pubmed/29551650.

100. Liang X-J, Chen C, Zhao Y, Wang PC. Circumventing tumor resistance to chemotherapy by nanotechnology. Methods Mol Biol [Internet]. 2010;596:467–88. Available from: http://www.ncbi.nlm.nih.gov/pubmed/19949937.

101. Furness S, Glenny A-M, Worthington H V, Pavitt S, Oliver R, Clarkson JE, et al. Interventions for the treatment of oral cavity and oropharyngeal cancer: chemotherapy. Cochrane database Syst Rev [Internet]. 2010;(9):CD006386. Available from: http://www.ncbi.nlm.nih.gov/pubmed/20824847.

102. Zhao C-Y, Cheng R, Yang Z, Tian Z-M. Nanotechnology for cancer therapy based on che-motherapy. Molecules [Internet]. 2018;23(4). Available from: http://www.ncbi.nlm.nih.gov/pubmed/29617302.

103. Ketabat F, Pundir M, Mohabatpour F, Lobanova L, Koutsopoulos S, Hadjiiski L, et al. Controlled drug delivery systems for oral cancer treatment-current status and future perspec-tives. Pharmaceutics [Internet]. 2019;11(7). Available from: http://www.ncbi.nlm.nih.gov/pubmed/31262096.

104. Marples B, Dhar S. Radiobiology and the renewed potential for nanoparticles. Int J Radiat Oncol Biol Phys [Internet]. 2017;98(3):489–91. Available from: http://www.ncbi.nlm.nih.gov/pubmed/28581384.

105. Zhou B, Wu Q, Wang M, Hoover A, Wang X, Zhou F, et al. Immunologically modified MnFe2O4 nanoparticles to synergize photothermal therapy and immunotherapy for cancer treatment. Chem Eng J [Internet]. 2020;396. Available from: http://www.ncbi.nlm.nih.gov/pubmed/32523422.

106. Hou X, Tao Y, Pang Y, Li X, Jiang G, Liu Y. Nanoparticle-based photothermal and photody-namic immunotherapy for tumor treatment. Int J cancer [Internet]. 2018;143(12):3050–60. Available from: http://www.ncbi.nlm.nih.gov/pubmed/29981170.

107. Buabeid MA, Arafa E-SA, Murtaza G. Emerging prospects for nanoparticle-enabled cancer immunotherapy. J Immunol Res [Internet]. 2020;2020:9624532. Available from: http://www.ncbi.nlm.nih.gov/pubmed/32377541.

108. Michot JM, Bigenwald C, Champiat S, Collins M, Carbonnel F, Postel-Vinay S, et al. Immune-related adverse events with immune checkpoint blockade: a comprehensive review. Eur J Cancer [Internet]. 2016;54:139–48. Available from: http://www.ncbi.nlm.nih.gov/pubmed/26765102.

109. Duan X, Chan C, Han W, Guo N, Weichselbaum RR, Lin W. Immunostimulatory nanomedi-cines synergize with checkpoint blockade immunotherapy to eradicate colorectal tumors. Nat Commun [Internet]. 2019;10(1):1899. Available from: http://www.ncbi.nlm.nih.gov/pubmed/31015397.

110. Blanco E, Shen H, Ferrari M. Principles of nanoparticle design for overcoming biological barriers to drug delivery. Nat Biotechnol [Internet]. 2015;33(9):941–51. Available from: http://www.ncbi.nlm.nih.gov/pubmed/26348965.

111. Zhang Y, Wang J, Xu M. A sensitive DNA biosensor fabricated with gold nanoparticles/poly (p-aminobenzoic acid)/carbon nanotubes modified electrode. Colloids Surf B Biointerfaces [Internet]. 2010;75(1):179–85. Available from: http://www.ncbi.nlm.nih.gov/pubmed/19740633.

112. Bonanni A, del Valle M. Use of nanomaterials for impedimetric DNA sensors: a review. Anal Chim Acta [Internet]. 2010;678(1):7–17. Available from: http://www.ncbi.nlm.nih.gov/pubmed/20869498.

113. Mahmoodi Chalbatani G, Dana H, Gharagouzloo E, Grijalvo S, Eritja R, Logsdon CD, et al. Small interfering RNAs (siRNAs) in cancer therapy: a nano-based approach. Int J Nanomedicine [Internet]. 2019;14:3111–28. Available from: http://www.ncbi.nlm.nih.gov/pubmed/31118626.

114. Babu A, Muralidharan R, Amreddy N, Mehta M, Munshi A, Ramesh R. Nanoparticles for siRNA-based gene silencing in tumor therapy. IEEE Trans Nanobioscience [Internet]. 2016;15(8):849–63. Available from: http://www.ncbi.nlm.nih.gov/pubmed/28092499.

115. Chaudhary V, Jangra S, Yadav NR. Nanotechnology based approaches for detection and delivery of microRNA in healthcare and crop protection. J Nanobiotechnology [Internet]. 2018;16(1):40. Available from: http://www.ncbi.nlm.nih.gov/pubmed/29653577.

116. Degliangeli F, Pompa PP, Fiammengo R. Nanotechnology-based strategies for the detection and quantification of microRNA. Chem Int. 2014;20(31):9476–92. Available from: http://www.ncbi.nlm.nih.gov/pubmed/24989446.

117. Li W, Ruan K. MicroRNA detection by microarray. Anal Bioanal Chem [Internet]. 2009;394(4):1117–24. Available from: http://www.ncbi.nlm.nih.gov/pubmed/19132354.

118. Longley DB, Johnston PG. Molecular mechanisms of drug resistance. J Pathol [Internet]. 2005;205(2):275–92. Available from: http://www.ncbi.nlm.nih.gov/pubmed/15641020.

119. Tekchandani P, Kurmi BD, Paliwal SR. Nanomedicine to deal with cancer cell biology in multi-drug resistance. Mini Rev Med Chem [Internet]. 2017;17(18):1793–810. Available from: http://www.ncbi.nlm.nih.gov/pubmed/26891930.

120. Dong X, Mumper RJ. Nanomedicinal strategies to treat multidrug-resistant tumors: current progress. Nanomedicine (Lond) [Internet]. 2010;5(4):597–615. Available from: http://www.ncbi.nlm.nih.gov/pubmed/20528455.

121. Meng H, Liong M, Xia T, Li Z, Ji Z, Zink JI, et al. Engineered design of mesoporous silica nanoparticles to deliver doxorubicin and P-glycoprotein siRNA to overcome drug resistance in a cancer cell line. ACS Nano [Internet]. 2010;4(8):4539–50. Available from: https://pubs.acs.org/doi/10.1021/nn100690m.

122. Sun T-M, Du J-Z, Yao Y-D, Mao C-Q, Dou S, Huang S-Y, et al. Simultaneous delivery of siRNA and paclitaxel via a "two-in-one" micelleplex promotes synergistic tumor suppression. ACS Nano [Internet]. 2011;5(2):1483–94. Available from: https://pubs.acs.org/doi/10.1021/nn103349h.

123. Rybinski B, Yun K. Addressing intra-tumoral heterogeneity and therapy resistance. Oncotarget [Internet]. 2016;7(44):72322–42. Available from: http://www.ncbi.nlm.nih.gov/pubmed/27608848.

124. Hu C-MJ, Zhang L. Nanoparticle-based combination therapy toward overcoming drug resistance in cancer. Biochem Pharmacol [Internet]. 2012;83(8):1104–11. Available from: http://www.ncbi.nlm.nih.gov/pubmed/22285912.

125. Wong HL, Rauth AM, Bendayan R, Manias JL, Ramaswamy M, Liu Z, et al. A new polymer-lipid hybrid nanoparticle system increases cytotoxicity of doxorubicin against multidrug-resistant human breast cancer cells. Pharm Res [Internet]. 2006;23(7):1574–85. Available from: http://www.ncbi.nlm.nih.gov/pubmed/16786442.

126. Tian Y, Jiang X, Chen X, Shao Z, Yang W. Doxorubicin-loaded magnetic silk fibroin nanoparticles for targeted therapy of multidrug-resistant cancer. Adv Mater [Internet]. 2014;26(43):7393–8. Available from: http://www.ncbi.nlm.nih.gov/pubmed/25238148.

127. Kang J-W, Cho H-J, Lee HJ, Jin H-E, Maeng H-J. Polyethylene glycol-decorated doxorubicin/carboxymethyl chitosan/gold nanocomplex for reducing drug efflux in cancer cells and extending circulation in blood stream. Int J Biol Macromol [Internet]. 2019;125:61–71. Available from: http://www.ncbi.nlm.nih.gov/pubmed/30521919.

128. Gu Y-J, Cheng J, Man CW-Y, Wong W-T, Cheng SH. Gold-doxorubicin nanoconjugates for overcoming multidrug resistance. Nanomedicine [Internet]. 2012;8(2):204–11. Available from: http://www.ncbi.nlm.nih.gov/pubmed/21704592.

129. Liu J, Zhao Y, Guo Q, Wang Z, Wang H, Yang Y, et al. TAT-modified nanosilver for combating multidrug-resistant cancer. Biomaterials [Internet]. 2012;33(26):6155–61. Available from: https://linkinghub.elsevier.com/retrieve/pii/S0142961212005765.

130. Wen Z-M, Jie J, Zhang Y, Liu H, Peng L-P. A self-assembled polyjuglanin nanoparticle loaded with doxorubicin and anti-Kras siRNA for attenuating multidrug resistance in human lung cancer. Biochem Biophys Res Commun [Internet]. 2017;493(4):1430–7. Available from: http://www.ncbi.nlm.nih.gov/pubmed/28958938.

131. Sakurai Y. Development of siRNA delivery targeting the tumor microenvironment with a new functional device. Yakugaku Zasshi [Internet]. 2019;139(11):1357–63. Available from: http://www.ncbi.nlm.nih.gov/pubmed/31685731.

132. Chen Y, Bathula SR, Li J, Huang L. Multifunctional nanoparticles delivering small interfering RNA and doxorubicin overcome drug resistance in cancer. J Biol Chem [Internet]. 2010;285(29):22639–50. Available from: http://www.ncbi.nlm.nih.gov/pubmed/20460382.

133. Forastiere A, Koch W, Trotti A, Sidransky D. Head and neck cancer. N Engl J Med [Internet]. 2001;345(26):1890–900. Available from: http://www.ncbi.nlm.nih.gov/pubmed/11756581.

134. Haddad RI, Shin DM. Recent advances in head and neck cancer. N Engl J Med [Internet]. 2008;359(11):1143–54. Available from: http://www.ncbi.nlm.nih.gov/pubmed/18784104.

135. Nör JE, Gutkind JS. Head and neck cancer in the new era of precision medicine. J Dent Res [Internet]. 2018;97(6):601–2. Available from: http://www.ncbi.nlm.nih.gov/pubmed/29771196.

136. Marur S, Forastiere AA. Head and neck cancer: changing epidemiology, diagnosis, and treatment. Mayo Clin Proc [Internet]. 2008;83(4):489–501. Available from: http://www.ncbi.nlm.nih.gov/pubmed/18380996.

137. Prince VM, Papagerakis S, Prince ME. Oral cancer and cancer stem cells: relevance to oral cancer risk factors, premalignant lesions, and treatment. Curr Oral Heal Reports [Internet]. 2016;3(2):65–73. Available from: http://link.springer.com/10.1007/s40496-016-0081-3.

138. Rivera C. Essentials of oral cancer. Int J Clin Exp Pathol [Internet]. 2015;8(9):11884–94. Available from: http://www.ncbi.nlm.nih.gov/pubmed/26617944.

139. Ramesh S, Tan CY, Hamdi M, Sopyan I, Teng WD. The influence of Ca/P ratio on the properties of hydroxyapatite bioceramics. In: Du S, Leng J, Asundi AK, editors. Proc. of SPIE Vol. 6423, 64233A, (2007); 2007. p. 64233A-1–6.

140. Xie X, O'Neill W, Pan Q. Immunotherapy for head and neck cancer: the future of treatment? Expert Opin Biol Ther [Internet]. 2017;17(6):701–8. Available from: http://www.ncbi.nlm.nih.gov/pubmed/28368668.

141. Grégoire V, Lefebvre J-L, Licitra L, Felip E, EHNS-ESMO-ESTRO Guidelines Working Group. Squamous cell carcinoma of the head and neck: EHNS-ESMO-ESTRO Clinical practice guidelines for diagnosis, treatment and follow-up. Ann Oncol Off J Eur Soc Med Oncol [Internet]. 2010;21 Suppl 5:v184–6. Available from: http://www.ncbi.nlm.nih.gov/pubmed/20555077.

142. De Felice F, Musio D, Tombolini V. Osteoradionecrosis and intensity modulated radiation therapy: an overview. Crit Rev Oncol Hematol [Internet]. 2016;107:39–43. Available from: http://www.ncbi.nlm.nih.gov/pubmed/27823650.

143. De Felice F, de Vincentiis M, Luzzi V, Magliulo G, Tombolini M, Ruoppolo G, et al. Late radiation-associated dysphagia in head and neck cancer patients: evidence, research and management. Oral Oncol [Internet]. 2018;77:125–30. Available from: http://www.ncbi.nlm.nih.gov/pubmed/29362118.

144. Kasahara Y, Endo K, Ueno T, Ueno H, Moriyama-Kita M, Odani A, et al. Bone invasion-targeted chemotherapy with a novel anionic platinum complex (3Pt) for oral squamous cell carcinoma. Cancer Sci [Internet]. 2019;110(10):3288–95. Available from: http://www.ncbi.nlm.nih.gov/pubmed/31348586.

145. Calixto G, Bernegossi J, Fonseca-Santos B, Chorilli M. Nanotechnology-based drug delivery systems for treatment of oral cancer: a review. Int J Nanomedicine [Internet]. 2014;9:3719–35. Available from: http://www.ncbi.nlm.nih.gov/pubmed/25143724.
146. Manaia EB, Abuçafy MP, Chiari-Andréo BG, Silva BL, Oshiro Junior JA, Chiavacci LA. Physicochemical characterization of drug nanocarriers. Int J Nanomedicine [Internet]. 2017;12:4991–5011. Available from: http://www.ncbi.nlm.nih.gov/pubmed/28761340.
147. De Felice F, Cavallini C, Barlattani A, Tombolini M, Brugnoletti O, Tombolini V, et al. Nanotechnology in oral cavity carcinoma: recent trends and treatment opportunities. Nanomaterials [Internet]. 2019;9(11):1546. Available from: https://www.mdpi.com/2079-4991/9/11/1546.
148. Moskovitz J, Moy J, Ferris RL. Immunotherapy for head and neck squamous cell carcinoma. Curr Oncol Rep [Internet]. 2018;20(2):22. Available from: http://www.ncbi.nlm.nih.gov/pubmed/29502288.
149. Farkona S, Diamandis EP, Blasutig IM. Cancer immunotherapy: the beginning of the end of cancer? BMC Med [Internet]. 2016;14:73. Available from: http://www.ncbi.nlm.nih.gov/pubmed/27151159.
150. Rapidis AD, Wolf GT. Immunotherapy of head and neck cancer: current and future considerations. J Oncol [Internet]. 2009;2009:346345. Available from: http://www.ncbi.nlm.nih.gov/pubmed/19680453.
151. Coley WB. II. Contribution to the knowledge of sarcoma. Ann Surg [Internet]. 1891;14(3):199–220. Available from: http://www.ncbi.nlm.nih.gov/pubmed/17859590.
152. Cheng C-T, Castro G, Liu C-H, Lau P. Advanced nanotechnology: an arsenal to enhance immunotherapy in fighting cancer. Clin Chim Acta [Internet]. 2019;492:12–9. Available from: http://www.ncbi.nlm.nih.gov/pubmed/30711524.
153. ClinicalTrials.gov U.S. National Library of Medicine. PARTNER: panitumumab added to regimen for treatment of head and neck cancer evaluation of response [Internet]. Available from: https://clinicaltrials.gov/ct2/show/NCT00454779.
154. ClinicalTrials.gov U.S. National Library of Medicine. Avelumab, cetuximab, and palbociclib in recurrent or metastatic head and neck squamous cell carcinoma [Internet]. Available from: https://clinicaltrials.gov/ct2/show/NCT03498378.
155. Kumar A, Chakravarty N, Bhatnagar S, Chowdhary GS. Efficacy and safety of concurrent chemoradiotherapy with or without Nimotuzumab in unresectable locally advanced squamous cell carcinoma of head and neck: prospective comparative study - ESCORT-N study. South Asian J cancer [Internet]. 8(2):108–11. Available from: http://www.ncbi.nlm.nih.gov/pubmed/31069191.
156. Bastholt L, Specht L, Jensen K, Brun E, Loft A, Petersen J, et al. Phase I/II clinical and pharmacokinetic study evaluating a fully human monoclonal antibody against EGFr (HuMax-EGFr) in patients with advanced squamous cell carcinoma of the head and neck. Radiother Oncol [Internet]. 2007;85(1):24–8. Available from: http://www.ncbi.nlm.nih.gov/pubmed/17602769.
157. Machiels J-P, Subramanian S, Ruzsa A, Repassy G, Lifirenko I, Flygare A, et al. Zalutumumab plus best supportive care versus best supportive care alone in patients with recurrent or metastatic squamous-cell carcinoma of the head and neck after failure of platinum-based chemotherapy: an open-label, randomised phase 3 trial. Lancet Oncol [Internet]. 2011;12(4):333–43. Available from: http://www.ncbi.nlm.nih.gov/pubmed/21377930.
158. Mesía R, Henke M, Fortin A, Minn H, Yunes Ancona AC, Cmelak A, et al. Chemoradiotherapy with or without panitumumab in patients with unresected, locally advanced squamous-cell carcinoma of the head and neck (CONCERT-1): a randomised, controlled, open-label phase 2 trial. Lancet Oncol [Internet]. 2015;16(2):208–20. Available from: http://www.ncbi.nlm.nih.gov/pubmed/25596660.
159. Giralt J, Trigo J, Nuyts S, Ozsahin M, Skladowski K, Hatoum G, et al. Panitumumab plus radiotherapy versus chemoradiotherapy in patients with unresected, locally advanced squamous-cell carcinoma of the head and neck (CONCERT-2): a randomised, controlled,

open-label phase 2 trial. Lancet Oncol [Internet]. 2015;16(2):221–32. Available from: http://www.ncbi.nlm.nih.gov/pubmed/25596659.

160. Rischin D, Spigel DR, Adkins D, Wein R, Arnold S, Singhal N, et al. PRISM: phase 2 trial with panitumumab monotherapy as second-line treatment in patients with recurrent or metastatic squamous cell carcinoma of the head and neck. Head Neck [Internet]. 2016;38 Suppl 1:E1756–61. Available from: http://www.ncbi.nlm.nih.gov/pubmed/26681429.

161. Vermorken JB, Stöhlmacher-Williams J, Davidenko I, Licitra L, Winquist E, Villanueva C, et al. Cisplatin and fluorouracil with or without panitumumab in patients with recurrent or metastatic squamous-cell carcinoma of the head and neck (SPECTRUM): an open-label phase 3 randomised trial. Lancet Oncol [Internet]. 2013;14(8):697–710. Available from: http://www.ncbi.nlm.nih.gov/pubmed/23746666.

162. Kozakiewicz P, Grzybowska-Szatkowska L. Application of molecular targeted therapies in the treatment of head and neck squamous cell carcinoma. Oncol Lett [Internet]. 2018;15(5):7497–505. Available from: http://www.ncbi.nlm.nih.gov/pubmed/29725456.

163. Chiu JW, Chan K, Chen EX, Siu LL, Abdul Razak AR. Pharmacokinetic assessment of dacomitinib (pan-HER tyrosine kinase inhibitor) in patients with locally advanced head and neck squamous cell carcinoma (LA SCCHN) following administration through a gastrostomy feeding tube (GT). Invest New Drugs [Internet]. 2015;33(4):895–900. Available from: http://www.ncbi.nlm.nih.gov/pubmed/25937431.

164. Elicin O, Ozsahin M. Current role of dacomitinib in head and neck cancer. Expert Opin Investig Drugs [Internet]. 2016;25(6):735–42. Available from: http://www.ncbi.nlm.nih.gov/pubmed/27070370.

165. Psyrri A, Rampias T, Vermorken JB. The current and future impact of human papillomavirus on treatment of squamous cell carcinoma of the head and neck. Ann Oncol Off J Eur Soc Med Oncol [Internet]. 2014;25(11):2101–15. Available from: http://www.ncbi.nlm.nih.gov/pubmed/25057165.

166. Abdul Razak AR, Soulières D, Laurie SA, Hotte SJ, Singh S, Winquist E, et al. A phase II trial of dacomitinib, an oral pan-human EGF receptor (HER) inhibitor, as first-line treatment in recurrent and/or metastatic squamous-cell carcinoma of the head and neck. Ann Oncol [Internet]. 2013;24(3):761–9. Available from: https://linkinghub.elsevier.com/retrieve/pii/S0923753419371315.

167. Machiels J-PH, Haddad RI, Fayette J, Licitra LF, Tahara M, Vermorken JB, et al. Afatinib versus methotrexate as second-line treatment in patients with recurrent or metastatic squamous-cell carcinoma of the head and neck progressing on or after platinum-based therapy (LUX-Head & Neck 1): an open-label, randomised phase 3 trial. Lancet Oncol [Internet]. 2015;16(5):583–94. Available from: http://www.ncbi.nlm.nih.gov/pubmed/25892145.

168. Clement PM, Gauler T, Machiels JP, Haddad RI, Fayette J, Licitra LF, et al. Afatinib versus methotrexate in older patients with second-line recurrent and/or metastatic head and neck squamous cell carcinoma: subgroup analysis of the LUX-Head & Neck 1 trial. Ann Oncol Off J Eur Soc Med Oncol [Internet]. 2016;27(8):1585–93. Available from: http://www.ncbi.nlm.nih.gov/pubmed/27084954.

169. Cohen EEW, Licitra LF, Burtness B, Fayette J, Gauler T, Clement PM, et al. Biomarkers predict enhanced clinical outcomes with afatinib versus methotrexate in patients with second-line recurrent and/or metastatic head and neck cancer. Ann Oncol Off J Eur Soc Med Oncol [Internet]. 2017;28(10):2526–32. Available from: http://www.ncbi.nlm.nih.gov/pubmed/28961833.

170. Harrington K, Temam S, Mehanna H, D'Cruz A, Jain M, D'Onofrio I, et al. Postoperative adjuvant lapatinib and concurrent chemoradiotherapy followed by maintenance lapatinib monotherapy in high-risk patients with resected squamous cell carcinoma of the head and neck: a phase III, randomized, double-blind, placebo-controlled study. J Clin Oncol [Internet]. 2015;33(35):4202–9. Available from: http://www.ncbi.nlm.nih.gov/pubmed/26527790.

171. Agulnik M, da Cunha SG, Hedley D, Nicklee T, Dos Reis PP, Ho J, et al. Predictive and pharmacodynamic biomarker studies in tumor and skin tissue samples of patients with recur-

rent or metastatic squamous cell carcinoma of the head and neck treated with erlotinib. J Clin Oncol [Internet]. 2007;25(16):2184–90. Available from: http://www.ncbi.nlm.nih.gov/pubmed/17538163.

172. Hainsworth JD, Spigel DR, Burris HA, Markus TM, Shipley D, Kuzur M, et al. Neoadjuvant chemotherapy/gefitinib followed by concurrent chemotherapy/radiation therapy/gefitinib for patients with locally advanced squamous carcinoma of the head and neck. Cancer [Internet]. 2009;115(10):2138–46. Available from: http://www.ncbi.nlm.nih.gov/pubmed/19288572.

173. Razak ARA, Ahn M-J, Yen C-J, Solomon BJ, Lee S-H, Wang H-M, et al. Phase Ib/II study of the PI3Kα inhibitor BYL719 in combination with cetuximab in recurrent/metastatic squamous cell cancer of the head and neck (SCCHN). J Clin Oncol [Internet]. 2014;32(15_suppl):6044. Available from: http://ascopubs.org/doi/10.1200/jco.2014.32.15_suppl.6044.

174. ClinicalTrials.gov U.S. National Library of Medicine. EACH: evaluating avelumab in combination with cetuximab in head and neck cancer (EACH) [Internet]. Available from: https://clinicaltrials.gov/ct2/show/NCT03494322.

175. ClinicalTrials.gov U.S. National Library of Medicine. Durvalumab, cetuximab and radiotherapy in head neck cancer (DUCRO-HN) [Internet]. Available from: https://clinicaltrials.gov/ct2/show/NCT03051906.

176. ClinicalTrials.gov U.S. National Library of Medicine. Durvalumab with or without tremelimumab in resectable locally advanced squamous cell carcinoma of the oral cavity (DUTRELASCO) [Internet]. Available from: https://clinicaltrials.gov/ct2/show/NCT03784066.

177. ClinicalTrials.gov U.S. National Library of Medicine. A study of atezolizumab (anti–Pd-L1 antibody) as adjuvant therapy after definitive local therapy in patients with high-risk locally advanced squamous cell carcinoma of the head and neck [Internet]. Available from: https://clinicaltrials.gov/ct2/show/NCT03452137.

178. ClinicalTrials.gov U.S. National Library of Medicine. Atezolizumab and bevacizumab in patients with recurrent or metastatic squamous-cell carcinoma of the head and neck (ATHENA) [Internet]. Available from: https://clinicaltrials.gov/ct2/show/NCT03818061.

179. Seiwert TY, Weiss J, Baxi SS, Ahn M-J, Fayette J, Gillison ML, et al. A phase 3, randomized, open-label study of first-line durvalumab (MEDI4736) ± tremelimumab versus standard of care (SoC; EXTREME regimen) in recurrent/metastatic (R/M) SCCHN: KESTREL. J Clin Oncol [Internet]. 2016;34(15_suppl):TPS6101. Available from: http://ascopubs.org/doi/10.1200/JCO.2016.34.15_suppl.TPS6101.

180. Bonomo P, Desideri I, Loi M, Mangoni M, Sottili M, Marrazzo L, et al. Anti PD-L1 DUrvalumab combined with Cetuximab and RadiOtherapy in locally advanced squamous cell carcinoma of the head and neck: a phase I/II study (DUCRO). Clin Transl Radiat Oncol [Internet]. 2018;9:42–7. Available from: http://www.ncbi.nlm.nih.gov/pubmed/29594250.

181. Peters S, Gettinger S, Johnson ML, Jänne PA, Garassino MC, Christoph D, et al. Phase II trial of atezolizumab as first-line or subsequent therapy for patients with programmed death-ligand 1-selected advanced non-small-cell lung cancer (BIRCH). J Clin Oncol [Internet]. 2017;35(24):2781–9. Available from: http://www.ncbi.nlm.nih.gov/pubmed/28609226.

182. ClinicalTrials.gov U.S. National Library of Medicine. A study to evaluate immune biomarker modulation in response to VTX-2337 in combination with an anti- PD-1 inhibitor in head and neck cancer [Internet]. Available from: https://clinicaltrials.gov/ct2/show/NCT03906526.

183. Moreno-Gonzalez A, Olson JM, Klinghoffer RA. Predicting responses to chemotherapy in the context that matters - the patient. Mol Cell Oncol [Internet]. 2016;3(1):e1057315. Available from: http://www.ncbi.nlm.nih.gov/pubmed/27308571.

184. Klinghoffer RA, Bahrami SB, Hatton BA, Frazier JP, Moreno-Gonzalez A, Strand AD, et al. A technology platform to assess multiple cancer agents simultaneously within a patient's tumor. Sci Transl Med [Internet]. 2015;7(284):284ra58. Available from: http://www.ncbi.nlm.nih.gov/pubmed/25904742.

185. Dey J, Kerwin WS, Grenley MO, Casalini JR, Tretyak I, Ditzler SH, et al. A platform for rapid, quantitative assessment of multiple drug combinations simultaneously in solid tumors

in vivo. PLoS One [Internet]. 2016;11(6):e0158617. Available from: http://www.ncbi.nlm.nih.gov/pubmed/27359113.

186. Frazier JP, Bertout JA, Kerwin WS, Moreno-Gonzalez A, Casalini JR, Grenley MO, et al. Multidrug analyses in patients distinguish efficacious cancer agents based on both tumor cell killing and immunomodulation. Cancer Res [Internet]. 2017;77(11):2869–80. Available from: http://www.ncbi.nlm.nih.gov/pubmed/28364003.

187. Dietsch GN, Lu H, Yang Y, Morishima C, Chow LQ, Disis ML, et al. Coordinated activation of toll-like Receptor8 (TLR8) and NLRP3 by the TLR8 agonist, VTX-2337, ignites tumoricidal natural killer cell activity. PLoS One [Internet]. 2016;11(2):e0148764. Available from: http://www.ncbi.nlm.nih.gov/pubmed/26928328.

188. Kong A, Good J, Kirkham A, Savage J, Mant R, Llewellyn L, et al. Phase I trial of WEE1 inhibition with chemotherapy and radiotherapy as adjuvant treatment, and a window of opportunity trial with cisplatin in patients with head and neck cancer: the WISTERIA trial protocol. BMJ Open [Internet]. 2020;10(3):e033009. Available from: http://bmjopen.bmj.com/lookup/doi/10.1136/bmjopen-2019-033009.

189. ClinicalTrials.gov U.S. National Library of Medicine. WEE1 inhibitor with cisplatin and radiotherapy: a trial in head and neck cancer (WISTERIA) [Internet]. Available from: https://clinicaltrials.gov/ct2/show/NCT03028766.

190. ClinicalTrials.gov U.S. National Library of Medicine. Abemaciclib + nivolumab in patients with recurrent/metastatic head and neck squamous cell carcinoma that progressed or recurred within six months after platinum-based chemotherapy [Internet]. Available from: https://clinicaltrials.gov/ct2/show/NCT03655444.

191. ClinicalTrials.gov U.S. National Library of Medicine. Clinical trial of abemaciclib in combination with pembrolizumab in patients with metastatic or recurrent head and neck cancer [Internet]. Available from: https://clinicaltrials.gov/ct2/show/NCT03938337.

192. ClinicalTrials.gov U.S. National Library of Medicine. TPST-1120 as monotherapy and in combination with nivolumab in subjects with advanced cancers [Internet]. Available from: https://clinicaltrials.gov/ct2/show/NCT03829436.

193. ClinicalTrials.gov U.S. National Library of Medicin. Sitravatinib (MGCD516) and nivolumab in oral cavity cancer window opportunity study (SNOW) [Internet]. Available from: https://clinicaltrials.gov/ct2/show/NCT03575598.

194. Kim Y, Lee SJ, Lee JY, Lee S-H, Sun J-M, Park K, et al. Clinical trial of nintedanib in patients with recurrent or metastatic salivary gland cancer of the head and neck: a multicenter phase 2 study (Korean Cancer study group HN14-01). Cancer [Internet]. 2017;123(11):1958–64. Available from: http://doi.wiley.com/10.1002/cncr.30537.

195. ClinicalTrials.gov U.S. National Library of Medicine. Trial of BIBF1120 (Nintedanib) in patients with recurrent or metastatic salivary gland cancer of the head and neck [Internet]. Available from: https://clinicaltrials.gov/ct2/show/NCT02558387.

196. ClinicalTrials.gov U.S. National Library of Medicine. Phase III open label study of MEDI 4736 With/without tremelimumab versus standard of care (SOC) in recurrent/metastatic head and neck cancer (KESTREL) [Internet]. Available from: https://clinicaltrials.gov/ct2/show/NCT02551159.

197. Swanson MS, Sinha UK. Rationale for combined blockade of PD-1 and CTLA-4 in advanced head and neck squamous cell cancer—review of current data. Oral Oncol [Internet]. 2015;51(1):12–5. Available from: http://www.ncbi.nlm.nih.gov/pubmed/25459157.

198. Wang D, Fei B, Halig LV, Qin X, Hu Z, Xu H, et al. Targeted iron-oxide nanoparticle for photodynamic therapy and imaging of head and neck cancer. ACS Nano [Internet]. 2014;8(7):6620–32. Available from: http://www.ncbi.nlm.nih.gov/pubmed/24923902.

199. ClinicalTrials.gov U.S. National Library of Medicine. A phase 1, bioavailability study of relatlimab in combination with nivolumab [Internet]. Available from: https://clinicaltrials.gov/ct2/show/NCT04112498.

200. ClinicalTrials.gov U.S. National Library of Medicine. Study of safety and tolerability of nivolumab treatment alone or in combination with relatlimab or ipilimumab in head and neck cancer [Internet]. Available from: https://clinicaltrials.gov/ct2/show/NCT04080804.
201. Maruhashi T, Okazaki I-M, Sugiura D, Takahashi S, Maeda TK, Shimizu K, et al. LAG-3 inhibits the activation of CD4+ T cells that recognize stable pMHCII through its conformation-dependent recognition of pMHCII. Nat Immunol [Internet]. 2018;19(12):1415–26. Available from: http://www.ncbi.nlm.nih.gov/pubmed/30349037.
202. ClinicalTrials.gov U.S. National Library of Medicine. Study to assess MEDI4736 with either AZD9150 or AZD5069 in advanced solid tumors & relapsed metastatic squamous cell carcinoma of head & neck [Internet]. Available from: https://clinicaltrials.gov/ct2/show/NCT02499328.
203. Cohen EEW, Harrington KJ, Hong DS, Mesia R, Brana I, Perez Segura P, et al. A phase Ib/II study (SCORES) of durvalumab (D) plus danvatirsen (DAN; AZD9150) or AZD5069 (CX2i) in advanced solid malignancies and recurrent/metastatic head and neck squamous cell carcinoma (RM-HNSCC): Updated results. Ann Oncol [Internet]. 2018;29:viii372. Available from: https://linkinghub.elsevier.com/retrieve/pii/S092375341949501X.
204. Adachi M, Cui C, Dodge CT, Bhayani MK, Lai SY. Targeting STAT3 inhibits growth and enhances radiosensitivity in head and neck squamous cell carcinoma. Oral Oncol [Internet]. 2012;48(12):1220–6. Available from: http://www.ncbi.nlm.nih.gov/pubmed/22770899.
205. Chan L-P, Wang L-F, Chiang F-Y, Lee K-W, Kuo P-L, Liang C-H. IL-8 promotes HNSCC progression on CXCR1/2-meidated NOD1/RIP2 signaling pathway. Oncotarget [Internet]. 2016;7(38):61820–31. Available from: http://www.ncbi.nlm.nih.gov/pubmed/27557518.
206. Forster MD, Devlin M-J. Immune checkpoint inhibition in head and neck cancer. Front Oncol [Internet]. 2018;8:310. Available from: http://www.ncbi.nlm.nih.gov/pubmed/30211111.
207. ClinicalTrials.gov U.S, National Library of Medicine. A study of epacadostat + pembroli-zumab in head and neck cancer patients, who failed prior PD-1/PD-L1 therapy.
208. ClinicalTrials.gov U.S. National Library of Medicine. Pembrolizumab plus epacadostat, pembrolizumab monotherapy, and the EXTREME regimen in recurrent or metastatic head and neck squamous cell carcinoma (KEYNOTE-669/ECHO-304) [Internet]. Available from: https://clinicaltrials.gov/ct2/show/NCT03358472.
209. Colevas AD, Yom SS, Pfister DG, Spencer S, Adelstein D, Adkins D, et al. NCCN guide-lines insights: head and neck cancers, version 1.2018. J Natl Compr Canc Netw [Internet]. 2018;16(5):479–90. Available from: http://www.ncbi.nlm.nih.gov/pubmed/29752322.
210. Lubek JE. Head and neck cancer research and support foundations. Oral Maxillofac Surg Clin North Am [Internet]. 2018;30(4):459–69. Available from: http://www.ncbi.nlm.nih.gov/pubmed/30266190.
211. Khalil DN, Budhu S, Gasmi B, Zappasodi R, Hirschhorn-Cymerman D, Plitt T, et al. The new era of cancer immunotherapy: manipulating T-cell activity to overcome malignancy. Adv Cancer Res [Internet]. 2015;128:1–68. Available from: http://www.ncbi.nlm.nih.gov/pubmed/26216629.
212. Zitvogel L, Kroemer G. Targeting PD-1/PD-L1 interactions for cancer immunotherapy. Oncoimmunology [Internet]. 2012;1(8):1223–5. Available from: http://www.ncbi.nlm.nih.gov/pubmed/23243584.
213. Benci JL, Xu B, Qiu Y, Wu TJ, Dada H, Twyman-Saint Victor C, et al. Tumor interferon signaling regulates a multigenic resistance program to immune checkpoint blockade. Cell [Internet]. 2016;167(6):1540–1554.e12. Available from: http://www.ncbi.nlm.nih.gov/pubmed/27912061.
214. Leventakos K, Mansfield AS. Advances in the treatment of non-small cell lung cancer: focus on nivolumab, pembrolizumab, and atezolizumab. BioDrugs [Internet]. 2016;30(5):397–405. Available from: http://www.ncbi.nlm.nih.gov/pubmed/27411930.
215. Gong J, Chehrazi-Raffle A, Reddi S, Salgia R. Development of PD-1 and PD-L1 inhibitors as a form of cancer immunotherapy: a comprehensive review of registration trials and future

considerations. J Immunother Cancer [Internet]. 2018;6(1):8. Available from: http://www.ncbi.nlm.nih.gov/pubmed/29357948.

216. Ferris RL. Immunology and immunotherapy of head and neck cancer. J Clin Oncol [Internet]. 2015;33(29):3293–304. Available from: http://www.ncbi.nlm.nih.gov/pubmed/26351330.

217. Ling DC, Bakkenist CJ, Ferris RL, Clump DA. Role of immunotherapy in head and neck cancer. Semin Radiat Oncol [Internet]. 2018;28(1):12–6. Available from: http://www.ncbi.nlm.nih.gov/pubmed/29173750.

218. Sim F, Leidner R, Bell RB. Immunotherapy for head and neck cancer. Oral Maxillofac Surg Clin North Am [Internet]. 2019;31(1):85–100. Available from: http://www.ncbi.nlm.nih.gov/pubmed/30449528.

219. Allison JP. Immune checkpoint blockade in cancer therapy: The 2015 Lasker-DeBakey Clinical Medical Research Award. JAMA [Internet]. 2015;314(11):1113–4. Available from: http://www.ncbi.nlm.nih.gov/pubmed/26348357.

220. Kerr WG, Chisholm JD. The next generation of immunotherapy for cancer: small molecules could make Big Waves. J Immunol [Internet]. 2019;202(1):11–9. Available from: http://www.ncbi.nlm.nih.gov/pubmed/30587569.

221. Cristina V, Herrera-Gómez RG, Szturz P, Espeli V, Siano M. Immunotherapies and future combination strategies for head and neck squamous cell carcinoma. Int J Mol Sci [Internet]. 2019;20(21):5399. Available from: https://www.mdpi.com/1422-0067/20/21/5399.

222. Wolchok JD, Kluger H, Callahan MK, Postow MA, Rizvi NA, Lesokhin AM, et al. Nivolumab plus ipilimumab in advanced melanoma. N Engl J Med [Internet]. 2013;369(2):122–33. Available from: http://www.ncbi.nlm.nih.gov/pubmed/23724867

223. Ferris RL, Haddad R, Even C, Tahara M, Dvorkin M, Ciuleanu TE, et al. Durvalumab with or without tremelimumab in patients with recurrent or metastatic head and neck squamous cell carcinoma: EAGLE, a randomized, open-label phase III study. Ann Oncol Off J Eur Soc Med Oncol [Internet]. 2020;31(7):942–50. Available from: http://www.ncbi.nlm.nih.gov/pubmed/32294530.

224. ClinicalTrials.gov U.S. National Library of Medicine. Study of MEDI4736 Monotherapy and in Combination With Tremelimumab Versus Standard of Care Therapy in Patients With Head and Neck Cancer (EAGLE) [Internet]. Available from: https://clinicaltrials.gov/ct2/show/NCT02369874.

225. ClinicalTrials.gov U.S. National Library of Medicine. Study of Nivolumab in Combination With Ipilimumab Versus Nivolumab in Combination With Ipilimumab Placebo in Patients With Recurrent or Metastatic Squamous Cell Carcinoma of the Head and Neck (CheckMate 714) [Internet]. Available from: https://clinicaltrials.gov/ct2/show/NCT02823574.

226. ClinicalTrials.gov U.S. National Library of Medicine. Study of Nivolumab in Combination With Ipilimumab Compared to the Standard of Care (Extreme Regimen) as First Line Treatment in Patients With Recurrent or Metastatic Squamous Cell Carcinoma of the Head and Neck (CheckMate 651) [Internet]. Available from: https://clinicaltrials.gov/ct2/show/NCT02741570.

227. Cristina V, Herrera-Gómez RG, Szturz P, Espeli V, Siano M. Immunotherapies and Future Combination Strategies for Head and Neck Squamous Cell Carcinoma. Int J Mol Sci [Internet]. 2019;20(21):PMC6862353. Available from: http://www.ncbi.nlm.nih.gov/pubmed/31671550.

228. Kang J, Demaria S, Formenti S. Current clinical trials testing the combination of immunotherapy with radiotherapy. J Immunother cancer [Internet]. 2016;4:51. Available from: http://www.ncbi.nlm.nih.gov/pubmed/27660705.

229. Demaria S, Formenti SC. Can abscopal effects of local radiotherapy be predicted by modeling T cell trafficking? J Immunother cancer [Internet]. 2016;4:29. Available from: http://www.ncbi.nlm.nih.gov/pubmed/27190630.

230. Sharabi AB, Lim M, DeWeese TL, Drake CG. Radiation and checkpoint blockade immunotherapy: radiosensitisation and potential mechanisms of synergy. Lancet Oncol [Internet]. 2015;16(13):e498–509. Available from: http://www.ncbi.nlm.nih.gov/pubmed/26433823.

231. Demaria S, Kawashima N, Yang AM, Devitt ML, Babb JS, Allison JP, et al. Immune-mediated inhibition of metastases after treatment with local radiation and CTLA-4 blockade in a mouse model of breast cancer. Clin Cancer Res [Internet]. 2005;11(2 Pt 1):728–34. Available from: http://www.ncbi.nlm.nih.gov/pubmed/15701862.

232. Deng L, Liang H, Burnette B, Beckett M, Darga T, Weichselbaum RR, et al. Irradiation and anti-PD-L1 treatment synergistically promote antitumor immunity in mice. J Clin Invest [Internet]. 2014;124(2):687–95. Available from: http://www.ncbi.nlm.nih.gov/pubmed/24382348.

233. Sharabi AB, Nirschl CJ, Kochel CM, Nirschl TR, Francica BJ, Velarde E, et al. Stereotactic radiation therapy augments antigen-specific PD-1-mediated antitumor immune responses via cross-presentation of tumor antigen. Cancer Immunol Res [Internet]. 2015;3(4):345–55. Available from: http://www.ncbi.nlm.nih.gov/pubmed/25527358.

234. ClinicalTrials.gov U.S. National Library of Medicine. Targeting PD-1 therapy resistance with focused high or high and low dose radiation in SCCHN. Available from: https://clinicaltrials.gov/ct2/show/NCT03085719.

235. ClinicalTrials.gov U.S. National Library of Medicine. Pembrolizumab in combination with cisplatin and intensity modulated radiotherapy (IMRT) in head and neck cancer. Available from: https://clinicaltrials.gov/ct2/show/NCT02777385.

236. ClinicalTrials.gov U.S. National Library of Medicine. Phase II trial of adjuvant cisplatin and radiation with pembrolizumab in resected head and neck squamous cell carcinoma. Available from: https://clinicaltrials.gov/ct2/show/NCT02641093.

237. ClinicalTrials.gov U.S. National Library of Medicine. Study of pembrolizumab (MK-3475) or placebo with chemoradiation in participants with locally advanced head and neck squamous cell carcinoma (MK-3475-412/KEYNOTE-412) [Internet]. Available from: https://clinicaltrials.gov/ct2/show/NCT03040999.

238. ClinicalTrials.gov U.S. National Library of Medicine. Study to compare avelumab in combination with standard of care chemoradiotherapy (SoC CRT) versus SoC CRT for definitive treatment in patients with locally advanced squamous cell carcinoma of the head and neck (JAVELIN HEAD AND NECK 100) [Internet]. Available from: https://clinicaltrials.gov/ct2/show/NCT02952586.

239. Machiels J-P, Tao Y, Burtness B, Tahara M, Licitra L, Rischin D, et al. Pembrolizumab given concomitantly with chemoradiation and as maintenance therapy for locally advanced head and neck squamous cell carcinoma: KEYNOTE-412. Future Oncol [Internet]. 2020;16(18):1235–43. Available from: http://www.ncbi.nlm.nih.gov/pubmed/32490686.

240. Powell SF, Gitau MM, Sumey CJ, Reynolds JT, Lohr M, McGraw S, et al. Safety of pembrolizumab with chemoradiation (CRT) in locally advanced squamous cell carcinoma of the head and neck (LA-SCCHN). J Clin Oncol [Internet]. 2017;35(15_suppl):6011. Available from: http://ascopubs.org/doi/10.1200/JCO.2017.35.15_suppl.6011.

241. Machiels J-P, Tao Y, Burtness B, Tahara M, Licitra L, Rischin D, et al. Pembrolizumab given concomitantly with chemoradiation and as maintenance therapy for locally advanced head and neck squamous cell carcinoma: KEYNOTE-412. Futur Oncol [Internet]. 2020;16(18):1235–43. Available from: https://www.futuremedicine.com/doi/10.2217/fon-2020-0184.

242. ClinicalTrials.gov U.S. National Library of Medicine. Pembrolizumab in Combination With CRT for LA-SCCHN. Available from: https://clinicaltrials.gov/ct2/show/NCT02586207.

243. Maeda H, Tominaga K, Iwanaga K, Nagao F, Habu M, Tsujisawa T, et al. Targeted drug delivery system for oral cancer therapy using sonoporation. J Oral Pathol Med [Internet]. 2009;38(7):572–9. Available from: http://www.ncbi.nlm.nih.gov/pubmed/19549112.

244. Hirabayashi F, Iwanaga K, Okinaga T, Takahashi O, Ariyoshi W, Suzuki R, et al. Epidermal growth factor receptor-targeted sonoporation with microbubbles enhances therapeutic efficacy in a squamous cell carcinoma model. PLoS One [Internet]. 2017;12(9):e0185293. Available from: http://www.ncbi.nlm.nih.gov/pubmed/28938010.

245. Kerr WG, Chisholm JD. The next generation of immunotherapy for cancer: small molecules could make big waves. J Immunol [Internet]. 2019;202(1):11–9. Available from: http://www.jimmunol.org/lookup/doi/10.4049/jimmunol.1800991.

246. Zhu H-F, Li Y. Small-Molecule Targets in tumor Immunotherapy. Nat Products Bioprospect [Internet]. 2018;8(4):297–301. Available from: http://link.springer.com/10.1007/s13659-018-0177-7.

247. Adams JL, Smothers J, Srinivasan R, Hoos A. Big opportunities for small molecules in immuno-oncology. Nat Rev Drug Discov [Internet]. 2015;14(9):603–22. Available from: http://www.ncbi.nlm.nih.gov/pubmed/26228631.

248. Weinmann H. Cancer immunotherapy: selected targets and small-molecule modulators. ChemMedChem [Internet]. 2016; 11(5):450–66. Available from: http://www.ncbi.nlm.nih.gov/pubmed/26836578.

249. Skalniak L, Zak KM, Guzik K, Magiera K, Musielak B, Pachota M, et al. Small-molecule inhibitors of PD-1/PD-L1 immune checkpoint alleviate the PD-L1-induced exhaustion of T-cells. Oncotarget [Internet]. 2017;8(42):72167–81. Available from: http://www.ncbi.nlm.nih.gov/pubmed/29069777.

250. ClinicalTrials.gov U.S. National Library of Medicine. A study of CA-170 (Oral PD-L1, PD-L2 and VISTA checkpoint antagonist) in patients with advanced tumors and lymphomas [Internet]. Available from: https://clinicaltrials.gov/ct2/show/NCT02812875

251. Huck BR, Kötzner L, Urbahns K. Small molecules drive big improvements in immuno-oncology therapies. Angew Chemie Int Ed [Internet]. 2018;57(16):4412–28. Available from: http://doi.wiley.com/10.1002/anie.201707816.

252. ClinicalTrials.gov U.S. National Library of Medicine. Topical or ablative treatment in preventing anal cancer in patients with HIV and Anal High-Grade Squamous Intraepithelial Lesions (ANCHOR) [Internet]. Available from: https://clinicaltrials.gov/ct2/show/NCT02135419.

253. ClinicalTrials.gov U.S. National Library of Medicine. Imiquimod, Fluorouracil, or Observation in Treating HIV-Positive Patients With High-Grade Anal Squamous Skin Lesions [Internet]. Available from: https://clinicaltrials.gov/ct2/show/NCT02059499.

254. ClinicalTrials.gov U.S. National Library of Medicine. Imiquimod and Pembrolizumab in Treating Patients With Stage IIIB-IV Melanoma [Internet]. Available from: https://clinicaltrials.gov/ct2/show/NCT03276832.

255. Bubna AK. Imiquimod - its role in the treatment of cutaneous malignancies. Indian J Pharmacol [Internet]. 2015;47(4):354–9. Available from: http://www.ncbi.nlm.nih.gov/pubmed/26288465.

256. ClinicalTrials.gov U.S. National Library of Medicine. Topical Resiquimod for the Treatment of Early Stage Cutaneous T Cell Lymphoma (CTCL) [Internet]. Available from: https://clinicaltrials.gov/ct2/show/NCT01676831.

257. ClinicalTrials.gov U.S. National Library of Medicine. Study of Immune Response Modifier in the Treatment of Hematologic Malignancies [Internet]. Available from: https://clinicaltrials.gov/ct2/show/NCT00276159.

258. ClinicalTrials.gov U.S. National Library of Medicine. Chemotherapy Plus Cetuximab in Combination With VTX-2337 in Patients With Recurrent or Metastatic Squamous Cell Carcinoma of the Head and Neck [Internet]. Available from: https://clinicaltrials.gov/ct2/show/NCT01836029.

259. ClinicalTrials.gov U.S. National Library of Medicine. Safety and Efficacy of MIW815 (ADU-S100) +/− Ipilimumab in Patients With Advanced/Metastatic Solid Tumors or Lymphomas [Internet]. Available from: https://clinicaltrials.gov/ct2/show/NCT02675439.

260. Weiss JM, Guérin M V, Regnier F, Renault G, Galy-Fauroux I, Vimeux L, et al. The STING agonist DMXAA triggers a cooperation between T lymphocytes and myeloid cells that leads to tumor regression. Oncoimmunology [Internet]. 2017;6(10):e1346765. Available from: http://www.ncbi.nlm.nih.gov/pubmed/29123960.

261. Sanchez Alberti A, Bivona AE, Cerny N, Schulze K, Weißmann S, Ebensen T, et al. Engineered trivalent immunogen adjuvanted with a STING agonist confers protection against

Trypanosoma cruzi infection. NPJ vaccines [Internet]. 2017;2:9. Available from: http://www. ncbi.nlm.nih.gov/pubmed/29263868.

262. ClinicalTrials.gov U.S. National Library of Medicine. Study of MK-1454 Alone or in Combination With Pembrolizumab (MK-3475) in Participants With Advanced/Metastatic Solid Tumors or Lymphomas (MK-1454-001) [Internet]. Available from: https://clinicaltrials.gov/ct2/show/NCT03010176.

263. Shi X, Song S, Ding Z, Fan B, Xu T, Huang W. Improving the Solubility and Dissolution of Ibrutinib by Preparing Solvates. J Pharm Innov [Internet]. 2019 Aug 27; Available from: http://link.springer.com/10.1007/s12247-019-09402-7.

264. Kim ES, Dhillon S. Ibrutinib: a review of its use in patients with mantle cell lymphoma or chronic lymphocytic leukaemia. Drugs [Internet]. 2015;75(7):769–76. Available from: http://link.springer.com/10.1007/s40265-015-0380-3.

265. Allegra A, Pioggia G, Tonacci A, Musolino C, Gangemi S. Cancer and SARS-CoV-2 infection: diagnostic and therapeutic challenges. cancers (Basel) [Internet]. 2020; 12(6):1581. Available from: https://www.mdpi.com/2072-6694/12/6/1581.

266. Treon SP, Castillo JJ, Skarbnik AP, Soumerai JD, Ghobrial IM, Guerrera ML, et al. The BTK inhibitor ibrutinib may protect against pulmonary injury in COVID-19–infected patients. Blood [Internet]. 2020;135(21):1912–5. Available from: https://ashpublications.org/blood/article/135/21/1912/454437/The-BTK-inhibitor-ibrutinib-may-protect-against.

267. Viernes DR, Choi LB, Kerr WG, Chisholm JD. Discovery and development of small molecule SHIP phosphatase modulators. Med Res Rev [Internet]. 2014;34(4):795–824. Available from: http://www.ncbi.nlm.nih.gov/pubmed/24302498.

268. Brooks R, Fuhler GM, Iyer S, Smith MJ, Park M-Y, Paraiso KHT, et al. SHIP1 inhibition increases immunoregulatory capacity and triggers apoptosis of hematopoietic cancer cells. J Immunol [Internet]. 2010;184(7):3582–9. Available from: http://www.ncbi.nlm.nih.gov/pubmed/20200281.

269. Kong D, Zhang Z. PI3K/AKT Inhibitors as Sensitizing Agents for Cancer Chemotherapy. In: Protein Kinase Inhibitors as Sensitizing Agents for Chemotherapy [Internet]. Elsevier; 2019. p. 187–205.. Available from: https://linkinghub.elsevier.com/retrieve/pii/B9780128164358000122.

270. Awan FT, Kharfan-Dabaja MA. Hematopoietic Cell Transplantation for Chronic Lymphocytic Leukemia. In: Hematopoietic Cell Transplantation for Malignant Conditions [Internet]. Elsevier; 2019. p. 185–190.. Available from: https://linkinghub.elsevier.com/retrieve/pii/B9780323568029000122.

271. Cheah CY, Fowler NH. Idelalisib in the management of lymphoma. Blood [Internet]. 2016;128(3):331–6. Available from: https://ashpublications.org/blood/article/128/3/331/35546/Idelalisib-in-the-management-of-lymphoma.

272. ClinicalTrials.gov U.S. National Library of Medicine. A Dose-Escalation Study to Evaluate the Safety, Tolerability, Pharmacokinetics, and Pharmacodynamics of IPI-549 [Internet]. Available from: https://clinicaltrials.gov/ct2/show/NCT02637531.

273. ClinicalTrials.gov U.S. National Library of Medicine. A Study to Assess Pharmacokinetics of Preladenant in Participants With Chronic Hepatic Impairment (P06513). Available from: https://clinicaltrials.gov/ct2/show/NCT01465412.

274. Pinna A. Adenosine A2A receptor antagonists in Parkinson's disease: progress in clinical trials from the newly approved istradefylline to drugs in early development and those already discontinued. CNS Drugs [Internet]. 2014;28(5):455–74. Available from: http://www.ncbi.nlm.nih.gov/pubmed/24687255.

275. Shin S-H, Park M-H, Byeon J-J, Lee B, Park Y, Kim N, et al. Analysis of vipadenant and its in vitro and in vivo Metabolites via liquid chromatography-quadrupole-time-of-flight mass spectrometry. Pharmaceutics [Internet]. 2018;10(4):260.. Available from: http://www.mdpi.com/1999-4923/10/4/260.

276. ClinicalTrials.gov U.S. National Library of Medicine. A Study to Assess Pharmacokinetics of Preladenant in Participants With Chronic Hepatic Impairment (P06513) [Internet]. Available from: https://clinicaltrials.gov/ct2/show/NCT01465412.

277. ClinicalTrials.gov U.S. National Library of Medicine. Study of Preladenant (MK-3814) Alone and With Pembrolizumab (MK-3475) in Participants With Advanced Solid Tumors (MK-3814A-062) [Internet]. Available from: https://clinicaltrials.gov/ct2/show/NCT03099161.

278. ClinicalTrials.gov U.S. National Library of Medicine. Oleclumab (MEDI9447) EGFRm NSCLC Novel Combination Study [Internet]. Available from: https://clinicaltrials.gov/ct2/show/NCT03381274.

279. Yingling JM, McMillen WT, Yan L, Huang H, Sawyer JS, Graff J, et al. Preclinical assessment of galunisertib (LY2157299 monohydrate), a first-in-class transforming growth factor-β receptor type I inhibitor. Oncotarget [Internet]. 2018;9(6):6659–77. Available from: http://www.ncbi.nlm.nih.gov/pubmed/29467918.

280. ClinicalTrials.gov U.S. National Library of Medicine. A Dose-finding Study of MK-8628 in Participants With Recurrent Glioblastoma Multiforme (MK-8628-002) [Internet]. Available from: https://clinicaltrials.gov/ct2/show/NCT02296476.

281. ClinicalTrials.gov U.S. National Library of Medicine. Study of CPI-0610 in Patients With Malignant Peripheral Nerve Sheath Tumors [Internet]. Available from: https://clinicaltrials.gov/ct2/show/NCT02986919.

282. ClinicalTrials.gov U.S. National Library of Medicine. Study of IDO Inhibitor and Temozolomide for Adult Patients With Primary Malignant Brain Tumors [Internet]. Available from: https://clinicaltrials.gov/ct2/show/NCT02052648.

283. ClinicalTrials.gov U.S. National Library of Medicine. Pediatric Trial of Indoximod With Chemotherapy and Radiation for Relapsed Brain Tumors or Newly Diagnosed DIPG [Internet]. Available from: https://clinicaltrials.gov/ct2/show/NCT04049669.

284. ClinicalTrials.gov U.S. National Library of Medicine. 1-Methyl-D-Tryptophan and Docetaxel in Treating Patients With Metastatic Solid Tumors [Internet]. Available from: https://clinicaltrials.gov/ct2/show/NCT01191216.

285. ClinicalTrials.gov U.S. National Library of Medicine. Study of the IDO Pathway Inhibitor, Indoximod, and Temozolomide for Pediatric Patients With Progressive Primary Malignant Brain Tumors [Internet]. Available from: https://clinicaltrials.gov/ct2/show/NCT02502708.

286. Opitz CA, Litzenburger UM, Opitz U, Sahm F, Ochs K, Lutz C, et al. The indoleamine-2,3-dioxygenase (IDO) inhibitor 1-methyl-D-tryptophan upregulates IDO1 in human cancer cells. PLoS One [Internet]. 2011;6(5):e19823. Available from: http://www.ncbi.nlm.nih.gov/pubmed/21625531.

287. ClinicalTrials.gov U.S. National Library of Medicine. Study of IDO Inhibitor in Combination With Checkpoint Inhibitors for Adult Patients With Metastatic Melanoma [Internet]. Available from: https://clinicaltrials.gov/ct2/show/NCT02073123.

288. Yue EW, Sparks R, Polam P, Modi D, Douty B, Wayland B, et al. INCB24360 (Epacadostat), a highly potent and selective indoleamine-2,3-dioxygenase 1 (IDO1) inhibitor for immuno-oncology. ACS Med Chem Lett [Internet]. 2017;8(5):486–91. Available from: https://pubs.acs.org/doi/10.1021/acsmedchemlett.6b00391.

289. Röhrig UF, Reynaud A, Majjigapu SR, Vogel P, Pojer F, Zoete V. Inhibition mechanisms of indoleamine 2,3-dioxygenase 1 (IDO1). J Med Chem [Internet]. 2019;62(19):8784–95. Available from: http://www.ncbi.nlm.nih.gov/pubmed/31525930.

290. Röhrig UF, Zoete V, Michielin O. The binding mode of N-hydroxyamidines to indoleamine 2,3-dioxygenase 1 (IDO1). biochemistry [Internet]. 2017;56(33):4323–5. Available from: http://www.ncbi.nlm.nih.gov/pubmed/28731684.

291. ClinicalTrials.gov U.S. National Library of Medicine. A Study of GDC-0919 and Atezolizumab Combination Treatment in Participants With Locally Advanced or Metastatic Solid Tumors [Internet]. Available from: https://clinicaltrials.gov/ct2/show/NCT02471846.

292. ClinicalTrials.gov U.S. National Library of Medicine. Indoleamine 2,3-Dioxygenase (IDO) Inhibitor in Advanced Solid Tumors. Available from: https://clinicaltrials.gov/ct2/show/NCT02048709.

293. Nayak-Kapoor A, Hao Z, Sadek R, Dobbins R, Marshall L, Vahanian NN, et al. Phase Ia study of the indoleamine 2,3-dioxygenase 1 (IDO1) inhibitor navoximod (GDC-0919) in patients with recurrent advanced solid tumors. J Immunother Cancer [Internet]. 2018 ;6(1):61. Available from: http://jitc.bmj.com/lookup/doi/10.1186/s40425-018-0351-9.

294. ClinicalTrials.gov U.S. National Library of Medicine. A Study of Chemo Only Versus Chemo Plus Nivo With or Without BMS-986205, Followed by Post- Surgery Therapy With Nivo or Nivo and BMS-986205 in Patients With MIBC [Internet]. Available from: https://clinicaltrials.gov/ct2/show/NCT03661320.

295. Crosignani S, Bingham P, Bottemanne P, Cannelle H, Cauwenberghs S, Cordonnier M, et al. Discovery of a novel and selective Indoleamine 2,3-dioxygenase (IDO-1) inhibitor 3-(5-Fluoro-1H-indol-3-yl)pyrrolidine-2,5-dione (EOS200271/PF-06840003) and its characterization as a potential Clinical candidate. J Med Chem [Internet]. 2017;60(23):9617–29. Available from: http://www.ncbi.nlm.nih.gov/pubmed/29111717.

296. Gomes B, Driessens G, Bartlett D, Cai D, Cauwenberghs S, Crosignani S, et al. Characterization of the selective Indoleamine 2,3-Dioxygenase-1 (IDO1) catalytic inhibitor EOS200271/PF-06840003 supports IDO1 as a critical resistance mechanism to PD-(L)1 Blockade Therapy. Mol Cancer Ther [Internet]. 2018;17(12):2530–42. Available from: http://www.ncbi.nlm.nih.gov/pubmed/30232146.

297. Karavasili C, Andreadis DA, Katsamenis OL, Panteris E, Anastasiadou P, Kakazanis Z, et al. Synergistic antitumor potency of a self-assembling peptide hydrogel for the local co-delivery of doxorubicin and curcumin in the treatment of head and neck cancer. Mol Pharm [Internet]. 2019;16(6):2326–41. Available from: http://www.ncbi.nlm.nih.gov/pubmed/31026168.

298. Chidambaram M, Manavalan R, Kathiresan K. Nanotherapeutics to overcome conventional cancer chemotherapy limitations. J Pharm Pharm Sci [Internet]. 2011;14(1):67. Available from: https://journals.library.ualberta.ca/jpps/index.php/JPPS/article/view/9199.

299. Pridgen EM, Alexis F, Farokhzad OC. Polymeric nanoparticle drug delivery technologies for oral delivery applications. Expert Opin Drug Deliv [Internet]. 2015;12(9):1459–73. Available from: http://www.tandfonline.com/doi/full/10.1517/17425247.2015.1018175.

300. Pignon J-P, le Maître A, Maillard E, Bourhis J, MACH-NC Collaborative Group. Meta-analysis of chemotherapy in head and neck cancer (MACH-NC): an update on 93 randomised trials and 17,346 patients. Radiother Oncol [Internet]. 2009;92(1):4–14. Available from: http://www.ncbi.nlm.nih.gov/pubmed/19446902.

301. Hanemaaijer SH, Kok IC, Fehrmann RSN, van der Vegt B, Gietema JA, Plaat BEC, et al. Comparison of carboplatin with 5-fluorouracil vs. cisplatin as concomitant chemoradiotherapy for locally advanced head and neck squamous cell carcinoma. Front Oncol [Internet]. 2020;10:761. Available from: http://www.ncbi.nlm.nih.gov/pubmed/32582534.

302. Puyo S, Montaudon D, Pourquier P. From old alkylating agents to new minor groove binders. Crit Rev Oncol Hematol [Internet]. 2014;89(1):43–61. Available from: https://linkinghub.elsevier.com/retrieve/pii/S1040842813001571.

303. Dasari S, Bernard Tchounwou P. Cisplatin in cancer therapy: molecular mechanisms of action. Eur J Pharmacol [Internet] 2014;740:364–378. Available from: https://linkinghub.elsevier.com/retrieve/pii/S0014299914005627.

304. Wang Z-Q, Liu K, Huo Z-J, Li X-C, Wang M, Liu P, et al. A cell-targeted chemotherapeutic nanomedicine strategy for oral squamous cell carcinoma therapy. J Nanobiotechnology [Internet]. 2015;13(1):63. Available from: http://www.jnanobiotechnology.com/content/13/1/63.

305. Specenier P, Vermorken JB. Cetuximab in the treatment of squamous cell carcinoma of the head and neck. Expert Rev Anticancer Ther [Internet]. 2011 Apr;11(4):511–24. Available from: http://www.ncbi.nlm.nih.gov/pubmed/21504318.

306. Specenier P, Vermorken JB. Biologic therapy in head and neck cancer: a road with hurdles. ISRN Oncol [Internet]. 2012;2012:163752. Available from: http://www.ncbi.nlm.nih.gov/pubmed/22745915.

307. Caster JM, Patel AN, Zhang T, Wang A. Investigational nanomedicines in 2016: a review of nanotherapeutics currently undergoing clinical trials. Wiley Interdiscip Rev Nanomedicine Nanobiotechnology [Internet]. 2017;9(1):e1416. Available from: http://doi.wiley.com/10.1002/wnan.1416.

308. Brannon-Peppas L, Blanchette JO. Nanoparticle and targeted systems for cancer therapy. Adv Drug Deliv Rev [Internet]. 2012;64:206–12. Available from: https://linkinghub.elsevier.com/retrieve/pii/S0169409X12002931.

309. Uchino H, Matsumura Y, Negishi T, Koizumi F, Hayashi T, Honda T, et al. Cisplatin-incorporating polymeric micelles (NC-6004) can reduce nephrotoxicity and neurotoxicity of cisplatin in rats. Br J Cancer [Internet]. 2005;93(6):678–87. Available from: http://www.ncbi.nlm.nih.gov/pubmed/16222314.

310. Endo K, Ueno T, Kondo S, Wakisaka N, Murono S, Ito M, et al. Tumor-targeted chemotherapy with the nanopolymer-based drug NC-6004 for oral squamous cell carcinoma. Cancer Sci [Internet]. 2013;104(3):369–74. Available from: http://doi.wiley.com/10.1111/cas.12079.

311. Desai KGH. Polymeric drug delivery systems for intraoral site-specific chemoprevention of oral cancer. J Biomed Mater Res Part B Appl Biomater [Internet]. 2018;106(3):1383–413. Available from: https://onlinelibrary.wiley.com/doi/abs/10.1002/jbm.b.33943

312. Mazzarino L, Travelet C, Ortega-Murillo S, Otsuka I, Pignot-Paintrand I, Lemos-Senna E, et al. Elaboration of chitosan-coated nanoparticles loaded with curcumin for mucoadhesive applications. J Colloid Interface Sci [Internet]. 2012;370(1):58–66. Available from: http://www.ncbi.nlm.nih.gov/pubmed/22284577.

313. Mazzarino L, Loch-Neckel G, Bubniak LDS, Mazzucco S, Santos-Silva MC, Borsali R, et al. Curcumin-loaded chitosan-coated nanoparticles as a new approach for the local treatment of oral cavity cancer. J Nanosci Nanotechnol [Internet]. 2015;15(1):781–91. Available from: http://www.ncbi.nlm.nih.gov/pubmed/26328442.

314. Khosa A, Reddi S, Saha RN. Nanostructured lipid carriers for site-specific drug delivery. Biomed Pharmacother [Internet]. 2018;103:598–613. Available from: https://linkinghub.elsevier.com/retrieve/pii/S0753332218313222.

315. Arulmozhi V, Pandian K, Mirunalini S. Ellagic acid encapsulated chitosan nanoparticles for drug delivery system in human oral cancer cell line (KB). Colloids Surf B Biointerfaces [Internet]. 2013;110:313–20. Available from: http://www.ncbi.nlm.nih.gov/pubmed/23732810.

316. Hoshyar N, Gray S, Han H, Bao G. The effect of nanoparticle size on in vivo pharmacokinetics and cellular interaction. Nanomedicine (Lond) [Internet]. 2016;11(6):673–92. Available from: http://www.ncbi.nlm.nih.gov/pubmed/27003448.

317. Kulkarni SA, Feng S-S. Effects of particle size and surface modification on cellular uptake and biodistribution of polymeric nanoparticles for drug delivery. Pharm Res [Internet]. 2013;30(10):2512–22. Available from: http://www.ncbi.nlm.nih.gov/pubmed/23314933.

318. Rizvi SAA, Saleh AM. Applications of nanoparticle systems in drug delivery technology. Saudi Pharm J SPJ Off Publ Saudi Pharm Soc [Internet]. 2018;26(1):64–70. Available from: http://www.ncbi.nlm.nih.gov/pubmed/29379334.

319. Sim RB, Wallis R. Surface properties: Immune attack on nanoparticles. Nat Nanotechnol [Internet]. 2011;6(2):80–1. Available from: http://www.ncbi.nlm.nih.gov/pubmed/21293484.

320. Lee SJ, Morrill AR, Moskovits M. Hot spots in silver nanowire bundles for surface-enhanced Raman spectroscopy. J Am Chem Soc [Internet]. 2006;128(7):2200–1. Available from: http://www.ncbi.nlm.nih.gov/pubmed/16478159.

321. Lee S, Jun B-H. Silver nanoparticles: synthesis and application for nanomedicine. Int J Mol Sci [Internet]. 2019;20(4):865. Available from: http://www.mdpi.com/1422-0067/20/4/865.

322. Doering WE, Piotti ME, Natan MJ, Freeman RG. SERS as a foundation for nanoscale, optically detected biological labels. Adv Mater [Internet]. 2007;19(20):3100–8. Available from: http://doi.wiley.com/10.1002/adma.200701984.
323. Schlinkert P, Casals E, Boyles M, Tischler U, Hornig E, Tran N, et al. The oxidative potential of differently charged silver and gold nanoparticles on three human lung epithelial cell types. J Nanobiotechnology [Internet]. 2015;13:1. Available from: http://www.ncbi.nlm.nih.gov/pubmed/25592092.
324. Thapa RK, Kim JH, Jeong J-H, Shin BS, Choi H-G, Yong CS, et al. Silver nanoparticle-embedded graphene oxide-methotrexate for targeted cancer treatment. Colloids Surf B Biointerfaces [Internet]. 2017;153:95–103. Available from:. http://www.ncbi.nlm.nih.gov/pubmed/28231500.
325. Suresh AK, Pelletier DA, Wang W, Morrell-Falvey JL, Gu B, Doktycz MJ. Cytotoxicity induced by engineered silver nanocrystallites is dependent on surface coatings and cell types. Langmuir [Internet]. 2012;28(5):2727–35. Available from: http://www.ncbi.nlm.nih.gov/pubmed/22216981.
326. Gurunathan S, Lee K-J, Kalishwaralal K, Sheikpranbabu S, Vaidyanathan R, Eom SH. Antiangiogenic properties of silver nanoparticles. Biomaterials [Internet]. 2009;30(31):6341–50. Available from: http://www.ncbi.nlm.nih.gov/pubmed/19698986.
327. Asharani P V, Hande MP, Valiyaveettil S. Anti-proliferative activity of silver nanoparticles. BMC Cell Biol [Internet]. 2009;10:65. Available from: http://www.ncbi.nlm.nih.gov/pubmed/19761582.
328. Satapathy SR, Siddharth S, Das D, Nayak A, Kundu CN. Enhancement of cytotoxicity and inhibition of angiogenesis in oral cancer stem cells by a hybrid nanoparticle of bioactive quinacrine and silver: implication of base excision repair cascade. Mol Pharm [Internet]. 2015;12(11):4011–25. Available from: http://www.ncbi.nlm.nih.gov/pubmed/26448277.
329. Kneipp J, Kneipp H, McLaughlin M, Brown D, Kneipp K. In vivo molecular probing of cellular compartments with gold nanoparticles and nanoaggregates. Nano Lett [Internet]. 2006;6(10):2225–31. Available from: http://www.ncbi.nlm.nih.gov/pubmed/17034088.
330. Sztandera K, Gorzkiewicz M, Klajnert-Maculewicz B. Gold nanoparticles in cancer treatment. Mol Pharm [Internet]. 2019;16(1):1–23. Available from: https://pubs.acs.org/doi/10.1021/acs.molpharmaceut.8b00810.
331. Elsayed I, Huang X, Elsayed M. Selective laser photo-thermal therapy of epithelial carcinoma using anti-EGFR antibody conjugated gold nanoparticles. Cancer Lett [Internet]. 2006;239(1):129–35. Available from: https://linkinghub.elsevier.com/retrieve/pii/S0304383505007378.
332. Lucky SS, Idris NM, Huang K, Kim J, Li Z, Thong PSP, et al. In vivo biocompatibility, biodistribution and therapeutic efficiency of titania coated upconversion nanoparticles for photodynamic therapy of solid oral cancers. Theranostics [Internet]. 2016;6(11):1844–65. Available from: http://www.ncbi.nlm.nih.gov/pubmed/27570555.
333. Marcazzan S, Varoni EM, Blanco E, Lodi G, Ferrari M. Nanomedicine, an emerging therapeutic strategy for oral cancer therapy. Oral Oncol [Internet]. 2018;76:1–7. Available from: https://linkinghub.elsevier.com/retrieve/pii/S1368837517303652.
334. Sato I, Umemura M, Mitsudo K, Fukumura H, Kim J-H, Hoshino Y, et al. Simultaneous hyperthermia-chemotherapy with controlled drug delivery using single-drug nanoparticles. Sci Rep [Internet]. 2016;6(1):24629. Available from: http://www.nature.com/articles/srep24629
335. Eguchi H, Umemura M, Kurotani R, Fukumura H, Sato I, Kim J-H, et al. A magnetic anti-cancer compound for magnet-guided delivery and magnetic resonance imaging. Sci Rep [Internet]. 2015;5:9194. Available from: http://www.ncbi.nlm.nih.gov/pubmed/25779357.
336. Wang D, Xu X, Zhang K, Sun B, Wang L, Meng L, et al. Codelivery of doxorubicin and MDR1-siRNA by mesoporous silica nanoparticles-polymerpolyethylenimine to improve oral squamous carcinoma treatment. Int J Nanomedicine [Internet]. 2018;13:187–98. Available from: http://www.ncbi.nlm.nih.gov/pubmed/29343957.

337. Shi X-L, Li Y, Zhao L-M, Su L-W, Ding G. Delivery of MTH1 inhibitor (TH287) and MDR1 siRNA via hyaluronic acid-based mesoporous silica nanoparticles for oral cancers treatment. Colloids Surf B Biointerfaces [Internet]. 2019;173:599–606. Available from: http://www.ncbi.nlm.nih.gov/pubmed/30352381.

338. Huang H-C, Barua S, Sharma G, Dey SK, Rege K. Inorganic nanoparticles for cancer imaging and therapy. J Control Release [Internet]. 2011;155(3):344–57. Available from: http://www.ncbi.nlm.nih.gov/pubmed/21723891.

339. Sato I, Umemura M, Mitsudo K, Fukumura H, Kim J-H, Hoshino Y, et al. Simultaneous hyperthermia-chemotherapy with controlled drug delivery using single-drug nanoparticles. Sci Rep [Internet]. 2016;6:24629. Available from: http://www.ncbi.nlm.nih.gov/pubmed/27103308.

340. Sah AK, Vyas A, Suresh PK, Gidwani B. Application of nanocarrier-based drug delivery system in treatment of oral cancer. Artif cells, nanomedicine, Biotechnol [Internet]. 2018;46(4):650–7. Available from: http://www.ncbi.nlm.nih.gov/pubmed/28880679.

341. Cavalli R, Soster M, Argenziano M. Nanobubbles: a promising efficienft tool for therapeutic delivery. Ther Deliv [Internet]. 2016;7(2):117–38. Available from: http://www.future-science.com/doi/10.4155/tde.15.92.

342. Fang C-L, Al-Suwayeh S, Fang J-Y. Nanostructured Lipid Carriers (NLCs) for drug delivery and targeting. Recent Pat Nanotechnol [Internet]. 2013;7(1):41–55. Available from: http://openurl.ingenta.com/content/xref?genre=article&issn=1872-2105&volume=7&issue=1&spage=41.

343. Zlotogorski A, Dayan A, Dayan D, Chaushu G, Salo T, Vered M. Nutraceuticals as new treatment approaches for oral cancer – I: Curcumin. Oral Oncol [Internet]. 2013;49(3):187–91. Available from: https://linkinghub.elsevier.com/retrieve/pii/S1368837512003181.

344. Beloqui A, Solinís MÁ, Rodríguez-Gascón A, Almeida AJ, Préat V. Nanostructured lipid carriers: Promising drug delivery systems for future clinics. Nanomedicine [Internet]. 2016;12(1):143–61. Available from: http://www.ncbi.nlm.nih.gov/pubmed/26410277.

345. Ghasemiyeh P, Mohammadi-Samani S. Solid lipid nanoparticles and nanostructured lipid carriers as novel drug delivery systems: applications, advantages and disadvantages. Res Pharm Sci [Internet]. 2018;13(4):288–303. Available from: http://www.ncbi.nlm.nih.gov/pubmed/30065762.

346. Sun M, Su X, Ding B, He X, Liu X, Yu A, et al. Advances in nanotechnology-based delivery systems for curcumin. Nanomedicine (Lond) [Internet]. 2012;7(7):1085–100. Available from: http://www.ncbi.nlm.nih.gov/pubmed/22846093.

347. Koutsopoulos S, Unsworth LD, Nagai Y, Zhang S. Controlled release of functional proteins through designer self-assembling peptide nanofiber hydrogel scaffold. Proc Natl Acad Sci U S A [Internet]. 2009;106(12):4623–8. Available from: http://www.ncbi.nlm.nih.gov/pubmed/19273853.

348. Karavasili C, Panteris E, Vizirianakis IS, Koutsopoulos S, Fatouros DG. Chemotherapeutic delivery from a self-assembling peptide nanofiber hydrogel for the management of glioblastoma. Pharm Res [Internet]. 2018;35(8):166. Available from: http://link.springer.com/10.1007/s11095-018-2442-1.

349. Sepantafar M, Maheronnaghsh R, Mohammadi H, Radmanesh F, Hasani-sadrabadi MM, Ebrahimi M, et al. Engineered hydrogels in cancer therapy and diagnosis. Trends Biotechnol [Internet]. 2017;35(11):1074–87. Available from: https://linkinghub.elsevier.com/retrieve/pii/S0167779917301646.

350. Coelho JF, Ferreira PC, Alves P, Cordeiro R, Fonseca AC, Góis JR, et al. Drug delivery systems: Advanced technologies potentially applicable in personalized treatments. EPMA J [Internet]. 2010;1(1):164–209. Available from: http://www.ncbi.nlm.nih.gov/pubmed/23199049.

351. Narayanaswamy R, Torchilin VP. Hydrogels and their applications in targeted drug delivery. Molecules [Internet]. 2019;24(3):603. Available from: http://www.mdpi.com/1420-3049/24/3/603.

352. Tian Y, Li S, Song J, Ji T, Zhu M, Anderson GJ, et al. A doxorubicin delivery platform using engineered natural membrane vesicle exosomes for targeted tumor therapy. Biomaterials [Internet]. 2014;35(7):2383–90. Available from: https://linkinghub.elsevier.com/retrieve/pii/S014296121301449X.

353. Batrakova E V, Kim MS. Using exosomes, naturally-equipped nanocarriers, for drug delivery. J Control Release [Internet]. 2015;219:396–405. Available from: http://www.ncbi.nlm.nih.gov/pubmed/26241750.

354. Bunggulawa EJ, Wang W, Yin T, Wang N, Durkan C, Wang Y, et al. Recent advancements in the use of exosomes as drug delivery systems. J Nanobiotechnology [Internet]. 2018 16(1):81. Available from: https://jnanobiotechnology.biomedcentral.com/articles/10.1186/s12951-018-0403-9.

355. Jiang X-C, Gao J-Q. Exosomes as novel bio-carriers for gene and drug delivery. Int J Pharm [Internet]. 2017;521(1–2):167–75. Available from: http://www.ncbi.nlm.nih.gov/pubmed/28216464.

356. Dehari H, Ito Y, Nakamura T, Kobune M, Sasaki K, Yonekura N, et al. Enhanced antitumor effect of RGD fiber-modified adenovirus for gene therapy of oral cancer. Cancer Gene Ther [Internet]. 2003;10(1):75–85. Available from: http://www.ncbi.nlm.nih.gov/pubmed/12489031.

357. Ha D, Yang N, Nadithe V. Exosomes as therapeutic drug carriers and delivery vehicles across biological membranes: current perspectives and future challenges. Acta Pharm Sin B [Internet]. 2016;6(4):287–96. Available from: http://www.ncbi.nlm.nih.gov/pubmed/27471669.

358. Suliman Y AO, Ali D, Alarifi S, Harrath AH, Mansour L, Alwasel SH. Evaluation of cytotoxic, oxidative stress, proinflammatory and genotoxic effect of silver nanoparticles in human lung epithelial cells. Environ Toxicol [Internet]. 2015;30(2):149–60. Available from:. http://www.ncbi.nlm.nih.gov/pubmed/23804405.

359. Ferris RL, Blumenschein G, Fayette J, Guigay J, Colevas AD, Licitra L, et al. Nivolumab for recurrent squamous-cell carcinoma of the head and neck. N Engl J Med [Internet]. 2016;375(19):1856–67. Available from: http://www.ncbi.nlm.nih.gov/pubmed/27718784.

360. Bertrand A, Kostine M, Barnetche T, Truchetet M-E, Schaeverbeke T. Immune related adverse events associated with anti-CTLA-4 antibodies: systematic review and meta-analysis. BMC Med [Internet]. 2015 ;13:211. Available from: http://www.ncbi.nlm.nih.gov/pubmed/26337719.

361. Panyam J, Labhasetwar V. Biodegradable nanoparticles for drug and gene delivery to cells and tissue. Adv Drug Deliv Rev [Internet]. 2003;55(3):329–47. Available from:. http://www.ncbi.nlm.nih.gov/pubmed/12628320.

362. Charrueau C, Zandanel C. Drug delivery by polymer nanoparticles: the challenge of controlled release and evaluation. In: Polymer nanoparticles for nanomedicines [Internet]. Cham: Springer International Publishing; 2016. p. 439–503. Available from: http://link.springer.com/10.1007/978-3-319-41421-8_14.

363. Wu L, Zhang J, Watanabe W. Physical and chemical stability of drug nanoparticles. Adv Drug Deliv Rev [Internet]. 2011;63(6):456–69. Available from: https://linkinghub.elsevier.com/retrieve/pii/S0169409X11000172.

364. Elsabahy M, Heo GS, Lim S-M, Sun G, Wooley KL. Polymeric nanostructures for imaging and therapy. chem rev [Internet]. 2015;115(19):10967–1011. Available from: http://www.ncbi.nlm.nih.gov/pubmed/26463640.

365. Metselaar JM, Lammers T. Challenges in nanomedicine clinical translation. Drug Deliv Transl Res [Internet]. 2020;10(3):721–5. Available from: http://www.ncbi.nlm.nih.gov/pubmed/32166632.

366. Duncan R, Gaspar R. Nanomedicine(s) under the microscope. Mol Pharm [Internet]. 2011;8(6):2101–41. Available from: https://pubs.acs.org/doi/10.1021/mp200394t.

367. Anselmo AC, Mitragotri S. Nanoparticles in the clinic: An update. Bioeng Transl Med [Internet]. 2019 4(3). Available from: https://onlinelibrary.wiley.com/doi/abs/10.1002/btm2.10143

368. Bobo D, Robinson KJ, Islam J, Thurecht KJ, Corrie SR. Nanoparticle-based medicines: A review of FDA-approved materials and Clinical trials to date. Pharm Res [Internet]. 2016;33(10):2373–87. Available from: http://link.springer.com/10.1007/s11095-016-1958-5.

369. Venditto VJ, Szoka FC. Cancer nanomedicines: so many papers and so few drugs! Adv Drug Deliv Rev [Internet]. 2013;65(1):80–8. Available from: https://linkinghub.elsevier.com/retrieve/pii/S0169409X12002992.

370. Kim H-M, Jeong S, Hahm E, Kim J, Cha MG, Kim K-M, et al. Large scale synthesis of surface-enhanced Raman scattering nanoprobes with high reproducibility and long-term stability. J Ind Eng Chem [Internet]. 2016 Jan;33:22–7. Available from: https://linkinghub.elsevier.com/retrieve/pii/S1226086X15004451.

371. Lin Y-W, Huang C-C, Chang H-T. Gold nanoparticle probes for the detection of mercury, lead and copper ions. Analyst [Internet]. 2011;136(5):863–71. Available from: http://www.ncbi.nlm.nih.gov/pubmed/21157604.

372. Ragelle H, Danhier F, Préat V, Langer R, Anderson DG. Nanoparticle-based drug delivery systems: a commercial and regulatory outlook as the field matures. Expert Opin Drug Deliv [Internet]. 2017;14(7):851–64. Available from: https://www.tandfonline.com/doi/full/10.1080/17425247.2016.1244187.

373. van der Meel R, Sulheim E, Shi Y, Kiessling F, Mulder WJM, Lammers T. Smart cancer nanomedicine. Nat Nanotechnol [Internet]. 2019;14(11):1007–17. Available from: http://www.nature.com/articles/s41565-019-0567-y.

374. Hare JI, Lammers T, Ashford MB, Puri S, Storm G, Barry ST. Challenges and strategies in anti-cancer nanomedicine development: an industry perspective. Adv Drug Deliv Rev [Internet]. 2017;108:25–38. Available from: https://linkinghub.elsevier.com/retrieve/pii/S0169409X16301351

375. Szebeni J, Simberg D, González-Fernández Á, Barenholz Y, Dobrovolskaia MA. Roadmap and strategy for overcoming infusion reactions to nanomedicines. Nat Nanotechnol [Internet]. 2018;13(12):1100–8. Available from: http://www.nature.com/articles/s41565-018-0273-1

376. Tainaka K, Kubota SI, Suyama TQ, Susaki EA, Perrin D, Ukai-Tadenuma M, et al. Whole-body imaging with single-cell resolution by tissue decolorization. Cell [Internet]. 2014 6;159(4):911–24. Available from: http://www.ncbi.nlm.nih.gov/pubmed/25417165.

377. Keller PJ, Dodt H-U. Light sheet microscopy of living or cleared specimens. Curr Opin Neurobiol [Internet]. 2012;22(1):138–43. Available from: http://www.ncbi.nlm.nih.gov/pubmed/21925871.

378. Sindhwani S, Syed AM, Wilhelm S, Chan WCW. Exploring passive clearing for 3D optical imaging of nanoparticles in intact tissues. Bioconjug Chem [Internet]. 2017;28(1):253–9. Available from: http://www.ncbi.nlm.nih.gov/pubmed/27801589.

379. Underwood JCE. More than meets the eye: the changing face of histopathology. Histopathology [Internet]. 2017;70(1):4–9. Available from: http://doi.wiley.com/10.1111/his.13047.

380. Jain PK, Lee KS, El-Sayed IH, El-Sayed MA. Calculated absorption and scattering properties of gold nanoparticles of different size, shape, and composition: applications in biological imaging and biomedicine. J Phys Chem B [Internet] 2006;110(14):7238–48. Available from: http://www.ncbi.nlm.nih.gov/pubmed/16599493.

381. Syed AM, Sindhwani S, Wilhelm S, Kingston BR, Lee DSW, Gommerman JL, et al. Three-dimensional imaging of transparent tissues via metal nanoparticle labeling. J Am Chem Soc [Internet]. 2017;139(29):9961–71. Available from: https://pubs.acs.org/doi/10.1021/jacs.7b04022.

382. Chauhan VP, Jain RK. Strategies for advancing cancer nanomedicine. Nat Mater [Internet]. 2013;12(11):958–62. Available from: http://www.ncbi.nlm.nih.gov/pubmed/24150413.

383. Sindhwani S, Syed AM, Wilhelm S, Glancy DR, Chen YY, Dobosz M, et al. Three-dimensional optical mapping of nanoparticle distribution in intact tissues. ACS Nano [Internet] 2016;10(5):5468–5478. Available from: https://pubs.acs.org/doi/10.1021/acsnano.6b01879.

384. De Felice F, Cavallini C, Barlattani A, Tombolini M, Brugnoletti O, Tombolini V, et al. Nanotechnology in oral cavity carcinoma: recent trends and treatment opportunities. Nanomater (Basel, Switzerland) [Internet]. 2019;9(11). Available from: http://www.ncbi. nlm.nih.gov/pubmed/31683582.

385. Mack MG, Balzer JO, Straub R, Eichler K, Vogl TJ. Superparamagnetic iron oxide-enhanced MR imaging of head and neck lymph nodes. Radiology [Internet]. 2002;222(1):239–44. Available from: http://www.ncbi.nlm.nih.gov/pubmed/11756732.

386. Mack MG, Rieger J, Baghi M, Bisdas S, Vogl TJ. Cervical lymph nodes. Eur J Radiol [Internet]. 2008;66(3):493–500. Available from: http://www.ncbi.nlm.nih.gov/pubmed/18337039.

387. Malam Y, Loizidou M, Seifalian AM. Liposomes and nanoparticles: nanosized vehicles for drug delivery in cancer. Trends Pharmacol Sci [Internet]. 2009;30(11):592–9. Available from: http://www.ncbi.nlm.nih.gov/pubmed/19837467.

388. Anzai Y, Piccoli CW, Outwater EK, Stanford W, Bluemke DA, Nurenberg P, et al. Evaluation of neck and body metastases to nodes with ferumoxtran 10-enhanced MR imaging: phase III safety and efficacy study. Radiology [Internet]. 2003;228(3):777–88. Available from: http:// www.ncbi.nlm.nih.gov/pubmed/12954896.

389. Wang Y-XJ, Hussain SM, Krestin GP. Superparamagnetic iron oxide contrast agents: physicochemical characteristics and applications in MR imaging. Eur Radiol [Internet]. 2001;11(11):2319–31. Available from: http://link.springer.com/10.1007/s003300100908.

390. Alex JC, Krag DN. Gamma-probe guided localization of lymph nodes. Surg Oncol [Internet]. 1993;2(3):137–43. Available from: https://linkinghub.elsevier.com/retrieve/ pii/096074049390001F.

391. Ramamurthy R, Kottayasamy Seenivasagam R, Shanmugam S, Palanivelu K. A prospective study on sentinel lymph node biopsy in early oral cancers Using methylene blue dye alone. Indian J Surg Oncol [Internet]. 2014;5(3):178–83. Available from: http://link.springer. com/10.1007/s13193-014-0337-0.

392. Vishnoi JR, Kumar V, Gupta S, Chaturvedi A, Misra S, Akhtar N, et al. Outcome of sentinel lymph node biopsy in early-stage squamous cell carcinoma of the oral cavity with methylene blue dye alone: a prospective validation study. Br J Oral Maxillofac Surg [Internet]. 2019;57(8):755–9. Available from: https://linkinghub.elsevier.com/retrieve/pii/ S0266435619302475.

393. Hutteman M, van der Vorst JR, Gaarenstroom KN, Peters AAW, Mieog JSD, Schaafsma BE, et al. Optimization of near-infrared fluorescent sentinel lymph node mapping for vulvar cancer. Am J Obstet Gynecol [Internet]. 2012;206(1):89.e1-5. Available from: http://www.ncbi. nlm.nih.gov/pubmed/21963099.

394. Jeong H-S, Lee C-M, Cheong S-J, Kim E-M, Hwang H, Na KS, et al. The effect of mannosylation of liposome-encapsulated indocyanine green on imaging of sentinel lymph node. J Liposome Res [Internet]. 2013;23(4):291–7. Available from: http://www.ncbi.nlm.nih.gov/ pubmed/23738810.

395. Zhang Z, Lee SH, Gan CW, Feng S-S. In vitro and in vivo investigation on PLA-TPGS nanoparticles for controlled and sustained small molecule chemotherapy. Pharm Res [Internet] 2008;25(8):1925–35. Available from: http://www.ncbi.nlm.nih.gov/pubmed/18509603.

396. Prashant C, Dipak M, Yang C-T, Chuang K-H, Jun D, Feng S-S. Superparamagnetic iron oxide--loaded poly(lactic acid)-D-alpha-tocopherol polyethylene glycol 1000 succinate copolymer nanoparticles as MRI contrast agent. Biomaterials [Internet]. 2010;31(21):5588–97. Available from: http://www.ncbi.nlm.nih.gov/pubmed/20434210.

397. Yan A, Von Dem Bussche A, Kane AB, Hurt RH. Tocopheryl polyethylene glycol succinate as a safe, antioxidant surfactant for processing carbon nanotubes and fullerenes. Carbon N Y [Internet]. 2007;45(13):2463–70. Available from: https://linkinghub.elsevier.com/retrieve/ pii/S0008622307004332.

398. di Cagno M, Stein PC, Styskala J, Hlaváč J, Skalko-Basnet N, Bauer-Brandl A. Overcoming instability and low solubility of new cytostatic compounds: a comparison of two approaches.

Eur J Pharm Biopharm [Internet]. 2012;80(3):657–62. Available from: http://www.ncbi.nlm. nih.gov/pubmed/22142591.

399. Xu H, Abe H, Naito M, Fukumori Y, Ichikawa H, Endoh S, et al. Efficient dispersing and shortening of super-growth carbon nanotubes by ultrasonic treatment with ceramic balls and surfactants. Adv Powder Technol [Internet] 2010;21(5):551–5. Available from: http://linkin-ghub.elsevier.com/retrieve/pii/S0921883110000269.

400. Mi Y, Liu Y, Feng S-S. Formulation of Docetaxel by folic acid-conjugated d-α-tocopheryl polyethylene glycol succinate 2000 (Vitamin E TPGS(2k)) micelles for targeted and synergistic chemotherapy. Biomaterials [Internet]. 2011;32(16):4058–66. Available from: http:// www.ncbi.nlm.nih.gov/pubmed/21396707.

401. Anbharasi V, Cao N, Feng S-S. Doxorubicin conjugated to D-alpha-tocopheryl polyethylene glycol succinate and folic acid as a prodrug for targeted chemotherapy. J Biomed Mater Res A [Internet]. 2010;94(3):730–43. Available from: http://www.ncbi.nlm.nih.gov/pubmed/20225211.

402. Guo Y, Luo J, Tan S, Otieno BO, Zhang Z. The applications of Vitamin E TPGS in drug delivery. Eur J Pharm Sci [Internet]. 2013;49(2):175–86. Available from: http://www.ncbi. nlm.nih.gov/pubmed/23485439.

403. Collnot E-M, Baldes C, Schaefer UF, Edgar KJ, Wempe MF, Lehr C-M. Vitamin E TPGS P-glycoprotein inhibition mechanism: influence on conformational flexibility, intracellular ATP levels, and role of time and site of access. Mol Pharm [Internet]. 2010;7(3):642–51. Available from: http://www.ncbi.nlm.nih.gov/pubmed/20205474.

404. Liu Y, Huang L, Liu F. Paclitaxel nanocrystals for overcoming multidrug resistance in cancer. Mol Pharm [Internet]. 2010;7(3):863–9. Available from: http://www.ncbi.nlm.nih.gov/pubmed/20420443.

405. Choudhury H, Gorain B, Pandey M, Kumbhar SA, Tekade RK, Iyer AK, et al. Recent advances in TPGS-based nanoparticles of docetaxel for improved chemotherapy. Int J Pharm [Internet]. 2017;529(1–2):506–22. Available from: https://linkinghub.elsevier.com/retrieve/pii/S0378517317306178.

406. Harney AS, Arwert EN, Entenberg D, Wang Y, Guo P, Qian B-Z, et al. Real-time Imaging reveals local, transient vascular permeability, and tumor cell intravasation stimulated by TIE2hi macrophage-derived VEGFA. Cancer Discov [Internet]. 2015;5(9):932–43. Available from: http://cancerdiscovery.aacrjournals.org/cgi/doi/10.1158/2159-8290.CD-15-0012.

407. Naumenko VA, Vlasova KY, Garanina AS, Melnikov PA, Potashnikova DM, Vishnevskiy DA, et al. Extravasating neutrophils open vascular barrier and improve liposomes delivery to tumors. ACS Nano [Internet]. 2019;13(11):12599–612. Available from: https://pubs.acs.org/doi/10.1021/acsnano.9b03848.

Chapter 5
The Role of Mass Cytometry in Early Detection, Diagnosis, and Treatment of Head and Neck Cancer

Amy S. Tsai, Jakob F. Einhaus, Julien Hedou, Eileen Tsai, Dyani Gaudilliere, and Brice Gaudilliere

Introduction

There have been increasingly more applications of single-cell technologies in the context of head and neck cancer (HNC) for detection, surveillance, treatment selection, and precision medicine. With clinical studies, in which the number of samples is low, the number of parameters measured per sample gains importance [1]. To this end, biological research continuously evolves to increase the resolution at which cellular features can be studied. Specifically, mass cytometry (cytometry by time-of-flight mass spectrometry, CyTOF), a highly multiplex flow cytometry technique, has revolutionized the way we can study complex human diseases, by utilizing metal-conjugated antibodies in lieu of fluorophores for the measurement of up to 50

A. S. Tsai
Stanford University School of Medicine, Department of Anesthesia, Stanford, CA, USA

University of California, Davis School of Medicine, Sacramento, CA, USA

J. F. Einhaus
Stanford University School of Medicine, Department of Anesthesia, Stanford, CA, USA

Eberhard Karls University of Tübingen, Tübingen, Germany

J. Hedou · B. Gaudilliere (✉)
Stanford University School of Medicine, Department of Anesthesia, Stanford, CA, USA
e-mail: gbrice@stanford.edu

E. Tsai
Stanford University School of Medicine, Department of Anesthesia, Stanford, CA, USA

Ohio State University College of Medicine, Columbus, OH, USA

D. Gaudilliere (✉)
Division of Plastic & Reconstructive Surgery, Department of Surgery, Stanford University School of Medicine, Palo Alto, CA, USA
e-mail: dyani.gaudilliere@stanford.edu

© Springer Nature Switzerland AG 2021
R. El Assal et al. (eds.), *Early Detection and Treatment of Head & Neck Cancers*, https://doi.org/10.1007/978-3-030-69859-1_5

parameters per single cell. Using inductively coupled plasma time-of-flight spectrometry, mass cytometry has significantly less confounding background activity and lacks the complications of spectral overlap compared to its predecessor, flow cytometry, and additional parameters are being added with the availability of new isotopes.

More recently, advancements in imaging modalities have taken advantage of the high dimensionality of mass spectrometry. Two such methods, collectively referred to as mass cytometry imaging (MCI), are imaging mass cytometry (IMC, Hyperion) and multiplexed ion beam imaging (MIBI), in which laser ablation of tissue samples stained with metal-conjugated antibodies allows for high-resolution imaging and spatial analysis of solid tissues [2]. High-dimensional imaging enables the investigation of tumor microenvironments that strongly contribute to pathological disease progression [3].

The ability of both suspension mass cytometry and MCI to simultaneously identify surface markers as well as the phosphorylation states of intracellular signaling markers on a single-cell basis allows for each individual cell phenotype to be identified in connection with its signaling function. Furthermore, exogenous perturbation of individual cells can offer better insight into the adaptive/dynamic scale of cell-type-specific responses. This is of particular significance in understanding cancer development, as pathway abnormalities can manifest not only in the basal expression of certain signaling molecules but also in pathological signaling intensity upon stimulation. Importantly, mass cytometry also allows for studying the dynamics of a cellular network, such as the immune landscape or the tumor microenvironment. The utility of mass cytometry has been demonstrated in many clinical settings, including identifying immune states in pre-eclampsia [4, 5], characterizing the immune response in surgical recovery [6, 7], discovering associations between systemic immune response and stroke recovery [8], and identifying immune features implicated in chronic periodontitis [9]. One of the most frequent applications has been in the field of cancer biology and clinical oncology.

In the field of solid tumors, HNC represents a particularly heterogeneous tumor entity in terms of location, originating tissue, structure, and histology. Here, high-parameter characterization of molecular tumor subtypes opens opportunities of unique diagnostic and prognostic value. In the case of head and neck squamous cell carcinoma (HNSCC), the most common form of head and neck cancer, the current diagnostic standard of morphological assessment of tumor histology has limited predictive value. Additionally, diagnosis of HNSCC trends toward later stages, precluding effective treatment. Recent studies suggest diverse cancer stem cell populations can coexist within a tumor, where the tumor initiation and metastatic properties of these cancer stem cells can be uncoupled [10]. Additionally, certain cancer stem cells present with therapy-resistant phenotypes that can relapse. A high-parameter assay could not only offer a potential solution to this dilemma but also offer insight into the pathophysiological process of disease progression, allowing for more targeted therapeutic efforts. The high-resolution information gained about tumor cell phenotype and function, as well as that of the systemic immune response to the tumor or treatment modalities, leads to numerous applications of these technologies in cancer biology.

In this chapter, we will discuss current applications of suspension mass cytometry and MCI in cancer biology research and therapy, followed by an outline of the process of collecting and analyzing tumor samples with these methods. Finally, we will discuss the bioinformatics techniques which have been developed alongside these technologies to analyze the resulting large datasets and develop predictive models which are of clinical significance.

Current Applications in Cancer Biology Research and Therapy

Two major applications of suspension mass cytometry and MCI in the study of cancer are in the identification of biomarkers of cancer progression and in the analysis of the host's response to treatments, such as immunotherapy or radiation therapy. Both applications will ultimately lead to major advances in the realm of precision medicine, as they allow for characterization of the implications of tumor heterogeneity on prognosis, impaired cellular processes, and treatment response.

Identifying Predictive Biomarkers

Studies identifying biomarkers relevant to the behavior of tumor cells or the host's immune response to the tumor have been illuminating [11–21]. In the context of tumor biology, regulation of cellular processes and progression of cellular differentiation are especially high-yield and relatively easily captured using the mass cytometry platform.

Providing effective therapeutics necessitates the understanding of biological processes driving the pathology of tumor progression or therapeutic resistance. In a study by Zunder et al., investigators were able to follow the dynamic process of reprogramming somatic cells into induced pluripotent stem cells (iPSCs) by simultaneously measuring differentiation, cell cycle, and signaling markers such as Oct4, Sox2, Klf4, and c-Myc [11]. Deriving molecular landmarks of dynamic biological processes with a time-resolved analysis of multiparameter mass cytometry data can provide an encouraging model for future studies on cancer progression. Identification of molecular pathways that promote cancer cell survival lays the foundation for new therapeutic developments.

Similar efforts have been translated to B-cell and T-cell maturation. Analysis of phosphoproteins, kinases, and phosphatases in signaling pathways shows patterns of activation that can be associated with disease. For example, STAT3 and STAT5 have been shown to be constitutively activated in AML [12–15]. Also in AML, Nolan et al. studied single-cell responses to exogenous stimulations using flow cytometry and found mutations in cancer cells that reorganized intracellular signaling pathways [16].

Specific to HNSCC, expression of CD10, a zinc-dependent metallopeptidase, has been found by FACS (fluorescence-activated cell sorting) analysis to be associated with cancer stem cell-like properties, such as an increased expression of Oct3/4. Such properties are implicated in higher resistance of HNSCC clones against chemotherapy and radiation [17]. The levels of CD10 correlate with the degree of metastasis, tumor grade, and rate of recurrence [18].

As stated above, understanding tumor heterogeneity is an important factor in individualizing treatment approaches to maximize the patient's treatment response and prognosis. Heterogeneity of cancers arises due to the different epigenetic, genetic, and microenvironmental influences during the evolution of the cancer. In follicular lymphoma, diverse HLA-DR expression was found through CyTOF analysis to have a strong contribution to tumor heterogeneity, potentially due to the influence of HLA-DR on PD-L1 checkpoint inhibitor therapy responsiveness [19]. When IMC is combined with phenogenomics, tumor heterogeneity can be linked to genomic subtypes of cancer. Bodenmiller et al. expanded the information content gained from IMC to describe patient-specific differences in mRNA-to-protein ratios for HER2 and CK19 in breast cancer samples that allow the detection of relevant pathological mechanisms in the regulation of translation, mRNA, and protein stability in tumor cells [20]. In breast cancer, combinations of cell phenotypes and cell-cell interactions were linked to different genomic subtypes with spatially arranged cellular neighborhoods being linked to prognosis [21].

Monitoring Response to Treatment

As a next step in the development or individualized prescription of targeted therapies, as well as in monitoring their effectiveness, mass cytometry has been used to study multiple therapies in several cancer types. A major goal in cancer therapy is to induce cancer cell apoptosis by interfering with cell signaling and/or mitosis. Single-cell methods are able to probe these pathways. Suspension mass cytometry has been used to study the response of cancer-related pathways to treatments for multiple myeloma, finding specific signaling proteins (CREB and MCL-1) that were associated with poor response [22]. CO-Detection by inDEXing (CODEX) multiplexed imaging has been used with tissue biopsies in cutaneous T cell lymphoma to study the response to a monoclonal antibody treatment (pembrolizumab), comparing tissue from patients who responded to the therapy to those who did not. Multiple differences were found between the two groups, including expression of PD-1 on tumor cells, changes in cell composition and frequency, as well as changes in cellular neighborhoods by spatial analysis. The implications for predicting the response to immunotherapy will allow improved selection of patients for certain therapies [23].

As immunotherapy, a treatment modality utilized in HNC therapy, leads to wide systemic immune changes in the host, suspension mass cytometry, which works well for studying leukocytes in whole blood or Peripheral Blood Mononuclear Cell (PBMCs), is particularly suited to study systemic immune changes resulting from cancer immunotherapy [24]. To this end, CyTOF was used to study the systemic immune response to urelumab (anti-CD137 antibody) therapy for patients with solid tumors and B-cell non-Hodgkin's lymphoma in serial blood samples taken at baseline and throughout treatment. The findings of increased CD8+ T cells and NK cells, a decrease in CD4+ T cells and regulatory CD4+ T cells, and cytokine changes were suggestive of an antitumor Th1 response [25].

In addition to immunotherapy, a treatment modality for HNSCC that is currently more important and more frequently utilized is radiation therapy. The sensitivity of a tumor to radiotherapy has a high impact in tumor control. For this reason, radio-sensitizing agents could improve the effectiveness of this treatment modality. Specifically, tepotinib, a MET receptor inhibitor, is used as a radiosensitizing agent as the MET receptor is involved in an aggressive phenotype of HNSCC and modulates DNA damage when exposed to ionizing radiation. By using CyTOF to study the molecular basis of radiosensitization by tepotinib, Nisa et al. found that after pretreatment with tepotinib, PI3K activity was modulated in radiosensitized cells but not in cells resistant to radiation [26].

Point-of-Care Diagnostics

There is also a precedent for using single-cell techniques for point-of-care diagnostics. HNCs often spread early to the cervical lymph nodes, making highly sensitive detection of lymph node metastasis a diagnostic priority. Specifically, fluorescence-activated cell sorting (FACS) in single-cell suspension used for rapid nodal staging was found to be sensitive, reliable, inexpensive, and fast in patients with HNSCC. This method was able to detect malignant cells in four cases not found by histopathology in addition to detecting all other studied cases of lymph node metastasis in a 3-hour time frame [27]. Expanding upon this method could prove invaluable in detecting early metastasis.

Technique for System-Level Analysis Using Mass Cytometry

Suspension Mass Cytometry Panel Design

Mass cytometry allows for a plethora of investigative studies, ranging from the exhaustion of a single biological process to the interrogation of an entire network of signaling components from a heterogeneous collection of cells. It allows for the establishment of disease progression as well as for identification of dysfunctional processes in diseased compared to healthy cohorts. The question answered depends on the design of the panel utilized for the study. Recently, a 40-parameter IMC panel for formalin-fixed, paraffin-embedded (FFPE) tissue sections was developed by Ijsselsteijin et al. for characterizing cancer immune microenvironments [28].

As previous studies in HNSCC have shown that CD10 correlates with prognostic factors, an optimized multicolor immunofluorescence panel (OMIP-045) was developed for mass cytometry analysis with the goal of studying features related to HNSCC prognosis [29]. The panel included metastatic, drug-resistant, stem cell, lineage, and activation markers associated with HNSCC progression (Table 5.1). A diverse panel of mutations has been identified in HNSCCs, thus mandating a broad panel with multiple prognostic markers. OMIP-045 was tested on (i) patient-matched HNSCC cell lines derived from primary and metastatic/recurrent lesions; (ii) a mixture of breast, skin, gastrointestinal, lung, and leukemic cancer cell lines with known mutations; and (iii) fresh tumor biopsies from patients with HNC [29].

Preparation of Solid Tumors for Suspension Mass Cytometry Analysis

Mass cytometry has the capacity to analyze solid tumors with two methods: single-cell suspension and solid tumor immunohistochemical sections, known as imaging mass cytometry (IMC) (Fig. 5.1). When considering single-cell suspension techniques, additional standardization steps can be employed for more consistent analysis.

Solid tumors can be either mechanically prepared for suspension or digested with various enzymes. Tonsils, for example, are easily prepared by mechanically dissociating the tissue, whereas other tumor type tissues may require enzymatic dissociation. Leelatian et al. standardized a technique to prepare viable single-cell suspensions using gliomas, melanomas, and small cell lung cancers [30].

The mechanical dissociation technique involves mincing the tissue with scalpels as well as filtration through a strainer. This step can be completed prior to enzymatic dissociation. The goal of the preparation protocol is to optimize the live cell count and the cell subset diversity, and according to Irish's study, combining the mechanical preparation with collagenase and DNase had high success to this end. They also optimized the timing of collagenase and DNase to 1 hour, with longer times leading to increases in cell death [30]. The result of these methods is that solid tissues or tumors, such as HNC, can be prepared in live, single-cell suspensions suited to mass cytometry analysis.

Preparation of Blood Samples for Suspension Mass Cytometry Analysis

In addition to studying the tumor tissue itself, suspension mass cytometry offers an ideal platform for studying the systemic immune system, which allows for system-level characterization of the host's immune response to immune therapy with a simple blood draw that can be repeated at multiple points throughout therapy.

Table 5.1 Antibodies used in OMIP-045

Specificity	Clone	Metal isotope	Purpose
Lineage markers			
CD45	HI30	89Y	Leukocytes
CD3	SK7	142Nd	T cells
CD31	390	145Nd	Endothelial cells
CD10	HI10A	156Gd	Cancer-associated fibroblasts
Vimentin	D21H3	154Sm	Mesenchymal cells
CD68	Y1/82A	171Yb	Macrophages and DCs
CD24	ML5	169Tm	B cells
CD324 (E-cadherin)	24E10	158Gd	Epithelial cells
Activation/suppression markers			
CD279 (PD-1)	EH12.2H7	155Gd	Tolerance promotion
CD274 (PD-L1)	29E.2A3	159Tb	Tolerance promotion
CD28	CD28.2	160Gd	T-cell activation
Ki-67	B56	161Dy	Proliferation
Signaling cascades associated with HNSCC			
pp53 (s15)	16G8	141Pr	Tumor suppressor protein
PARP (cleaved)	F21-852	143Nd	Repair of single-stranded DNA
pERK 1/2 [T202/Y204]	D13.14.4E	167Er	Proliferation
pEGFR Ty845	D7A5	146Nd	Proliferation
HER2	29D8	148Nd	Proliferation
pAkt [S473]	D9E	152Sm	Survival
pMET Ty1234/1235	Polyclonal rabbit IgG	162Dy	Proliferation
DDR2	290804	163Dy	Proliferation
TRAF3	B1–6	168Er	Associated with HNSCC
EGFR	AY13	170Er	Proliferation
YAP1	867711	172Yb	Proliferation
HES1	4H1HES1	173Yb	Transcription suppressor
EPHA2	SHM16	174Yb	Migration and proliferation
pS6 [S235/S236]	N7-548	175Lu	Increased translation
MET	D1C2	176Yb	Proliferation
Metastasis and drug resistance			
CD29	TS2/16	147Sm	Metastasis
MMP-9	4H3	150Nd	Metastasis
TIMP3	277128	153Eu	Metastasis inhibitor
MDR1	UIC2	151Eu	Drug resistance
Cancer stem cells			
ALDH1(A1)	703410	144Nd	Associated with cancer stem cells
CD166	3A6	164Dy	Associated with cancer stem cells
CD44	PJ18	166Er	Associated with cancer stem cells

Reproduced with copy right permission from [29]

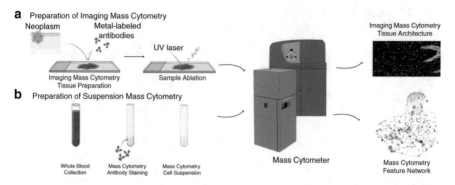

Fig. 5.1 Workflow of imaging and suspension mass cytometry

For this purpose, patient blood samples can be processed after isolation of PBMCs or as whole blood samples in selectable conditions with or without in vitro stimulation. In unstimulated samples, the endogenous activation of the patient's immune system at the time of blood draw can be grasped for physiological assessment of a certain treatment or condition. Alternatively, samples can be stimulated in vitro with various stimuli such as interleukins, growth factors, or other cytokines to capture the dynamic potential of immunological responses. After in vitro stimulation, the cells are fixed using a proteomic stabilizer. If whole blood samples are used, erythrocytes in the cell suspension are lysed using an appropriate lysis buffer prior to the staining process.

Barcoding to Preserve Reagents and to Minimize Batch Effects

Once the solid tumor tissue, whole blood, or PBMCs have been prepared for suspension mass cytometry analysis, the samples can be barcoded. Mass cytometry's capacity for high-resolution analysis allows for the introduction of palladium-based barcoding reagents. Pooled sample analysis not only decreases the quantity of expensive reagents required but also minimizes experimental errors, which is integral in high-dimensional analysis. Unique combinatorial sets of 3 out of 6 stable purified palladium isotopes (Pd102, 104, 105, 106, 108, and 110) allow for the simultaneous analysis of up to 20 samples run together (Fig. 5.2). Once samples have been properly barcoded and pooled, each sample is introduced to the same concentration of antibodies. Upon completion of data collection, a de-barcoding algorithm [11] allows for samples to be separated on the basis of the tag as well as on the removal of any doublets.

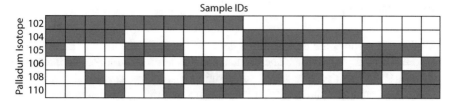

Fig. 5.2 Palladium isotope combination for barcoding in suspension mass cytometry

Staining for Suspension Mass Cytometry

Isotopically pure metal-conjugated antibodies, the most common affinity reagents, are the backbone of mass cytometry. Upon binding to the target of interest, the attached metal ions serve as reporters for subsequent evaluation. Cell suspensions are incubated with metal-conjugated antibodies to tag surface antigens, which are used primarily for phenotypic identification of cell types. To assess intracellular proteins of interest, cells are permeabilized with methanol to allow for penetration of the bulky antibodies. Together, the two rounds of incubation allow for high-resolution functional assessment of a broad spectrum of immune cells on a single-cell basis.

Suspension Mass Cytometry Run with Normalization

Barcoded and antibody-stained single suspension cells are analyzed on the Helios mass cytometer (Fluidigm, Inc.) at a rate of 600 to 1000 events per second with normalization "beads" consisting of polymers conjugated with metal ions that can be used to standardize the concentration of cells and the signal intensity across experimental days. The resulting data are normalized using Normalizer v0.1 MATLAB Compiler Runtime (MathWorks) [31]. Files are then de-barcoded with a single-cell MATLAB debarcoding tool [11]. Files are uploaded to CellEngine for two-dimensional gating based on abundance of measured isotopes.

Preparation of Tissue Samples for Imaging Mass Cytometry Analysis

Fresh tissue samples from patients are obtained and fixed in optimal cutting temperature compound (OCT compound) for frozen samples or 10% formalin solution overnight and then transferred to a 70% ethanol in 4 degrees until tissue processing for FFPE samples.

IMC Processing

FFPE tissue sections are dewaxed in xylene, hydrated in ethanol, and incubated in antigen retrieval (AR) buffer. The tissue sample is blocked with 3% bovine serum albumin (BSA) to decrease nonspecific antibody binding. Tissues are incubated with metal-conjugated antibodies and then stained with an iridium intercalator stain. Similarly, fresh frozen tissue can also be processed for analysis. Detailed methods are outlined by Ijsselsteijin et al. [28]. It is important to note a hematoxylin and eosin (H&E) section can be prepared in addition to the metal-conjugated antibody-labeled section to help with co-registration and setting of fiducials. These sections should be consecutive.

IMC Run

Machine optimization is performed using a three-element tuning slide to standardize data analysis across experimental days (Fluidigm). The H&E section can be used to identify regions of interest (ROIs) in the consecutive IMC slide. Alternatively, the IMC slide itself can be used for co-registration. As each tissue type has its own optimal laser power for ablation, in each study, the appropriate laser power is determined by ablating six adjacent ROIs (dimensions 50–50 μm; 0-1-2-3-4-5 dB). The set laser power will be used for all tissue slides in that set of runs. Upon optimizing the machine, samples can be analyzed without direct supervision, which is beneficial in the event of large tissue sections or prolonged runs. Tissue samples are ablated with a UV laser at 1 μm resolution at a speed of 1 mm^2 every 2 hours. Each $μm^2$ unit of tissue is aerosolized, atomized, and ionized before entering a time-of-flight mass spectrometer for the measurement of isotype abundance. The isotype abundance is used to build a high-resolution image of the tissue sample, akin to immunohistochemistry stains.

Cell Segmentation

IMC raw data are converted files compatible with further analysis using open-source Python scripts or MCD viewer (v.1.0.560, Fluidigm). CellProfiler [32] then removes outlier pixels, denoises the data, and crops the images to reduce the file size for ilastik [33], a pixel classifier that can be used to perform cell segmentation. Segmentation is completed based on the abundance of measured isotopes, generating a probability map of chosen cellular organelles, such as nuclei, cytoplasm, and background compartments. Obtained probability masks are imported back to CellProfiler to generate cell segmentation masks. HistoCAT [34] is used to annotate, or phenotypically classify, each cell type, either manually via marker expression or with PhenoGraph clustering [35]. Frequency and median values are exported, and a neighborhood analysis can be performed to identify cellular relationships and microenvironments.

Bioinformatics Methods to Identify Predictive Biomarkers

Goals of the Analysis

Clearly defined study or clinical goals must be established prior to any panel design or sample acquisition with the computational methods in mind from the beginning. Depending on the objective, analyses usually focus on identifying differences between phenotypes in a classic differential expression analysis or using statistical learning framework. Examples of research goals for applying these mass cytometry methods to the study of HNC may be to identify tumor features predicting tumor activity, host immune features predicting tumor prognosis or spread, or tumor or host features predicting favorable response to chemotherapy or immunotherapy. Depending on the goals of the study, each framework offers elements of biological interpretation on a wide range of intracellular pathways at the single-cell level of granularity. However, for the statistical analysis, the precision of the technique brings a limitation from the number of information obtained per sample. In order to achieve both statistical and model trainings, the data must be processed into robust features that represent the data extensively in a summarized manner.

Feature Extraction from Single-Cell Raw Data

In order to translate the single-cell data gained from mass cytometry analysis into a usable set of features for the analysis, the first step is to identify each cell and group them into cell types in a meaningful way. Two ways to do this include manual gating and unsupervised clustering algorithms. Gates are manually created by using the expression of phenotypic and functional markers to identify cell types in a literature evidence-based setting. An example of a gating strategy can be seen in Fig. 5.3. Unsupervised clustering uses unbiased algorithms to identifying populations that cluster together with algorithms such as k-means clustering or k-nearest neighbor.

While a predefined list of cell types is traditionally characterized from human blood and tissue samples, the single-cell informational content gained from detection of surface proteins and intracellular signaling states allows for agnostic identification of phenotypically and functionally distinct cell subtypes. For example, in the human monocyte system, three cell types are traditionally described including classical monocytes ($CD14^+CD16^-$), non-classical monocytes ($CD14^-CD16^+$), and intermediate monocytes ($CD14^+CD16^+$). However, in a study using mass cytometry

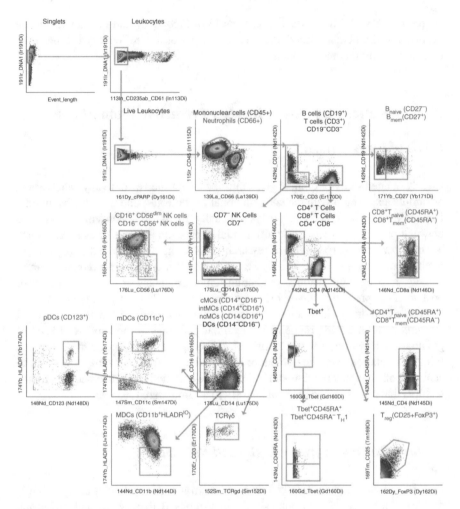

Fig. 5.3 Example of a traditional manual gating strategy

analysis of patient blood before and after surgery, eight distinct monocyte subsets were detectable [36]. Several powerful unsupervised methods have been developed that allow agnostic identification of immune cell subset without the need for a priori biological knowledge. These can be broadly categorized into clustering algorithms or dimension reduction algorithms. One clustering algorithm, spanning-tree progression analysis of density-normalized events (SPADE) [37], automatically groups cells obtained from flow or mass cytometry into populations and projects them into a tree as shown in Fig. 5.4. Alternatively, t-distributed stochastic neighbor embedding (t-SNE) is a nonlinear dimension reduction technique for high-dimensional data that allows for determining the relationship between datapoints on a two- or three-dimensional map [38].

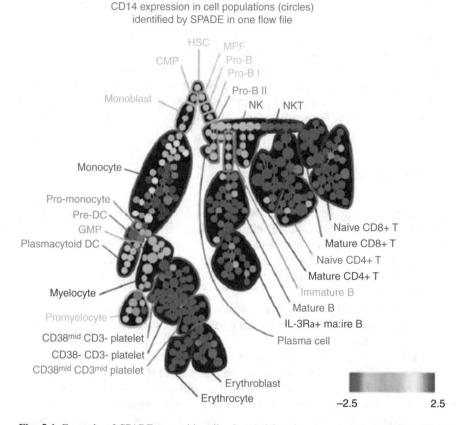

CD14 expression in cell populations (circles) identified by SPADE in one flow file

Fig. 5.4 Example of SPADE tree with cells clustered by phenotype based on surface CD14 expression. (Reproduced with copy right permission from [39])

Creating a Predictive Model

Single-cell methods measuring multiple parameters per cell generate datasets with an overwhelming number of features compared to the number of samples, which tax the limits of traditional statistical tools. Therefore, a number of statistical learning algorithms have been developed to deal with the complexity of high-dimensional datasets. In particular, algorithms featuring the sparsity properties of the L1 regularization such as the lasso (least absolute shrinkage and selection operator) and the elastic net have been successful in creating models that are able to classify disease status and clinical outcomes, such as surgical outcomes and chronic periodontal disease. Classical analyses use manually gated cell populations from which frequency and medians of the intracellular markers of individual cell types are extracted. Alternatively, algorithms like SPADE (Spanning-tree Progression Analysis of Density-normalized Events) (Fig. 5.4) and Citrus (cluster identification, characterization, and regression) have been developed to allow for autonomic clustering and feature extraction.

The simultaneous analysis provided by mass cytometry allows for analysis of each parameter as well as analysis of the dynamics of how multiple parameters evolve together during the progression of the disease. A predictive model generated using the above methods has high value in cancer research involving biomarker identification or monitoring of immunotherapy. However, a lower-cost, efficient, focused assay would improve the translation of these techniques to be used at the bedside. For this reason, model reduction strategies can be used to determine the simplest model that would include key features that still give high predictive or diagnostic value [40].

Limitations and Future Directions

Mass cytometry is subject to some caveats. For one, cells must be ionized, meaning that not only are a high volume of cells required but also the cells cannot be recovered after analysis, as they can be in FACS. The throughput of mass cytometry is also significantly lower than flow cytometry, and metal reporters often have lower sensitivity than fluorophores, precluding the study of cellular markers that are extremely low in number.

As with flow cytometry, mass cytometry uses predetermined reporters that require investigators to consider markers prior to data collection; thus, novel features may have been excluded. Regardless, the ability to uncover novel dynamics of cellular cross talk is a strength that mass cytometry offers.

The application of suspension mass cytometry and MCI in HNC has been limited, leaving room for future studies to expand our knowledge of tumor biology and its interaction with the host's biology and therapeutic interventions, both conventional and novel. By combining these methods with proteomics and metabolomics methods, a high level of content can be obtained to allow for system-level understanding of tumor activity and treatment susceptibility, which eventually can be adapted with the methods outlined in section "Bioinformatics Methods to Identify Predictive Biomarkers" of this chapter to focus on the most biologically relevant targets in the development of future HNC therapeutic strategies.

Acknowledgments We would like to extend our gratitude to the Nolan Lab for developing the mass cytometry technologies, the Gaudilliere Lab for developing study protocols for application in clinical studies, the Aghaeepour Lab for their innovative data analysis tools, and the Angst Lab for coordinating clinical studies to which mass cytometry can be directly applied.

References

1. Spitzer MH, Nolan GP. Mass cytometry: single cells, many features. Cell. 2016;165(4):780–91.
2. Ptacek J, et al. Multiplexed ion beam imaging (MIBI) for characterization of the tumor microenvironment across tumor types. Lab Investig. 2020;100(8):1111–23.
3. Giesen C, et al. Highly multiplexed imaging of tumor tissues with subcellular resolution by mass cytometry. Nat Methods. 2014;11(4):417–22.

4. Han X, et al. Differential dynamics of the maternal immune system in healthy pregnancy and preeclampsia. Front Immunol. 2019;10:1305.
5. Aghaeepour N, et al. An immune clock of human pregnancy. Sci Immunol. 2017;2(15):eaan2946.
6. Aghaeepour N, et al. Deep immune profiling of an arginine-enriched nutritional intervention in patients undergoing surgery. J Immunol. 2017;199:2171.
7. Gaudillière B, et al. Clinical recovery from surgery correlates with single-cell immune signatures. Sci Transl Med. 2014;6(255):255ra131.
8. Tsai AS, et al. A year-long immune profile of the systemic response in acute stroke survivors. Brain. 2019;142(4):978–91.
9. Gaudilliere DK, et al. Systemic immunologic consequences of chronic periodontitis. J Dent Res. 2019;98(9):985–93.
10. Jian Z, et al. Cancer stem cells in squamous cell carcinoma. J Invest Dermatol. 2017;137(1):31–7.
11. Zunder ER, et al. Palladium-based mass tag cell barcoding with a doublet-filtering scheme and single-cell deconvolution algorithm. Nat Protoc. 2015;10(2):316–33.
12. Benekli M, et al. Constitutive activity of signal transducer and activator of transcription 3 protein in acute myeloid leukemia blasts is associated with short disease-free survival. Blood. 2002;99(1):252–7.
13. Birkenkamp KU, et al. Regulation of constitutive STAT5 phosphorylation in acute myeloid leukemia blasts. Leukemia. 2001;15(12):1923–31.
14. Turkson J, Jove R. STAT proteins: novel molecular targets for cancer drug discovery. Oncogene. 2000;19(56):6613–26.
15. Xia Z, et al. Expression of signal transducers and activators of transcription proteins in acute myeloid leukemia blasts. Cancer Res. 1998;58(14):3173–80.
16. Irish JM, et al. Single cell profiling of potentiated phospho-protein networks in cancer cells. Cell. 2004;118(2):217–28.
17. Fukusumi T, et al. CD10 as a novel marker of therapeutic resistance and cancer stem cells in head and neck squamous cell carcinoma. Br J Cancer. 2014;111(3):506–14.
18. Dionne LK, Driver ER, Wang XJ. Head and neck cancer stem cells: from identification to tumor immune network. J Dent Res. 2015;94(11):1524–31.
19. Wogsland CE, et al. Mass cytometry of follicular lymphoma tumors reveals intrinsic heterogeneity in proteins including HLA-DR and a deficit in nonmalignant plasmablast and germinal center B-cell populations. Cytometry B Clin Cytom. 2017;92(1):79–87.
20. Schulz D, et al. Simultaneous multiplexed imaging of mRNA and proteins with subcellular resolution in breast cancer tissue samples by mass cytometry. Cell Syst. 2018;6(1):25–36.e5.
21. Jackson HW, et al. The single-cell pathology landscape of breast cancer. Nature. 2020;578(7796):615–20.
22. Teh CE, et al. Deep profiling of apoptotic pathways with mass cytometry identifies a synergistic drug combination for killing myeloma cells. Cell Death Differ. 2020;27(7):2217–33.
23. Schuerch CM, et al. Dynamics of the cutaneous T cell lymphoma microenvironment in patients treated with pembrolizumab revealed by highly multiplexed tissue imaging. Blood. 2019;134(1521).
24. Sahaf B, et al. High-parameter immune profiling with CyTOF. Methods Mol Biol. 2020;2055:351–68.
25. Chester C, et al. Biomarker characterization using mass cytometry in a phase 1 trial of urelumab (BMS-663513) in subjects with advanced solid tumors and relapsed/refractory B-cell non-Hodgkin lymphoma. J Clin Oncol. 2014;32(15_suppl):3017–3017.
26. Nisa L, et al. Targeting the MET receptor tyrosine kinase as a strategy for radiosensitization in locoregionally advanced head and neck squamous cell carcinoma. Mol Cancer Ther. 2020;19(2):614–26.
27. Häyry V, et al. Rapid nodal staging of head and neck cancer surgical specimens with flow cytometric analysis. Br J Cancer. 2018;118(3):421–7.
28. Ijsselsteijn ME, et al. A 40-marker panel for high dimensional characterization of cancer immune microenvironments by imaging mass cytometry. Front Immunol. 2019;10:2534.

29. Brodie TM, Tosevski V, Medová M. OMIP-045: characterizing human head and neck tumors and cancer cell lines with mass cytometry. Cytometry A. 2018;93(4):406–10.
30. Leelatian N, et al. Single cell analysis of human tissues and solid tumors with mass cytometry. Cytometry B Clin Cytom. 2017;92(1):68–78.
31. Finck R, et al. Normalization of mass cytometry data with bead standards. Cytometry A. 2013;83(5):483–94.
32. Carpenter AE, et al. CellProfiler: image analysis software for identifying and quantifying cell phenotypes. Genome Biol. 2006;7(10):R100.
33. Berg S, et al. ilastik: interactive machine learning for (bio)image analysis. Nat Methods. 2019;16(12):1226–32.
34. Schapiro D, et al. histoCAT: analysis of cell phenotypes and interactions in multiplex image cytometry data. Nat Methods. 2017;14(9):873–6.
35. Levine JH, et al. Data-driven phenotypic dissection of AML reveals progenitor-like cells that correlate with prognosis. Cell. 2015;162(1):184–97.
36. Hamers AAJ, et al. Human monocyte heterogeneity as revealed by high-dimensional mass cytometry. Arterioscler Thromb Vasc Biol. 2019;39(1):25–36.
37. Qiu P, et al. Extracting a cellular hierarchy from high-dimensional cytometry data with SPADE. Nat Biotechnol. 2011;29(10):886–91.
38. van der Maaten LJ, Hinton GE. Visualizing high-dimensional data using t-SNE. J Mach Learn Res. 2008;9(nov):2579–605.
39. Bendall SC, et al. Single-cell mass cytometry of differential immune and drug responses across a human hematopoietic continuum. Science. 2011;332(6030):687–96.
40. Aghaeepour N, et al. GateFinder: projection-based gating strategy optimization for flow and mass cytometry. Bioinformatics. 2018;34(23):4131–3.

Chapter 6
Deep Learning-Based Cancer Region Segmentation from H&E Slides for HPV-Related Oropharyngeal Squamous Cell Carcinomas

Cheng Lu, Can Koyuncu, Andrew Janowczyk, Christopher C. Griffith, Deborah J. Chute, James S. Lewis Jr, and Anant Madabhushi

Introduction

Human papillomavirus-related (p16-positive) oropharyngeal squamous cell carcinoma (OPSCC) patients are usually cured with some combination of surgery, radiation, and chemotherapy, but approximately 10–20% of these patients will develop recurrent disease. Patients who are cured, however, may have major comorbidity from radiation and chemotherapy. Consequently, identifying those patients with aggressive versus indolent tumors is critical. Biomarkers, which separate less from more aggressive cancers, could aid in identifying the appropriate patients for de-intensification of therapy [1].

Tissue-based morphologic data is plentiful and carries with it large amounts of valuable information about tumor biology and behavior across myriad histologic types [2–5]. Classically, tumor morphology is visually assessed by pathologists using established staging and grading criteria [6]. However, for many cancers, the visual assessment of nuclear morphology may not directly correlate with disease

C. Lu · C. Koyuncu · A. Janowczyk
Department of Biomedical Engineering, Case Western Reserve University,
Cleveland, OH, USA

C. C. Griffith · D. J. Chute
Department of Pathology, Cleveland Clinic, Cleveland, OH, USA

J. S. Lewis Jr
Vanderbilt University Medical Center, Department of Pathology, Microbiology and Immunology, Nashville, TN, USA

A. Madabhushi (✉)
Department of Biomedical Engineering, Case Western Reserve University,
Cleveland, OH, USA

Louis Stokes Cleveland Veterans Administration Medical Center, Cleveland, OH, USA
e-mail: anant.madabhushi@case.edu

© Springer Nature Switzerland AG 2021
R. El Assal et al. (eds.), *Early Detection and Treatment of Head & Neck Cancers*, https://doi.org/10.1007/978-3-030-69859-1_6

prognosis and patient outcome. Even though some of the traditional clinical and staging parameters have been shown to have prognostic value [7, 8], there continues to be a need for better assessment of tumor morphology quantitatively for better prognosticating disease outcome. The computational interrogation of histologic image primitives and their corresponding morphology measurements (e.g., nuclear shape, diversity, arrangement) have been shown to be associated with disease outcome and treatment response [3, 9–14].

In previous work of oropharyngeal cancer, our group has shown that the complexity of clusters of proximally located nuclei can reflect disease aggressiveness and potentially help in improved risk stratification of patients to appropriately manage their therapeutic strategies [15]. However, an important prerequisite for these approaches is the definition of the tumor region on whole slide images. Unfortunately, manually annotating tumor regions is both time-consuming and tedious due to the vast size of whole-mount tissue images. Therefore, development of algorithms for automated tumor detection is a critical first step in this process.

While this is an area that has been investigated by a number of groups [5, 16–18] including ours [19–22], little work specifically in the context of oropharyngeal cancers has been done for automated tumor delineation. Deep learning models have been successfully applied in a wide range of medical image analysis tasks [5, 23]. The convolutional neural network (CNN) [24] stacks the input image with several convolutional layers, which extract and learn the underlying abstract patterns from the image to perform the detection, classification, and segmentation tasks. In the context of breast cancer, Cruz-Roa et al. [25] proposed a CNN method to detect the invasive ductal carcinoma regions from hematoxylin and eosin (H&E)-stained whole slide image with an accuracy of 84%. Wang et al. [18] utilized deep learning system to localize the tumor regions on metastatic breast cancer slides with an area under the receiver operating curve (AUC) of 0.71. There are other successful examples of utilizing deep learning models for tumor detection in the context of skin cancer [26–28] and a non-deep learning-based approach for prostate cancer [5] from whole slide pathology images.

In this book chapter, we present an automated deep learning tumor segmentation model for automated tumor extent delineation in whole slide tissue images of p16-positive oropharyngeal squamous cell carcinomas. A total of 248 digital whole slide images (WSIs) from 248 patients were used in this study. To ease annotation burden, coarse annotations (i.e., polygon-style bounding box annotations) were employed, thereby reducing the total amount of effort needed for creating training exemplars for the deep learning model. To further reduce the workload for the annotators, the training images were intentionally non-exhaustively annotated. One of the key things we sought to demonstrate in this study was that satisfactory segmentation results could be achieved even when using non-exhaustive tumor annotations for training the model.

The remainder of this book chapter is organized as follows. We first introduce the patient selection, annotation, and deep learning model in *Method and Materials*. We then present the results of the model and discuss our findings.

Method and Materials

Patient Selection

With approval from the Human Research Protection Offices of Washington University in St. Louis, Johns Hopkins University, and Case Western Reserve University, primary tumor specimens from 248 consecutive patients with newly diagnosed, p16-positive OPSCC from February 2009 to April 2013 were identified. The tumor's p16 status was determined via immunohistochemistry, using the currently recommended threshold of $\geq 70\%$ of tumor cells positive with nuclear and cytoplasmic staining at a strong (3+) staining level. All cases from each institution were reviewed to confirm the diagnosis of SCC by the respective study pathologists at each institution, and then one representative H&E-stained slide was selected from each case. Whole slides were digitally scanned on a Philips Ultra-Fast Digital Scanner (Philips North America Corporation, Andover, MD; serial no. FMT0099) at 40× magnification (0.25 µm/pixel resolution).

Tumor/Non-tumor Annotations

All digitized whole slide tissue images were hosted on an institutional web-based server, named Bisque [29], and were annotated for tumor-containing regions by one study pathologist (JSL). Figure 6.1 shows the annotated tumor regions overlaid on H&E-stained images. Note that a polygon-style annotation approach was taken by the pathology readers to provide an approximate delineation of the tumor confined region. None of the tumors were exhaustively annotated for all foci of disease. The preparation of negative training samples proceeded similarly, with 30 whole slide tissue images being annotated for regions absent of tumor. To provide an accurate assessment of our approach, the test set consisted of five held-out whole slide images which were exhaustively annotated for tumor presence with precise pixel-level boundary markings.

Deep Learning Model for Tumor Detection

The architecture chosen for this work was a popular 34-layer patch-wise residual convolutional neural network [30] termed ResNet (see Table 6.1 for layout). Each residual block contained two convolutional layers of kernel size (3, 3) with a ReLu activation function and batch normalization [31] between them. Taken together, this architecture resulted in a total of 26 trainable layers with 646,353 trainable parameters. The Adam optimization algorithm with binary cross-entropy loss from Keras [32], with a TensorFlow backend, was used for training.

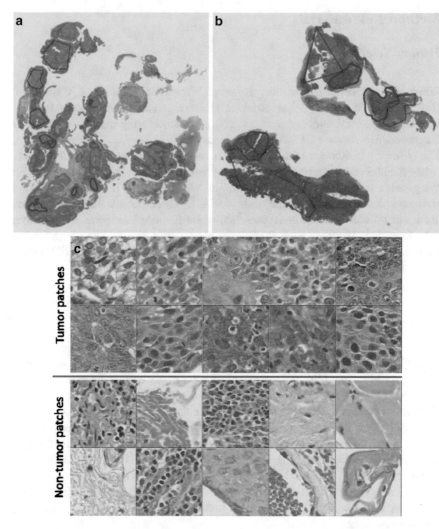

Fig. 6.1 (**a**) and (**b**) Two exemplary annotated tumor regions (red) and non-tumor regions (blue), overlaid on H&E-stained images. (**c**) Example of tumor and non-tumor patches extracted from (red) and (green) regions, which were used for training the model

In this study, all the WSIs were scanned at 40× magnification, and the associated annotations were made at 40× magnification. Considering the computational efficiency and model accuracy, we down-sampled the images to 20× (0.5 μm/pixel) and extracted image patches of size 128 by 128 pixels of the annotated tumor and non-tumor regions for training the model. Image patches that contained white background, or insufficient tissue (patches containing less than 50% of tissue area), were excluded.

Image data augmentation is an efficient way to reduce overfitting on models by increasing the amount and diversity of the training data [32, 33]. During the training process, patches were augmented via random left-right flipping and rotation by 90°

Table 6.1 Description of the tumor detection model (ResNet). It is a 34-layer cascaded CNN model. Each residual block contains two convolutional layers of kernel size (3, 3) with a ReLu activation function and batch normalization between them. Max pooling layer down-sampled the input representation to obtain an abstraction of the underlying image. The dropout (32) is used to prevent overfitting by randomly ignoring a certain portion of parameters to be updated

Layer no.	Layer description
1	Input layer
2–3	Residual block of 16 feature maps
4–5	Residual block of 16 feature maps
6	Max pooling layer of size (2, 2)
	Dropout 10%
7–8	Residual block of 32 feature maps
9–10	Residual block of 32 feature maps
11	Max pooling layer of size (2, 2)
	Dropout 10%
12–13	Residual block of 64 feature maps
14–15	Residual block of 64 feature maps
16	Max pooling layer of size (2, 2)
	Dropout 10%
17–18	Residual block of 64 feature maps
19–20	Residual block of 64 feature maps
21	Max pooling layer of size (2, 2)
	Dropout 10%
22–23	Residual block of 64 feature maps
24–25	Residual block of 64 feature maps
26	Max pooling layer of size (2, 2)
	Dropout 10%
27–28	Residual block of 64 feature maps
29–30	Residual block of 64 feature maps
31	Max pooling layer of size (2, 2)
	Flattening layer converting the tensor to a vector
32	Dense layer of 64 nodes with ReLu activation
33	Dense layer of one node with sigmoid activation
34	Output layer

as histology images do not have a canonical orientation. To compensate for possible stain differences during the slide preparation process, patches were additionally augmented by perturbing their brightness and contrast.

The image brightness of a patch was adjusted by a random factor between [−0.5, 0.5], in which negative/positive factors make the image darker/lighter, respectively. Contrast adjustment similarly proceeded with a random factor between [0.3, 2], in which higher values result in higher contrast between the lightest and darkest portions of an image.

Tumor/Non-tumor Annotations

A flowchart depicting the construction and evaluation of our tumor detection model is shown in Fig. 6.2. A cohort of 243 WSIs with tumor annotations was used to train and validate the model to recognize the tumor region in the image. This cohort was

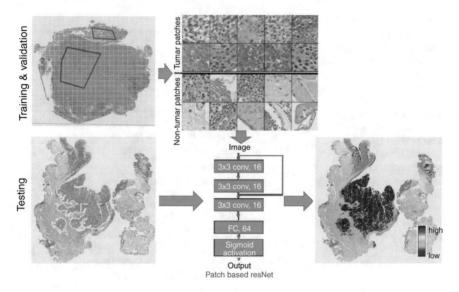

Fig. 6.2 The overall flowchart of the tumor detection model construction and evaluation. A set of 243 WSIs were used for training and validation purpose, in which the tumor and non-tumor patches were extracted from the annotated regions and fed into the ResNet model. In the testing phase, five independent WSIs were used to evaluate the tumor segmentation performance

divided into 80% ($n = 194$) training and 20% ($n = 49$) validation sets. The annotated regions in the WSIs were cropped and subsequently split into non-overlapping image patches of 128 × 128 pixels resulting in 1,894,928 training patches and 210,737 validation patches. The model was then trained for 100 epochs with the validation set being employed at the end of each epoch to track model convergence. The final model was selected in a way to minimize the error on the validation set (epoch number 78) and was subsequently locked down. The model was then evaluated using sensitivity, specificity, and accuracy as metrics on the five held-out WSI test images. These test images were exhaustively annotated for all tumors.

Results and Discussion

On the validation set ($n = 49$), the model yielded an 88.53% sensitivity, a 91.56% specificity, and a 90.04% accuracy. These performance metrics reflect the pixel-level detection accuracy with respect to the manually delineated ground-truth cancer masks from the pathologist. On the held-out testing set ($n = 5$), the model yielded an 81.36% sensitivity, a 95.14% specificity, and an 88.25% accuracy. Three representative test images are shown in Fig. 6.3 where the first column displays the patch-wise probability of tumor presence (note: only probabilities >0.5 were shown) of the ResNet classifier and the second column shows the corresponding manually produced ground truth of tumor extent. Most of the tumor regions appear to have been successfully delineated by the model, as evidenced both visually and quantitatively. A few regions appeared to be false-positive regions (green arrows in Fig. 6.3). We checked the "false-positive" regions generated by the deep learning model and found that a portion of these regions appear to be normal epithelium tissue which is

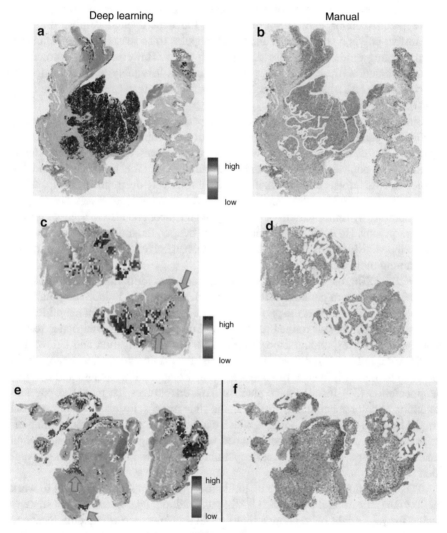

Fig. 6.3 Qualitative comparison between the patch-wise tumor detection model output (left column) and the manual annotation (right column) on the testing images. The tumor heat maps are overlaid on top of the image (note: only probabilities >0.5 were shown). Most of the tumor regions appear to be successfully delineated by the model; green arrows indicate the false-positive regions compared to the manually annotated tumor regions

similar in appearance to the cancer region. Additionally, more than half of these "false-positive" regions were indeed genuine tumor regions that were unintentionally missed by the annotator. In other words, most of these were "false-negative" ground-truthing errors by the expert reader.

In this study, two kinds of annotations were prepared: one involved non-exhaustive polygon shape annotation which requires less time to obtain and the second set of annotations were more exhaustive and labor intensive and yielded more precise tumor delineation. Based on the experimental results, the non-exhaustive polygon shape-based annotation appears to be reasonable for training a deep learning model for disease detection on WSIs. However, when it comes to model evaluation, the performance of the model is inevitably underestimated on account of the lack of sufficient granularity associated with the ground-truth annotation on a per-pixel basis.

Since we have a fairly large number of patches for training a model, nearly 2,000,000 patches at 20× magnification (not accounting for the augmentation patches), we chose a popular network architecture, ResNet [30]. This model at median size comprises 646,353 trainable parameters. The rationale behind the choice of ResNet was that we wanted to use a relatively deep model, compared to the traditional AlexNet [24] which contains five convolutional layers [19, 24], to learn complexity tumor pattern of oropharyngeal cancer and also to account for the stain variations. However, as the network goes deeper, the training becomes harder due to the vanishing gradient problem [30]. ResNet solves this problem and makes the training more efficient.

We chose 20× magnification as the image resolution for training the model since our goal was to learn patterns of the tumor in detail and thus reduce computational complexity. We found that the performance of a model trained at 40× magnification was comparable to that trained at 20× magnification and achieved better results compared to corresponding models trained at 10× magnification and below. The WSIs were collected from two different sites; thus stain variation was present. In order to avoid the influence of stain variation, we applied brightness and contrast augmentation [34] for all image patches. This encourages the model to pay less attention to color-specific information in the slide images. Instead it encourages the model to focus on learning patterns which can better discriminate tumor from non-tumor regions. In fact, our model trained with color augmentation resulted in an accuracy of 90% compared to corresponding models trained without augmentation (86%).

This study did, however, have its limitations: (i) by employing a model to work at 20× magnification, the approach is still computationally expensive. One strategy going forward might be to adopt a multi-resolution approach where only locations identified as suspicious at much lower magnifications are interrogated at 20× [35]. (ii) The test set only comprised five WSIs. Clearly before this approach can be deployed in a clinical context, much larger independent multisite testing is warranted.

Perspectives and Future Directions

In this study, we presented an automated tumor detection model for p16+ oropharyngeal squamous cell carcinomas using H&E-stained whole slide images. The tumor detection model yielded an accuracy of about 90% in both of the validation and test cohorts. A notable takeaway of this study is the fact that the high accuracy was achieved by using a training set comprised of non-exhaustive polygon shape annotations of the tumor. Such an accurate and efficient tumor detection model could be used for early detection of disease and the prediction of aggressiveness in OPSCC, which could improve the patients' survival to manage their therapeutic strategies appropriately. One future work will entail coupling this automated tumor detection approach with downstream quantitative histomorphometric-based digital biomarker for risk stratification and prognosis prediction.

References

1. Yom SS, Gillison ML, Trotti AM. Dose de-escalation in human papillomavirus-associated oropharyngeal cancer: first tracks on powder. Int J Radiat Oncol Biol Phys. 2015;93(5):986–8.
2. Bera K, Schalper K, Rimm D, Velcheti V, Madabhushi A. Artificial intelligence in digital pathology: New tools for diagnosis and precision oncology. Nat Rev Clin Oncol. 2019;16:703; Accepted.
3. Lu C, Lewis JS, Dupont WD, Plummer WD, Janowczyk A, Madabhushi A. An oral cavity squamous cell carcinoma quantitative histomorphometric-based image classifier of nuclear morphology can risk stratify patients for disease-specific survival. Mod Pathol. 2017;30:1655.
4. Vamathevan J, Clark D, Czodrowski P, Dunham I, Ferran E, Lee G, et al. Applications of machine learning in drug discovery and development. Nat Rev Drug Discov. 2019;18(6):463–77.
5. Campanella G, Hanna MG, Geneslaw L, Miraflor A, Silva VWK, Busam KJ, et al. Clinical-grade computational pathology using weakly supervised deep learning on whole slide images. Nat Med. 2019;25(8):1301–9.
6. Li Y, Bai S, Carroll W, Dayan D, Dort JC, Heller K, et al. Validation of the risk model: high-risk classification and tumor pattern of invasion predict outcome for patients with low-stage oral cavity squamous cell carcinoma. Head Neck Pathol. 2013;7(3):211–23.
7. Barletta JA, Yeap BY, Chirieac LR. Prognostic significance of grading in lung adenocarcinoma. Cancer. 2010;116(3):659–69.
8. Chang Y-C, Nieh S, Chen S-F, Jao S-W, Lin Y-L, Fu E. Invasive pattern grading score designed as an independent prognostic indicator in oral squamous cell carcinoma: Invasive pattern grading score in OSCC. Histopathology. 2010;57(2):295–303.
9. Lee G, Veltri RW, Zhu G, Ali S, Epstein JI, Madabhushi A. Nuclear shape and architecture in benign fields predict biochemical recurrence in prostate cancer patients following radical prostatectomy: preliminary findings. Eur Urol Focus. 2016;3:457.
10. Corredor G, Wang X, Zhou Y, Lu C, Fu P, Syrigos K, et al. Spatial architecture and arrangement of tumor-infiltrating lymphocytes for predicting likelihood of recurrence in early-stage non-small cell lung cancer. Clin Cancer Res. 2019;25(5):1526–34.
11. Lu C, Romo-Bucheli D, Wang X, Janowczyk A, Ganesan S, Gilmore H, et al. Nuclear shape and orientation features from H&E images predict survival in early-stage estrogen receptor-positive breast cancers. Lab Invest [Internet]. 2018 [cited 2018 Jul 30]; Available from: http://www.nature.com/articles/s41374-018-0095-7.

12. Lu C, Wang X, Prasanna P, Corredor G, Sedor G, Bera K, et al. Feature driven local cell graph (FeDeG): predicting overall survival in early stage lung cancer. In: Medical image computing and computer assisted intervention – MICCAI 2018 – 21st International Conference, 2018, Proceedings [Internet]. Springer Verlag; 2018 [cited 2019 Jan 1]. p. 407–16. Available from: https://cwru.pure.elsevier.com/en/publications/feature-driven-local-cell-graph-fedeg-predicting-overall-survival.

13. Beck AH, Sangoi AR, Leung S, Marinelli RJ, Nielsen TO, van de Vijver MJ, et al. Systematic analysis of breast cancer morphology uncovers stromal features associated with survival. Sci Transl Med. 2011;3(108):108–13.

14. Yuan Y. Modelling the spatial heterogeneity and molecular correlates of lymphocytic infiltration in triple-negative breast cancer. J R Soc Interface. 2015;12(103):20141153.

15. Lewis JS, Ali S, Luo J, Thorstad WL, Madabhushi A. A quantitative histomorphometric classifier (QuHbIC) identifies aggressive versus indolent p16-positive oropharyngeal squamous cell carcinoma. Am J Surg Pathol. 2014;38(1):128–37.

16. Fedorov A, Penzkofer T, Hirsch MS, Flood TA, Vangel MG, Masry P, et al. The role of pathology correlation approach in prostate cancer index lesion detection and quantitative analysis with multiparametric MRI. Acad Radiol. 2015;22(5):548–55.

17. Haas GP, Delongchamps NB, Jones RF, Chandan V, Serio AM, Vickers AJ, et al. Needle biopsies on autopsy prostates: sensitivity of cancer detection based on true prevalence. J Natl Cancer Inst. 2007;99(19):1484–9.

18. Wang D, Khosla A, Gargeya R, Irshad H, Beck AH. Deep learning for identifying metastatic breast cancer. arXiv:160605718 [cs, q-bio] [Internet]. 2016 [cited 2019 Sep 14]; Available from: http://arxiv.org/abs/1606.05718.

19. Cruz-Roa A, Gilmore H, Basavanhally A, Feldman M, Ganesan S, Shih NNC, et al. Accurate and reproducible invasive breast cancer detection in whole-slide images: a deep learning approach for quantifying tumor extent. Sci Rep. 2017;7:46450.

20. Janowczyk A, Madabhushi A. Deep learning for digital pathology image analysis: a comprehensive tutorial with selected use case. J Pathol Inform. 2016;7:29.

21. Monaco JP, Tomaszewski JE, Feldman MD, Hagemann I, Moradi M, Mousavi P, et al. High-throughput detection of prostate cancer in histological sections using probabilistic pairwise Markov models. Med Image Anal. 2010;14(4):617–29.

22. Janowczyk A, Madabhushi A. Deep learning for digital pathology image analysis: A comprehensive tutorial with selected use cases. J Pathol Inform [Internet]. 2016 [cited 2017 Aug 7];7. Available from: http://www.ncbi.nlm.nih.gov/pmc/articles/PMC4977982/.

23. Bychkov D, Linder N, Turkki R, Nordling S, Kovanen PE, Verrill C, et al. Deep learning based tissue analysis predicts outcome in colorectal cancer. Sci Rep. 2018;8(1):3395.

24. Krizhevsky A, Sutskever I, Hinton GE. ImageNet classification with deep convolutional neural networks. Commun ACM. 2017;60(6):84–90.

25. Cruz-Roa A, Basavanhally A, González F, Gilmore H, Feldman M, Ganesan S, et al. Automatic detection of invasive ductal carcinoma in whole slide images with convolutional neural networks. In: Gurcan MN, Madabhushi A, editors. 2014 [cited 2016 Sep 6]. p. 904103. Available from: http://proceedings.spiedigitallibrary.org/proceeding.aspx?doi=10.1117/12.2043872.

26. Esteva A, Kuprel B, Novoa RA, Ko J, Swetter SM, Blau HM, et al. Dermatologist-level classification of skin cancer with deep neural networks. Nature. 2017;542(7639):115–8.

27. Xie P, Zuo K, Zhang Y, Li F, Yin M, Lu K. Interpretable classification from skin cancer histology slides using deep learning: a retrospective multicenter study. arXiv:190406156 [cs, q-bio] [Internet]. 2019 12 [cited 2019 Sep 14]; Available from: http://arxiv.org/abs/1904.06156.

28. Lu C, Mandal M. Automated analysis and diagnosis of skin melanoma on whole slide histopathological images. Pattern Recogn. 2015;48(8):2738–50.

29. Kvilekval K, Fedorov D, Obara B, Singh A, Manjunath BS. Bisque: a platform for bioimage analysis and management. Bioinformatics. 2010;26(4):544–52.

30. He K, Zhang X, Ren S, Sun J. Deep residual learning for image recognition. In: 2016 IEEE conference on computer vision and pattern recognition (CVPR). 2016. p. 770–8.

31. Ioffe S, Szegedy C. Batch normalization: accelerating deep network training by reducing internal covariate shift. In: Proceedings of the 32nd international conference on international conference on machine learning – Volume 37. 2015. p. 448–56.
32. Chollet, Francois and others. Keras [Internet]. 2015. Available from: https://keras.io.
33. Hinton GE, Srivastava N, Krizhevsky A, Sutskever I, Salakhutdinov RR. Improving neural networks by preventing co-adaptation of feature detectors. arXiv:12070580 [cs] [Internet]. 2012 [cited 2019 Sep 4]; Available from: http://arxiv.org/abs/1207.0580.
34. Perez L, Wang J. The effectiveness of data augmentation in image classification using deep learning. arXiv:171204621 [cs] [Internet]. 2017 [cited 2019 Sep 12]; Available from: http://arxiv.org/abs/1712.04621.
35. Doyle S, Feldman M, Tomaszewski J, Madabhushi A. A boosted Bayesian multiresolution classifier for prostate cancer detection from digitized needle biopsies. IEEE Trans Biomed Eng. 2012;59(5):1205–18.

Chapter 7
Salivary Biomarkers for Non-invasive Early Detection of Head and Neck Cancer

Shilpa Kusampudi and Nagarjun Konduru

Introduction

The gold standard for tumor detection and its genetic profiling involves the use of tissue biopsies. The limitations associated with tissue biopsies include their invasive nature, patient risk, sample preparation, procedural costs, and sensitivity in detecting a tumor. The accuracy of various biopsy modalities is affected by a lack of ability to cover the clinical heterogeneity spectrum [2].

Due to the inherent limitations of tissue biopsies, current research in cancer diagnostics is striving toward the development and use of liquid biopsies for tumor detection. Liquid biopsies use relatively accessible biological sources such as blood, urine, saliva, stool, pleural effusions, and cerebrospinal fluid [2, 3]. Tumor-derived genetic information for cancer diagnosis, screening, and prognosis is obtained while performing liquid biopsy from circulating tumor cells (CTCs), circulating tumor DNA (ctDNA), and exosomes [1]. Establishment of liquid biopsies would enable early tumor detection, monitoring, and recognition of resistance mutations.

Liquid biopsies analyze circulating tumor-derived material, which is called the *tumor circulome*. Tumor circulome includes circulating tumor proteins, ctDNA, CTCs, tumor-derived extracellular vehicles (EVs), and their constituents, including circulating tumor (ct) RNAs and tumor-educated platelets (TEPs) (Fig. 7.1). ctDNA provides information on mutations, deletions, gene amplification, methylation patterns, and translocations. CTCs are a rich source of genomic, proteomic, transcriptomic, and cytogenetic information and can be cultured ex vivo. EVs provide a molecular fingerprint for the tumor cells based on origin. DNA, RNA, and protein (both surface and intraluminal) of EVs serve as cancer biomarkers. These molecular constituents (nanobiopsies) of the EVs reflect the makeup of the tumor cell and

S. Kusampudi · N. Konduru (✉)
Department of Cellular and Molecular Biology, University of Texas Health Science Center at Tyler, Tyler, TX, USA
e-mail: nagarjun.konduruvenkata@uthct.edu

© Springer Nature Switzerland AG 2021
R. El Assal et al. (eds.), *Early Detection and Treatment of Head & Neck Cancers*, https://doi.org/10.1007/978-3-030-69859-1_7

149

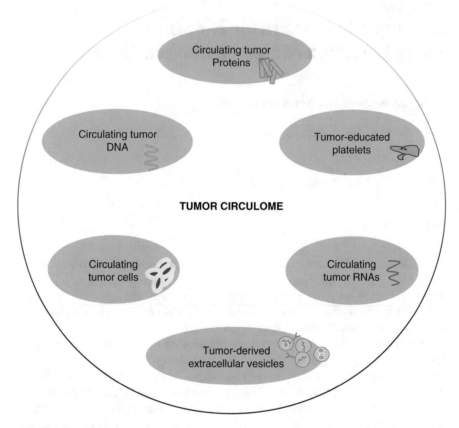

Fig. 7.1 Components of tumor circulome

origin. ctRNAs include micro-(mi)RNA expression panels, long non-coding (lnc) RNA expression, and circulating RNA associated with EV. They provide quantitative biomarker information such as tumor-specific alternative splicing and gene fusions. TEPs contain tumor-derived RNAs and tumor-induced, alternatively spliced transcripts and, hence, act as a source of biomarker information [2].

The first significant milestone in this field was reached with the US Food and Drug Administration (FDA) approval for ctDNA and CTCs [2]. Lung cancer diagnosis through liquid biopsy using ctDNA was approved in 2016 by the US FDA [4]. The main drawback with CTCs, however, is the need for extremely sensitive and specific approaches for their detection and analyses [5]. In head and neck oncology, development of non-invasive diagnostic tools is a challenge. Circulating tumor derivatives such as ctDNA, CTC, and exosomes in a patient's blood are explored for analysis [6–8]. Research on biological activity and molecular function of EVs has been scant in head and neck cancers (HNCs) [9]. Therefore, this chapter would discuss the role of EVs in the diagnosis of HNC.

Patients with HNC are often diagnosed at an advanced stage of the disease. The HNC burden is measured through sophisticated imaging and clinical examination, but there is a dearth of available biomarkers. Implementation of a liquid biopsy through serial blood sampling has the potential to detect metastatic events at the earliest stages in HNC and, therefore, would enable monitoring of ongoing treatments and residual disease posttreatment [8, 10].

Extracellular Vesicles

EVs include different vesicles based on their biogenesis and release pathway, such as exosomes, microvesicles (MVs) (deciduous MVs, particles, ectosomes), shedding MVs, apoptotic blebs, virus particles, virus-like particles, and oncosomes [9, 11]. EVs have a diameter ranging between 30 and 1000 nm [12]. They are known to carry mRNA, miRNA, DNA, protein, lipids, membrane lipids, membrane proteins, cytoskeletal proteins, protein chaperones, and virus miRNA [9]. EVs are easy to isolate from plasma [13], urine [14], cerebrospinal fluid [15], amniotic membrane fluid [16], bronchoalveolar lavage fluid [17], synovial fluid [18], malignant ascites [19], breast milk [20], and saliva [21].

EVs are involved in various cellular processes such as intercellular communication, cellular homeostasis, coagulation, and waste management and have specialized functions [22]. These vesicles have also been reported to influence recombination of the extracellular matrix as well as angiopoiesis. They also create a microenvironment that helps in transformation and transferring of tumor cells, leading to cancer drug resistance and metastasis [9, 23]. The potential of EVs as a novel source for biomarkers in diagnosis, prognosis, and therapy in modern preventive and precision medicine has been discussed by several researchers [9, 24, 25]. The properties and functional mechanisms of some EVs, such as exosomes, deciduous MVs, ectosomes, particles, virus particles, virus-like particles, and oncosomes, are not entirely elucidated [9].

Two main types of EVs include exosomes and MVs. Both vesicle types are membranous high-density vesicles which exhibit similarity in cytoskeletal proteins, membrane lipids, and external phosphatidylserine composition, but the vesicular structures exhibit differences in morphology, shape, size, density, and their biogenesis [9, 26].

Exosomes

These small lipid bilayer membrane vesicles with diameters ranging from 40 to 150 nm [27, 28] exhibit an enriched surface of proteins, including components of the endosomal sorting complexes required for transport complexes (ESCRT complexes); fusion and transport proteins (Rab GTPases, annexins, and flotillin), some of which are involved in multivesicular endosome (MVE) biogenesis (e.g., Alix and Tsg101); integrins; tetraspanins (CD9, CD63, CD81, CD82); and heat shock proteins (HSP70, HSP90) [28–30]. The presence of exosomes in the tumor microenvironment suggests their importance in tumorigenesis, tumor invasion, and metastasis since they can act as promoters of tumor progression or possess an anti-tumor function [28, 31]. Based on the mode of biogenesis, cell type, and physiological conditions, exosomes are a source of numerous types of cell-derived biological molecules, such as proteins, lipids, mRNAs, miRNAs, lncRNAs, genomic DNA, cDNA, and mitochondrial DNA (mtDNA) [32] (Table 7.1). Exosomes can be released abundantly by different types of cells into the body fluids, such as amniotic fluid, ascites, bile, blood, breast milk, cerebrospinal fluid, lymph, semen, saliva, tears, and urine, in both healthy and diseased conditions [33]. Exosomes form when MVEs fuse with the cytomembrane after inward budding of MVEs via regulation of various signal molecules (Fig. 7.2). Exosome protein components vary from cell tissues to a large extent, and they share some standard essential components consistent with the cellular tissues from which they are mostly derived. Exosomes recognize and fuse with recipient cells specifically, transport autologous substances into them, and lead to changes in biological function [9].

Microvesicles

MVs form as cytomembrane blisters outward [34] through changes in the intracellular calcium ion concentration and cytoskeletal reconstitution. They have diameters ranging between 100 and 1000 nm [9, 34]. The formation of MVs depends on

Table 7.1 Differences between exosomes and microvesicles

	Exosomes	Microvesicles
Origin	Endocytic pathway	Plasma membrane
Formation	Exosomes form when multivesicular endosomes (MVEs) fuse with the cytomembrane after inward budding of MVEs via regulation of various signal molecules	Microvesicle (MV) formation depends on the activation of cell surface receptors, and cytomembrane blisters outward to form MVs through changes in the intracellular calcium ion concentration and cytoskeletal reconstitution
Size	40–150 nm	100–1000 nm
Markers	ESCRT complexes; Rab GTPases, annexins, and flotillin; Alix and Tsg101; integrins; CD9, CD63, CD81, and CD82; and HSP70 and HSP90	Phosphatidylserines, integrins, selectins, and CD40 ligands
Differential centrifugation	100,000 g	10,000 g

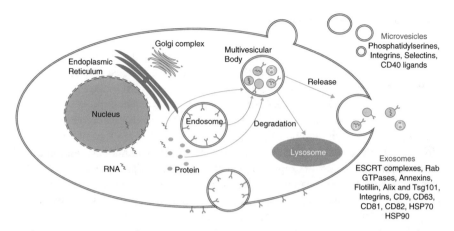

Fig. 7.2 Biogenesis of exosomes and microvesicles

the activation of cell surface receptors, and their dynamic molecular organizations depend on the cell type and its activated state. Phosphatidylserines, integrins, selectins, and CD40 ligands are the surface markers distinguishing them based on cell origin [9, 29] (Table 7.1 and Fig. 7.2).

The significance of human tumor-derived vesicles (TDVs) in the diagnosis of several types of cancers, including breast, lung, ovarian, prostate, colon, and gastric cancer, has been reported [9]. However, based on the source of the extracted body fluids, TDVs have different properties, such as their complexity, range, and viscosity. They include exosomes and MVs secreted via different kinds of cells, including malignant cells, healthy cells, and immune cells.

Differential centrifugation is the most common method for extraction of exosomes and MVs. The initial step involves removal of cell debris and contaminants followed by either 10,000 g or 100,000 g high-speed centrifugation to obtain MVs or exosomes, respectively [29, 35]. The body fluids and cell culture supernatants are generally contaminated by other apoptotic vesicles, cell debris, and protein aggregates; hence, additional filtering steps post centrifugation or density gradient centrifugation are performed [9, 36]. As MVs also have 100 nm size range which overlaps with the size range of exosomes (40–150 nm) [29, 37], confirmatory tests need to be performed [38]. The identification of biomarkers specific for exosomes and MVs has allowed efficient differentiation and purification of the two EVs. The identity of the isolated EV type is further confirmed through immunoblotting, mass spectrometry, and imaging techniques. Recent advances in technology also allow separation and quantification of exosomes and MVs via high-throughput analysis of immunolabeled vesicles using a high-resolution flow cytometry-based method, which was not possible using the conventional flow cytometers, as they could separate only vesicles smaller than 300 nm [29].

Diagnosis of Head and Neck Cancers

Cancers of the head and neck are among the top 10 cancers occurring globally based on the 2018 GLOBOCAN data, and their incidences are increasing every year. The term HNC refers to many anatomical sites of occurrence, such as the lip, oral cavity, salivary glands, oropharynx, nasopharynx, hypopharynx, paranasal sinus, and larynx. The two most common HNCs are oral cavity squamous cell carcinoma (SCC) and oropharyngeal carcinoma [9]. Though lifestyle factors are a common cause of HNC, viral infections can also cause these cancers [9], with human papillomavirus (HPV) commonly causing oropharyngeal carcinoma and Epstein-Barr virus (EBV) causing nasopharyngeal carcinoma. Exosomes are used by cancer cells and virus-infected cells to regulate the microenvironment, and viruses possibly use exosomes to spread infection and escape acquired immunity [9].

HNCs are mostly diagnosed at an advanced stage due to the lack of awareness about the early symptoms, which are often confused with benign disorders leading to delayed diagnosis and higher mortality rates. Contemplating the challenge associated with diagnosis of HNC, there is a strong rationale to consider exosomes as potential diagnostic markers for HNC. Protocols need to be further optimized to isolate and purify exosomes via non-invasive methods. As liquid biopsy samples are mostly viscous, depletion of albumin from urine or serum samples and dilution of viscous specimens, such as plasma and saliva, are considered [39]. The source of the exosomes and their role in HNC is outlined in Table 7.2.

Table 7.2 Source of exosome

Sample source of EVs	EV markers	Cancer	Reference
Serum	FasL+ microvesicles	OCSS	[40]
Serum	LMP1	EBV-infected nasopharynx cancer	[41]
Plasma of patients	Galectin-9	Nasopharynx cancers	[42]
Blood, plasma	BART miRNA	Nasopharynx cancer cells	[43]
Serum	CD63	Laryngeal carcinomas	[44]
Serum	miR-21 and HOTAIR	Laryngeal carcinoma lymph node metastasis	[44]
Saliva	PD-L1	Oral cancers	[45]
Serum	miR-24-3p	Nasopharyngeal carcinoma	[46]
Plasma	MMP13-containing exosomes	Nasopharyngeal carcinoma	[47]
Saliva	miR-196a/b	HNSCC	[48]
Peripheral blood	Viral BART miRNAs	Nasopharyngeal carcinoma	[43]
Plasma	PD-L1	HNC	[49]
Blood	miR-21, miR-205, and miR-148b	Hypoxic oral cavity SCC	[50]
Saliva	CD63	Oral cancer	[51]

Micro-RNAs

miRNAs are small non-coding RNA of 18–24 base pairs and are the most common genetic material in exosomes. Cancer researchers consider miRNA as a new promising class of potential diagnostic biomarkers due to their association with almost all kinds of cancers [9, 52, 53]. miRNA is regarded as an essential regulator of mRNA and protein expression, and it is actively secreted into the extracellular environment and within exosomes [54]. miRNAs are produced by apoptotic and necrotic cells at times. They are thought to play an important role in cell-to-cell communication. miRNAs exhibit tumor suppression and affect oncogenes [55]. For example, miR-21 is one of the most common miRNAs in human cancers; it can suppress apoptosis genes and PTEN, thus increasing the survival rates of cells [9].

Upon exposure to salivary ribonucleases, endogenous salivary miRNA degrades at a slower rate in comparison to non-salivary miRNA [56, 57], as miRNAs are packed in exosomes, which protect miRNAs against degradation [58, 59].

Protection of circulatory miRNA against degradation is proposed by forming ribonucleoprotein complexes (i.e., with AGO2 or HDL proteins) or by being incorporated into extracellular vesicles, such as apoptotic bodies, shedding vesicles, and exosomes [60]. Also, circulating miRNAs encapsulated in MVs are protected against the activity of the RNases present in the blood, representing a more reliable method for evaluating circulating tumor miRNA signatures [33, 61].

Saliva as a Source of Biomarkers for Diagnosis of HNC

In cancer biomarker research, it is essential to use standardized methods that allow for multiple collections with minimum variability and fluctuations, thereby facilitating early diagnosis, monitoring of disease progression, or treatment response [62]. The methods of sample collection also influence the proteomic screening for biomarkers [39].

Saliva is preferred for biomarker studies due to its ease of collection [63], and detection of secreted molecules directly from the saliva of patients with HNC provides opportunities toward the development of non-invasive diagnostics. However, using saliva for diagnosis has its limitations. The concentration of biomarkers and the composition of saliva may be influenced by circadian fluctuations [64], or it may vary based on the method of saliva collection [65]. The oral microenvironment and patient conditions mostly influence the protein composition of whole saliva. These hurdles limit the use of saliva in the circumstances requiring multiple sample collections for disease monitoring. Therefore, sample collection from individual salivary glands would provide specific information for the examination of particular gland diseases. In the case of the salivary exosome, viscosity and cellular contamination of the whole saliva (WS) versus glandular saliva make it a less than ideal medium for exosomal isolation [39].

Saliva is a biological fluid that originates from three pairs of major salivary glands located near the upper posterior teeth (parotid), under the tongue (sublingual, SL), and on the floor of the mouth (submandibular, SM) [66]. Saliva is a complex mixture consisting of 99% water and less than 1% proteins (i.e., immunoglobulins, hydrolases, mucins), lipids, carbohydrates, electrolytes, and other low-molecular-weight components (e.g., urea and ammonia) [67].

WS is a combination of secretions produced from the parotids and SM and SL glands. The parotids produce serous secretions, whereas the SM and SL glands produce mixed secretions that are both serous and mucinous. Of the proteins found in saliva, 65% are synthesized from the SM glands [68], and 20–30% are transported from blood capillaries into the saliva [69]. WS consists of proteins such as amylase, mucins, histatins, and cystatins, microorganisms, cellular debris, gingival crevicular fluid (GCF), and serum components [39, 70].

Saliva collection is a relatively simple and non-invasive procedure and can be performed in two different ways: unstimulated WS (UWS) and stimulated WS (SWS). UWS is collected by spitting, suction, drool, or swab, whereas the SWS is obtained using a stimulant, such as citric acid, or with the reflex masticatory response of a standardized bolus (e.g., paraffin or a gum base) [70]. The yield of SWS is threefold higher in volume compared to UWS [71]. The two methods of saliva collection (UWS and SWS) exhibit differences in protein ratios, ions, and water content that might give rise to the discovery of different biomarker subsets [39]. UWS is used majorly for diagnostic biomarker studies. The main advantage of UWS is that it is less influenced by salivary gland function and provides a more precise reflection of an equilibrated state with the systemic clinical condition [39]. In contrast, SWS is less suitable for diagnostic applications due to the use of a stimulant agent which changes salivary composition (i.e., pH) and might dilute the biomarker concentration as a result of increased water production in the saliva [72]. However, the use of SWS for diagnosis is suggested to allow biomarker detection, and this field is still evolving [39, 73].

Investigation of saliva as an alternative biological matrix remains a potentially useful paradigm in oral cavity SCC due to the direct contact with the diseased tissue. Early diagnosis of HNC would improve survival; hence, the use of salivary biomarkers may help in early-stage tumor detection. Because of the ready availability of saliva and ease in processing, a saliva-based diagnostic approach would be advantageous in understanding the molecular basis of oral diseases [39].

Salivary Markers in HNC

Mass spectrometry-based salivary proteomic analyses have been applied to HNC [74], and so far more than 3000 proteins have been identified in saliva [39, 72, 75].

- It has been observed that during HNC, alpha-1-B glycoprotein and complement factor B were found to be present in patients, but not in healthy controls [62].

- Salivary endothelin levels [76] and fibrin, S100 calcium-binding protein, trans-ferrin, Ig heavy chain constant region, and cofilin-1 levels increased in saliva of patients with head and neck (HN) SCC in comparison to the control group [77]. The differences in protein expression are associated with tumor progression and metastasis, making it a potential tool in monitoring patients at risk for oral neo-plasms [39].
- Soluble CD44 is the most promising candidate in the detection of HNSCC and can differentiate between malignant and benign lesions [78].
- Cytokeratin 19 fragment (Cyfra21-1), tissue polypeptide-specific antigen (TPS), and cancer antigen 125 (CA-125) levels increase by fourfold in the saliva of patients with oral cavity SCC [39, 79].

Saliva is a compound fluid containing several proteins (amylase ~60%) [80], proline-rich proteins (acidic, basic, and glycosylated), statherins, and histatins [81]. These abundant proteins may mask the important biomarkers present at rela-tively low concentrations [39, 77]. Salivary exosomes are believed to overcome this problem in oral tumors. The exosome/MV subfraction reduces the complexity of the whole fluid and also enriches the cancer-specific antigen concentration. Saliva is expected to be enriched with tumor-secreted biomarkers as a result of direct contact with both premalignant and malignant oral neoplasms. Moreover, tumor cells shed salivary vesicles containing oncogenic surface molecules such as CD44 and CD95L, which are even soluble in saliva and serve as HNC biomark-ers [39].

Zlotogorski-Hurvitz et al. (2019) conducted a study to determine the Fourier-transform infrared (FTIR) spectra of salivary exosomes from patients with oral can-cer and healthy individuals (HI) as infrared (IR) spectroscopy is a non-destructive method that can investigate solid tissues, fluids, and cells [82]. It acts on the prin-ciple of vibrating molecular bonds, and the resulting absorption wavelengths, which depend on the involved atoms and the strength of intermolecular interactions, deter-mine the chemical profile of a specific material. FTIR spectroscopy coupled with computational methods can provide fingerprint spectra of benign tissues and their counterpart malignant tumors with a high rate of accuracy [83–85]. Oral cancer sali-vary exosomes display a specific IR spectral signature, which is distinguished from HI exosomes based on subtle changes in the conformations of biomolecules such as proteins, lipids, and nucleic acids. This non-invasive method should be further investigated for the diagnosis of oral cancer at its very early stages or in oral lesions with potential for malignant transformation [82].

Characterization of MVs and Exosomes in Saliva

As stated above, saliva is said to be an ideal fluid for oral cancer diagnostics [86]. Exosome isolation from saliva has been optimized [87, 88], and this small fraction reduces the overall complexity of oral fluid caused due to local and systemic sources

[89]. Non-neoplastic epithelial cells from salivary glands release exosomes [90], and constitutive exosome production has also been reported in cultures of various neoplastic cells [27].

Due to the versatile and dynamic nature of the exosomes, pathological conditions have been found to influence the exosome composition. Saliva-derived vesicles of oral cancer show variation in size, density, and CD63 expression in comparison to the saliva of individuals without cancer. Exosomes from individuals with HNSCC range from 20 to 400 nm in size. They exhibit aggregation and display an increased expression of the CD63 membrane marker [51].

Unlike exosomes isolated from urine or blood, large datasets of cancer-derived exosomes from saliva are not available. Proteomic analysis of exosomes derived from saliva reduces the complexity in comparison to WS [91]. Exosomes would be specific in a study involving certain salivary gland disorders, whereas WS would be more informative for oral cancer detection [92]. Fractionation of human WS using gel exclusion chromatography [93] exposed the presence of exosome I and exosome II. Both exosomes display protein markers like CD63, Alix, Tsg101, and HSP70 but differ in size, density, and protein content, reflecting the heterogeneity of salivary exosomes. Ogawa et al. (2011) found exosome I to have an electron-dense structure with larger size in comparison to exosome II [93]. Exosome II has size and shape similar to the exosomes from other sources [93]. These differences in salivary exosomes may imply origin of exosomes from different salivary glands which might be the reason for the variance in the two salivary exosomes [93]. The differences and commonalities of exosome I and II are discussed in Table 7.3. Characterization of salivary vesicles needs to be improved in order to define the function of these vesicles in the oral cavity. Low concentrations of exosomes in saliva stand as a limitation for functional studies with translational applications; on the other hand, the protein yield from MVs is eight times greater than that of exosomes, and both are collected from an equal volume of WS [39, 94].

Though there is a significant overlap of both salivary exosomes and MV proteins, salivary MVs contain specific proteins, which may perhaps be potentially informative for early detection of various oral diseases. Therefore, the identification of promising markers in salivary exosomes or MVs will possibly provide a valid screening tool for early disease onset in oral cancer [39].

As oral cancer is a complex disease, several factors should be considered when investigating oral cancer exosomes in saliva. The tumor site may have a profound impact on the route of entry for cancer exosomes. For example, among tumors on the tonsils, buccal mucosa, and tongue, tonsillar tumor exosomes may not be detectable in the patient's saliva in comparison to tumors on the buccal mucosa or the tongue. Due to the anatomical complexity of the oral compartment, cancer exosomes found in very low abundance at early stages of tumor development pose a challenge to the researchers [95]. Identification of specific early cancer-specific exosomal markers may offer a solution for early cancer detection.

Table 7.3 Differences and commonalities in exosome I and exosome II

	Exosome I	Exosome II	Reference
Average diameter	83.5 nm	40.5 nm	[110]
Exosomal biomarkers	Alix, tumor susceptibility gene 101 (TSG101), and heat shock protein (HSP) 7, immunoglobulin (Ig) A and the polymeric Ig receptor (pIgR), CD63	Alix, tumor susceptibility gene 101 (TSG101), and heat shock protein (HSP) 7, immunoglobulin (Ig) A and the polymeric Ig receptor (pIgR)	[93]
Number of proteins identified	101	154	[93, 110]
Proteins highly expressed	Ezrin, moesin, radixin, Rab GDP dissociation inhibitor β, α-enolase, guanine nucleotide-binding protein Gi/Gs/Gt subunit β-1, and annexins, mucin 5B	DPP IV, carbonic anhydrase 6, cystatin family proteins, IgG, Fc-binding protein, and galectin-3-binding protein	[93, 110]
Moesin expression	Yes	No	[93]
Properties	Proteomic properties	Proteomic properties, exhibit better immunogenicity, metabolically active in cleaving chemokines (CXCL11 and CXCL12), degradation of polypeptides	[93, 110]
Possible origin	Ductal, acinar, or both cell types; sublingual gland, B cells	Ductal, acinar, or both cell types; parotid gland and submandibular glands	[93]
Commonality	Contain cell surface and cytoskeletal proteins; Alix, tumor susceptibility gene 101 (TSG101), and HSP70, immunoglobulin (Ig) A and the polymeric Ig receptor (pIgR), GW182, CD63, actin, DPP IV, and galectin-3 Alpha-amylase and proline-rich proteins were detected in small amount or not detected at all 68 proteins overlap		[93, 110]

Treatment of Cancers Using Exosomes

Exosome-Based Immunotherapy Exosomes of dendritic cell origin have been developed as immunotherapeutic anticancer agents [96].

Exosome Removal for Cancer Therapy Inhibition of exosome formation has been observed using a drug named amiloride [97].

Exosomes as Anticancer Drug Delivery Vehicles Due to the excellent biodistribution and biocompatibility of exosomes, their use as nucleic acid or drug delivery vehicles has gained interest [98]. Exosomes can be utilized as capable vehicles for drug delivery and have been tested to deliver active drugs such as paclitaxel [99, 100].

Exosome-Mediated Delivery of Therapeutic Short Interfering (si) RNA Delivery of siRNA to the target cells induces cell death in recipient cancer cells via effective posttranscriptional gene silencing [101, 102].

A Novel Therapeutic Strategy

siRNA Liquid biopsies provide information about the biomarker mRNAs as cancer cells exhibit increased expression of specific mRNAs. These mRNAs can be blocked by a chosen exosomal siRNA-based targeted therapy [103].

miRNA This highly conserved class of small (18–22 nucleotide) non-coding RNA molecules controls all gene expression through the targeted suppression of mRNA translation [104]. Inhibiting cancer-specific miRNAs with anti-sense oligonucleotides, or mimicking miRNAs with tumor suppressor function, has therefore long been muted as a potential therapeutic strategy in cancer [103].

lncRNA This class of regulatory non-coding RNA that exceeds 200 nucleotides in length acts simultaneously with DNA-binding proteins and other elements to epigenetically regulate DNA transcription [105]. The lncRNAs have been found to participate in crucial biological processes of both physiology and disease, and during malignant transformation, lncRNA expression is found to be dysregulated [106]. Exosomes have been found to contain lncRNAs [107]. Cellular sorting of lncRNAs into exosomes is a highly regulated process, which is disrupted as a response to paracrine signals from the tumor microenvironment [103].

Research Perspective

We are far from fully understanding the fundamental biology of salivary biomarkers; some achievements have been made aiming at developing a device for specific salivary biomarker detection [60]. Protein polymorphisms in saliva and degradation due to protein instability in stored samples have made saliva a difficult source for biomarker research [108], due to low concentrations of saliva substrate (thousand-fold less than those in the blood) [109]. Further research is required to translate salivary diagnostics into routine clinical practice to improve cancer diagnosis and reduce mortality [60].

Identification of biomarkers that predict the onset of HNC or response to therapy is of clinical importance. Exosomal ncRNAs provide relevant biological information on cancer, which would aid in the development of therapies specific to varied types of cancers. Further large-scale and randomized studies are required to better define the potential role of exosomes as diagnostic or prognostic markers for cancer [103]. Salivary exosome would prove to be a perfect source for finding a biomarker that can aid in early detection of oral cancer through a simple saliva test.

References

1. Bai Y, Zhao H. Liquid biopsy in tumors: opportunities and challenges. Ann Transl Med. 2018;6(Suppl 1):S89.
2. De Rubis G, Rajeev Krishnan S, Bebawy M. Liquid biopsies in cancer diagnosis, monitoring, and prognosis. Trends Pharmacol Sci. 2019;40(3):172–86.
3. Siravegna G, Marsoni S, Siena S, Bardelli A. Integrating liquid biopsies into the management of cancer. Nat Rev Clin Oncol. 2017;14(9):531–48.
4. Kwapisz D. The first liquid biopsy test approved. Is it a new era of mutation testing for non-small cell lung cancer? Ann Transl Med. 2017;5(3):46.
5. Christou N, Meyer J, Popeskou S, David V, Toso C, Buchs N, et al. Circulating tumour cells, circulating tumour DNA and circulating tumour miRNA in blood assays in the different steps of colorectal cancer management, a review of the evidence in 2019. Biomed Res Int. 2019;2019:5953036.
6. Ignatiadis M, Lee M, Jeffrey SS. Circulating tumor cells and circulating tumor DNA: challenges and opportunities on the path to clinical utility. Clin Cancer Res. 2015;21(21):4786–800.
7. Gold B, Cankovic M, Furtado LV, Meier F, Gocke CD. Do circulating tumor cells, exosomes, and circulating tumor nucleic acids have clinical utility? A report of the association for molecular pathology. J Mol Diagn. 2015;17(3):209–24.
8. Schmidt H, Kulasinghe A, Kenny L, Punyadeera C. The development of a liquid biopsy for head and neck cancers. Oral Oncol. 2016;61:8–11.
9. Jia YJ, Zhou ML, Zhou SH. Exosomes, microvesicles, and head and neck cancers. Int J Clin Exp Med. 2016;9(8):15040–9.
10. Visacri MB, Ferrari GB, Dias P, Pimentel R, de Souza CM, Costa AP, et al. Quality of life of patients with squamous cell carcinoma of the head and neck receiving high-dose cisplatin chemotherapy and radiotherapy. South Med J. 2015;108(6):343–9.
11. Shah R, Patel T, Freedman JE. Circulating extracellular vesicles in human disease. N Engl J Med. 2018;379(10):958–66.
12. Pap E, Pallinger E, Falus A. The role of membrane vesicles in tumorigenesis. Crit Rev Oncol Hematol. 2011;79(3):213–23.
13. Grant R, Ansa-Addo E, Stratton D, Antwi-Baffour S, Jorfi S, Kholia S, et al. A filtration-based protocol to isolate human plasma membrane-derived vesicles and exosomes from blood plasma. J Immunol Methods. 2011;371(1–2):143–51.
14. Pisitkun T, Shen RF, Knepper MA. Identification and proteomic profiling of exosomes in human urine. Proc Natl Acad Sci U S A. 2004;101(36):13368–73.
15. Street JM, Barran PE, Mackay CL, Weidt S, Balmforth C, Walsh TS, et al. Identification and proteomic profiling of exosomes in human cerebrospinal fluid. J Transl Med. 2012;10:5.
16. Keller S, Rupp C, Stoeck A, Runz S, Fogel M, Lugert S, et al. CD24 is a marker of exosomes secreted into urine and amniotic fluid. Kidney Int. 2007;72(9):1095–102.
17. Prado N, Marazuela EG, Segura E, Fernandez-Garcia H, Villalba M, Thery C, et al. Exosomes from bronchoalveolar fluid of tolerized mice prevent allergic reaction. J Immunol. 2008;181(2):1519–25.
18. Skriner K, Adolph K, Jungblut PR, Burmester GR. Association of citrullinated proteins with synovial exosomes. Arthritis Rheum. 2006;54(12):3809–14.

19. Runz S, Keller S, Rupp C, Stoeck A, Issa Y, Koensgen D, et al. Malignant ascites-derived exosomes of ovarian carcinoma patients contain CD24 and EpCAM. Gynecol Oncol. 2007;107(3):563–71.
20. Admyre C, Johansson SM, Qazi KR, Filen JJ, Lahesmaa R, Norman M, et al. Exosomes with immune modulatory features are present in human breast milk. J Immunol. 2007;179(3):1969–78.
21. Ogawa Y, Kanai-Azuma M, Akimoto Y, Kawakami H, Yanoshita R. Exosome-like vesicles with dipeptidyl peptidase IV in human saliva. Biol Pharm Bull. 2008;31(6):1059–62.
22. van der Pol E, Boing AN, Harrison P, Sturk A, Nieuwland R. Classification, functions, and clinical relevance of extracellular vesicles. Pharmacol Rev. 2012;64(3):676–705.
23. Xie C, Ji N, Tang Z, Li J, Chen Q. The role of extracellular vesicles from different origin in the microenvironment of head and neck cancers. Mol Cancer. 2019;18(1):83.
24. Gonzalez E, Falcon-Perez JM. Cell-derived extracellular vesicles as a platform to identify low-invasive disease biomarkers. Expert Rev Mol Diagn. 2015;15(7):907–23.
25. Cufaro MC, Pieragostino D, Lanuti P, Rossi C, Cicalini I, Federici L, et al. Extracellular vesicles and their potential use in monitoring cancer progression and therapy: the contribution of proteomics. J Oncol. 2019;2019:1639854.
26. Gyorgy B, Modos K, Pallinger E, Paloczi K, Pasztoi M, Misjak P, et al. Detection and isolation of cell-derived microparticles are compromised by protein complexes resulting from shared biophysical parameters. Blood. 2011;117(4):e39–48.
27. Thery C, Zitvogel L, Amigorena S. Exosomes: composition, biogenesis and function. Nat Rev Immunol. 2002;2(8):569–79.
28. Kalluri R. The biology and function of exosomes in cancer. J Clin Invest. 2016;126(4):1208–15.
29. Raposo G, Stoorvogel W. Extracellular vesicles: exosomes, microvesicles, and friends. J Cell Biol. 2013;200(4):373–83.
30. Ruivo CF, Adem B, Silva M, Melo SA. The biology of cancer exosomes: insights and new perspectives. Cancer Res. 2017;77(23):6480–8.
31. Zhang W, Xia W, Lv Z, Ni C, Xin Y, Yang L. Liquid biopsy for cancer: circulating tumor cells, circulating free DNA or exosomes? Cell Physiol Biochem. 2017;41(2):755–68.
32. Abels ER, Breakefield XO. Introduction to extracellular vesicles: biogenesis, RNA cargo selection, content, release, and uptake. Cell Mol Neurobiol. 2016;36(3):301–12.
33. Lousada-Fernandez F, Rapado-Gonzalez O, Lopez-Cedrun JL, Lopez-Lopez R, Muinelo-Romay L, Suarez-Cunqueiro MM. Liquid biopsy in oral cancer. Int J Mol Sci. 2018;19(6):1704.
34. Thery C, Ostrowski M, Segura E. Membrane vesicles as conveyors of immune responses. Nat Rev Immunol. 2009;9(8):581–93.
35. Thery C, Amigorena S, Raposo G, Clayton A. Isolation and characterization of exosomes from cell culture supernatants and biological fluids. Curr Protoc Cell Biol. 2006;Chapter 3:Unit 3 22.
36. Taylor DD, Zacharias W, Gercel-Taylor C. Exosome isolation for proteomic analyses and RNA profiling. Methods Mol Biol. 2011;728:235–46.
37. Gould SJ, Raposo G. As we wait: coping with an imperfect nomenclature for extracellular vesicles. J Extracell Vesicles. 2013;2
38. Thery C, Witwer KW, Aikawa E, Alcaraz MJ, Anderson JD, Andriantsitohaina R, et al. Minimal information for studies of extracellular vesicles 2018 (MISEV2018): a position statement of the International Society for Extracellular Vesicles and update of the MISEV2014 guidelines. J Extracell Vesicles. 2018;7(1):1535750.
39. Principe S, Hui AB, Bruce J, Sinha A, Liu FF, Kislinger T. Tumor-derived exosomes and microvesicles in head and neck cancer: implications for tumor biology and biomarker discovery. Proteomics. 2013;13(10–11):1608–23.
40. Kim JW, Wieckowski E, Taylor DD, Reichert TE, Watkins S, Whiteside TL. Fas ligand-positive membranous vesicles isolated from sera of patients with oral cancer induce apoptosis of activated T lymphocytes. Clin Cancer Res. 2005;11(3):1010–20.

41. Houali K, Wang X, Shimizu Y, Djennaoui D, Nicholls J, Fiorini S, et al. A new diagnostic marker for secreted Epstein-Barr virus encoded LMP1 and BARF1 oncoproteins in the serum and saliva of patients with nasopharyngeal carcinoma. Clin Cancer Res. 2007;13(17):4993–5000.
42. Keryer-Bibens C, Pioche-Durieu C, Villemant C, Souquère S, Nishi N, Hirashima M, et al. Exosomes released by EBV-infected nasopharyngeal carcinoma cells convey the viral latent membrane protein 1 and the immunomodulatory protein galectin 9. BMC Cancer. 2006;6(1):283.
43. Gourzones C, Gelin A, Bombik I, Klibi J, Verillaud B, Guigay J, et al. Extra-cellular release and blood diffusion of BART viral micro-RNAs produced by EBV-infected nasopharyngeal carcinoma cells. Virol J. 2010;7:271.
44. Wang J, Zhou Y, Lu J, Sun Y, Xiao H, Liu M, et al. Combined detection of serum exosomal miR-21 and HOTAIR as diagnostic and prognostic biomarkers for laryngeal squamous cell carcinoma. Med Oncol. 2014;31(9):148.
45. Yu J, Lin Y, Xiong X, Li K, Yao Z, Dong H, et al. Detection of exosomal PD-L1 RNA in saliva of patients with periodontitis. Front Genet. 2019;10:202.
46. Ye SB, Zhang H, Cai TT, Liu YN, Ni JJ, He J, et al. Exosomal miR-24-3p impedes T-cell function by targeting FGF11 and serves as a potential prognostic biomarker for nasopharyngeal carcinoma. J Pathol. 2016;240(3):329–40.
47. You Y, Shan Y, Chen J, Yue H, You B, Shi S, et al. Matrix metalloproteinase 13-containing exosomes promote nasopharyngeal carcinoma metastasis. Cancer Sci. 2015; 106(12):1669–77.
48. Alvarez-Teijeiro S, Menendez ST, Villaronga MA, Rodrigo JP, Manterola L, de Villalain L, et al. Dysregulation of Mir-196b in head and neck cancers leads to pleiotropic effects in the tumor cells and surrounding stromal fibroblasts. Sci Rep. 2017;7(1):17785.
49. Theodoraki MN, Yerneni SS, Hoffmann TK, Gooding WE, Whiteside TL. Clinical significance of PD-L1(+) exosomes in plasma of head and neck cancer patients. Clin Cancer Res. 2018;24(4):896–905.
50. Li L, Li C, Wang S, Wang Z, Jiang J, Wang W, et al. Exosomes derived from hypoxic oral squamous cell carcinoma cells deliver miR-21 to normoxic cells to elicit a prometastatic phenotype. Cancer Res. 2016;76(7):1770–80.
51. Sharma S, Gillespie BM, Palanisamy V, Gimzewski JK. Quantitative nanostructural and single-molecule force spectroscopy biomolecular analysis of human-saliva-derived exosomes. Langmuir. 2011;27(23):14394–400.
52. Esquela-Kerscher A, Slack FJ. Oncomirs – microRNAs with a role in cancer. Nat Rev Cancer. 2006;6(4):259–69.
53. Schwarzenbach H. The clinical relevance of circulating, exosomal miRNAs as biomarkers for cancer. Expert Rev Mol Diagn. 2015;15(9):1159–69.
54. Taylor DD, Gercel-Taylor C. MicroRNA signatures of tumor-derived exosomes as diagnostic biomarkers of ovarian cancer. Gynecol Oncol. 2008;110(1):13–21.
55. Chen K, Rajewsky N. The evolution of gene regulation by transcription factors and microRNAs. Nat Rev Genet. 2007;8(2):93–103.
56. Park NJ, Li Y, Yu T, Brinkman BM, Wong DT. Characterization of RNA in saliva. Clin Chem. 2006;52(6):988–94.
57. Park NJ, Zhou H, Elashoff D, Henson BS, Kastratovic DA, Abemayor E, et al. Salivary microRNA: discovery, characterization, and clinical utility for oral cancer detection. Clin Cancer Res. 2009;15(17):5473–7.
58. Etheridge A, Lee I, Hood L, Galas D, Wang K. Extracellular microRNA: a new source of biomarkers. Mutat Res. 2011;717(1–2):85–90.
59. John K, Wu J, Lee BW, Farah CS. MicroRNAs in head and neck cancer. Int J Dent. 2013;2013:650218.
60. Rapado-Gonzalez O, Majem B, Muinelo-Romay L, Alvarez-Castro A, Santamaria A, Gil-Moreno A, et al. Human salivary microRNAs in cancer. J Cancer. 2018;9(4):638–49.

61. Kai K, Dittmar RL, Sen S. Secretory microRNAs as biomarkers of cancer. Semin Cell Dev Biol. 2018;78:22–36.
62. Ohshiro K, Rosenthal DI, Koomen JM, Streckfus CF, Chambers M, Kobayashi R, et al. Pre-analytic saliva processing affect proteomic results and biomarker screening of head and neck squamous carcinoma. Int J Oncol. 2007;30(3):743–9.
63. Lee JM, Garon E, Wong DT. Salivary diagnostics. Orthod Craniofac Res. 2009;12(3):206–11.
64. Henson BS, Wong DT. Collection, storage, and processing of saliva samples for downstream molecular applications. Methods Mol Biol. 2010;666:21–30.
65. Topkas E, Keith P, Dimeski G, Cooper-White J, Punyadeera C. Evaluation of saliva collection devices for the analysis of proteins. Clin Chim Acta. 2012;413(13–14):1066–70.
66. Lamy E, Mau M. Saliva proteomics as an emerging, noninvasive tool to study livestock physiology, nutrition and diseases. J Proteome. 2012;75(14):4251–8.
67. Soini HA, Klouckova I, Wiesler D, Oberzaucher E, Grammer K, Dixon SJ, et al. Analysis of volatile organic compounds in human saliva by a static sorptive extraction method and gas chromatography-mass spectrometry. J Chem Ecol. 2010;36(9):1035–42.
68. Drake RR, Cazare LH, Semmes OJ, Wadsworth JT. Serum, salivary and tissue proteomics for discovery of biomarkers for head and neck cancers. Expert Rev Mol Diagn. 2005;5(1):93–100.
69. Yeh CK, Christodoulides NJ, Floriano PN, Miller CS, Ebersole JL, Weigum SE, et al. Current development of saliva/oral fluid-based diagnostics. Tex Dent J. 2010;127(7):651–61.
70. Chiappin S, Antonelli G, Gatti R, De Palo EF. Saliva specimen: a new laboratory tool for diagnostic and basic investigation. Clin Chim Acta. 2007;383(1–2):30–40.
71. Liu J, Duan Y. Saliva: a potential media for disease diagnostics and monitoring. Oral Oncol. 2012;48(7):569–77.
72. Yan W, Apweiler R, Balgley BM, Boontheung P, Bundy JL, Cargile BJ, et al. Systematic comparison of the human saliva and plasma proteomes. Proteomics Clin Appl. 2009;3(1):116–34.
73. Streckfus CF, Dubinsky WP. Proteomic analysis of saliva for cancer diagnosis. Expert Rev Proteomics. 2007;4(3):329–32.
74. Bigler LR, Streckfus CF, Dubinsky WP. Salivary biomarkers for the detection of malignant tumors that are remote from the oral cavity. Clin Lab Med. 2009;29(1):71–85.
75. Amado FM, Ferreira RP, Vitorino R. One decade of salivary proteomics: current approaches and outstanding challenges. Clin Biochem. 2013;46(6):506–17.
76. Pickering V, Jordan RC, Schmidt BL. Elevated salivary endothelin levels in oral cancer patients--a pilot study. Oral Oncol. 2007;43(1):37–41.
77. Dowling P, Wormald R, Meleady P, Henry M, Curran A, Clynes M. Analysis of the saliva proteome from patients with head and neck squamous cell carcinoma reveals differences in abundance levels of proteins associated with tumour progression and metastasis. J Proteome. 2008;71(2):168–75.
78. Franzmann EJ, Reategui EP, Pereira LH, Pedroso F, Joseph D, Allen GO, et al. Salivary protein and solCD44 levels as a potential screening tool for early detection of head and neck squamous cell carcinoma. Head Neck. 2012;34(5):687–95.
79. Nagler R, Bahar G, Shpitzer T, Feinmesser R. Concomitant analysis of salivary tumor markers--a new diagnostic tool for oral cancer. Clin Cancer Res. 2006;12(13):3979–84.
80. Deutsch O, Fleissig Y, Zaks B, Krief G, Aframian DJ, Palmon A. An approach to remove alpha amylase for proteomic analysis of low abundance biomarkers in human saliva. Electrophoresis. 2008;29(20):4150–7.
81. Amado F, Lobo MJ, Domingues P, Duarte JA, Vitorino R. Salivary peptidomics. Expert Rev Proteomics. 2010;7(5):709–21.
82. Zlotogorski-Hurvitz A, Dekel BZ, Malonek D, Yahalom R, Vered M. FTIR-based spectrum of salivary exosomes coupled with computational-aided discriminating analysis in the diagnosis of oral cancer. J Cancer Res Clin Oncol. 2019;145(3):685–94.
83. Baker MJ, Gazi E, Brown MD, Shanks JH, Gardner P, Clarke NW. FTIR-based spectroscopic analysis in the identification of clinically aggressive prostate cancer. Br J Cancer. 2008;99(11):1859–66.

84. Li Q, Hao C, Kang X, Zhang J, Sun X, Wang W, et al. Colorectal cancer and colitis diagnosis using Fourier transform infrared spectroscopy and an improved K-nearest-neighbour classifier. Sensors. 2017;17(12):2739.
85. Simonova D, Karamancheva I. Application of Fourier transform infrared spectroscopy for tumor diagnosis. Biotechnol Biotechnol Equip. 2013;27(6):4200–7.
86. Elashoff D, Zhou H, Reiss J, Wang J, Xiao H, Henson B, et al. Prevalidation of salivary biomarkers for oral cancer detection. Cancer Epidemiol Biomark Prev. 2012;21(4):664–72.
87. Michael A, Bajracharya SD, Yuen PS, Zhou H, Star RA, Illei GG, et al. Exosomes from human saliva as a source of microRNA biomarkers. Oral Dis. 2010;16(1):34–8.
88. Lasser C, Alikhani VS, Ekstrom K, Eldh M, Paredes PT, Bossios A, et al. Human saliva, plasma and breast milk exosomes contain RNA: uptake by macrophages. J Transl Med. 2011;9:9.
89. Al-Tarawneh SK, Border MB, Dibble CF, Bencharit S. Defining salivary biomarkers using mass spectrometry-based proteomics: a systematic review. OMICS. 2011;15(6):353–61.
90. Gonzalez-Begne M, Lu B, Han X, Hagen FK, Hand AR, Melvin JE, et al. Proteomic analysis of human parotid gland exosomes by multidimensional protein identification technology (MudPIT). J Proteome Res. 2009;8(3):1304–14.
91. Hirtz C, Chevalier F, Centeno D, Egea JC, Rossignol M, Sommerer N, et al. Complexity of the human whole saliva proteome. J Physiol Biochem. 2005;61(3):469–80.
92. de Jong EP, Xie H, Onsongo G, Stone MD, Chen XB, Kooren JA, et al. Quantitative proteomics reveals myosin and actin as promising saliva biomarkers for distinguishing premalignant and malignant oral lesions. PLoS One. 2010;5(6):e11148.
93. Ogawa Y, Miura Y, Harazono A, Kanai-Azuma M, Akimoto Y, Kawakami H, et al. Proteomic analysis of two types of exosomes in human whole saliva. Biol Pharm Bull. 2011;34(1):13–23.
94. Xiao H, Wong DT. Proteomic analysis of microvesicles in human saliva by gel electrophoresis with liquid chromatography-mass spectrometry. Anal Chim Acta. 2012;723:61–7.
95. Teh MT. Is salivary exosome the answer to early detection of oral cancer. Dent Open J. 2015;2(2):e3–4.
96. Pitt JM, Charrier M, Viaud S, Andre F, Besse B, Chaput N, et al. Dendritic cell-derived exosomes as immunotherapies in the fight against cancer. J Immunol. 2014;193(3):1006–11.
97. Zhang X, Yuan X, Shi H, Wu L, Qian H, Xu W. Exosomes in cancer: small particle, big player. J Hematol Oncol. 2015;8:83.
98. Reiners KS, Dassler J, Coch C, Pogge von Strandmann E. Role of exosomes released by dendritic cells and/or by tumor targets: regulation of NK cell plasticity. Front Immunol. 2014;5:91.
99. Pascucci L, Cocce V, Bonomi A, Ami D, Ceccarelli P, Ciusani E, et al. Paclitaxel is incorporated by mesenchymal stromal cells and released in exosomes that inhibit in vitro tumor growth: a new approach for drug delivery. J Control Release. 2014;192:262–70.
100. Smyth T, Kullberg M, Malik N, Smith-Jones P, Graner MW, Anchordoquy TJ. Biodistribution and delivery efficiency of unmodified tumor-derived exosomes. J Control Release. 2015;199:145–55.
101. Shtam TA, Kovalev RA, Varfolomeeva EY, Makarov EM, Kil YV, Filatov MV. Exosomes are natural carriers of exogenous siRNA to human cells in vitro. Cell Commun Signal. 2013;11:88.
102. Zhang Y, Li L, Yu J, Zhu D, Zhang Y, Li X, et al. Microvesicle-mediated delivery of transforming growth factor beta1 siRNA for the suppression of tumor growth in mice. Biomaterials. 2014;35(14):4390–400.
103. Bullock MD, Silva AM, Kanlikilicer-Unaldi P, Filant J, Rashed MH, Sood AK, et al. Exosomal non-coding RNAs: diagnostic, prognostic and therapeutic applications in cancer. Noncoding RNA. 2015;1(1):53–68.
104. Iorio MV, Croce CM. MicroRNAs in cancer: small molecules with a huge impact. J Clin Oncol. 2009;27(34):5848–56.

105. Ponting CP, Oliver PL, Reik W. Evolution and functions of long noncoding RNAs. Cell. 2009;136(4):629–41.
106. Ling H, Vincent K, Pichler M, Fodde R, Berindan-Neagoe I, Slack FJ, et al. Junk DNA and the long non-coding RNA twist in cancer genetics. Oncogene. 2015;34(39):5003–11.
107. Huang X, Yuan T, Tschannen M, Sun Z, Jacob H, Du M, et al. Characterization of human plasma-derived exosomal RNAs by deep sequencing. BMC Genomics. 2013;14:319.
108. Schulz BL, Cooper-White J, Punyadeera CK. Saliva proteome research: current status and future outlook. Crit Rev Biotechnol. 2013;33(3):246–59.
109. Christodoulides N, Mohanty S, Miller CS, Langub MC, Floriano PN, Dharshan P, et al. Application of microchip assay system for the measurement of C-reactive protein in human saliva. Lab Chip. 2005;5(3):261–9.
110. Yineng Han, Lingfei Jia, Yunfei Zheng, Weiran Li, Salivary Exosomes: Emerging Roles in Systemic Disease. International Journal of Biological Sciences 2018;14(6):633–43.

Chapter 8
Surgical Ablative Treatment of Head and Neck Cancers

Robin T. Wu, Vasu Divi, and Karl C. Bruckman

Introduction

Head and neck anatomy centers on function and aesthetics. Structures such as the mandible and the larynx, while millimeters in separation, serve vastly disparate occupations. As such, tumor extirpation can be particularly morbid.

Transoral excision of superficial tumors in the oral cavity was reported as early as the fifth century. In the 1800s, Billroth and Von Langenbeck described the lower lip split and mandibulotomy for access to elaborate tumors [1]. Kocher then pioneered the submandibular resection, allowing proximal vascular control and reduced need for mandibulotomy. A great advancement in surgical visualization came when Garcia refined the indirect laryngoscopy by experimenting on his own larynx. In 1873, Billroth initiated the first laryngectomy for cancer, albeit with profound mortality rates due to aspiration and sepsis [2].

The forefather of modern head and neck surgery was George Crile, who published his extensive experience in the early 1900s. After reviewing his cases from 1899 to 1906, Crile advocated for en bloc resection of neck lymphatics, improving survival rates from 19% to 75% [3, 4]. Martin added the level I–V modified radical neck dissection for metastatic neck disease.

Towards the late twentieth century, new technological advances have allowed for decreased morbidity. In rapid succession, Jako and Kleinsasser developed microlaryngoscopy [5], Polanyi invented the CO_2 laser [6], and Jako and Strong reported using the two in combination [7].

R. T. Wu · K. C. Bruckman (✉)
Division of Plastic & Reconstructive Surgery, Department of Surgery, Stanford University School of Medicine, Stanford, CA, USA
e-mail: Bruckman@stanford.edu

V. Divi
Division of Head & Neck Surgery, Department of Otolaryngology, Stanford University School of Medicine, Stanford, CA, USA

© Springer Nature Switzerland AG 2021
R. El Assal et al. (eds.), *Early Detection and Treatment of Head & Neck Cancers*, https://doi.org/10.1007/978-3-030-69859-1_8

While techniques have flourished, the principles are steadfast. Tumor ablation is the primary modality to prevent progression and metastasis. Resection with clean margins must weigh multi-functional morbidities of the head and neck. Perhaps paramount of which is lengthy discussion with the patient regarding individual goals. Ninety percent of head and neck cancers are squamous cell carcinomas (SCC) [8]; thus the focus of this chapter will be the ablative management of head and neck SCC, upon which resection of other malignancies are often mirrored.

General Principles

Elective Tracheostomy

Aspiration and airway edema, risking loss of airway, are serious sequelae of head and neck cancer resection. Guidelines for elective tracheotomies are controversial. Grading systems exist such as the clinical assessment scoring system for tracheostomy (CASST) including a variety of surgical and patient factors (Table 8.1) [9].

Generally, those with increased secretions such as patients with chronic aspiration, patients with posterior tongue tumors with potential of tongue fall, and those with a free or pedicle flaps for airway reconstruction will require prolonged airway control with a tracheotomy. Those with large tumors encroaching on the airway will often need an urgent tracheotomy or urgent surgical resection with elective tracheotomy in anticipation of postoperative swelling. Generally speaking, the most common indication for tracheostomy is in patients diagnosed with laryngeal cancer [10].

Tracheotomies are performed prior to tumor resection. An open tracheotomy is performed, and an endotracheal tube is advanced for ventilation during the

Table 8.1 Gupta et al. developed the CASST grading system to predict the need for tracheostomy with a sensitivity of 95.5% and a negative predictive value of 99.3% [9]

Major criteria	Points
Previous radiation in same region of surgery	2
Resection of two more sub-site of oral cavity or oropharynx	2
Bilateral neck dissection	2
Extended hemi- or central-arch mandibulectomy	2
Bulky flap used for reconstruction	2
Flap causing compression (e.g., use of a reconstruction plate, intact mandibular rim)	2
Minor criteria	
Age > 65 years	1
Previously operation at the same site	1
Trismus	1
Pathological CT chest findings (e.g., COPD, emphysema)	1
Total score < 6	No need for tracheostomy
Total score > 7	Likely need for tracheostomy

procedure. Decannulation rates are high, studies reporting up to 88.5%, and should be carried out when secretions are controlled and mechanical ventilation is no longer required [11].

Feeding

High rates of dysphagia exist after head and neck cancer surgery, further compounded by treatment- and disease-related cachexia. Malnutrition complicates curative goals and increases morbidity with each treatment step. Thus, many clinicians opt for prophylactic feeding tube placement at the time of surgical resection or at the onset of swallowing compromise [12].

One review from Moffitt Cancer Center identifies body mass index below 25, tumor stage three or greater, and a cumulative cisplatin dose great than 200 mg/m² as the factors most associated with percutaneous endoscopic gastrostomy tube placement [13]. As high as 60% of patients undergoing chemoradiation for head and neck cancer undergo feeding tube placement which remain for a median of 9 months. However, most studies fail to find significant improvements in morbidity or survival with feeding tube placement [14–19].

There is little consensus among institutions regarding practices for prophylactic feeding tube placement. At this juncture, authors do not recommend prophylactic placement without identified patient comorbidities. National Comprehensive Cancer Network (NCCN) guidelines currently identify (i) severe weight loss, (ii) symptomatic patients, (iii) risk for aspiration, and (iv) high-dose radiation as strong considerations for percutaneous endoscopic gastrostomy (PEG) placement (Table 8.2). The ease of modern endoscopic placement allows swift enteric feeding once malnutrition is identified. Likewise, open discussion should ensue prior to surgical resection to determine patient preference for feeding.

Reconstruction

Head and neck reconstruction principles are complex and beyond the scope of this chapter, and it is been covered in the subsequent chapter in this volume. In general, surgical principles follow the reconstructive ladder. Small defects in the alveolar arch or hard palate can be allowed to granulate by secondary intention as scar contracture is negligible. On the opposite spectrum, the free fibula flap has arisen as the work horse of mandibular reconstruction, with excellent aesthetic results and minimal donor site morbidity.

A plastic surgery team should be involved early in surgical planning. Aesthetic and functional goals must be discussed thoroughly as final reconstruction may take years to complete.

Table 8.2 Taken from the NCCN guidelines for head and neck cancer. With a copyright permission, the content adopted from [125]

Global nutrition recommendations for patients receiving (chemo)radiotherapy	
Utilize oral intake as much as possible when maintaining safety	
Monitor for the lifetime of the patient even well after therapy	
Factors predicting limited enteral feeding requirement	**Factors suggesting strong consideration of prophylactic PEG**
Very good performance status as measured by the Eastern Cooperative Oncology Group (ECOG/WHO/Zubrod) score	Severe weight loss prior to treatment
	5% past 1 month
	10% past 6 months
No significant	Symptoms includes
Pretreatment weight loss	Ongoing dehydration
5% past 1 month	Severe dysphagia
10% past 6 months	Anorexia
Airway obstruction	Odynophagia interfering with oral intake
Dysphagia	Significant comorbidities requiring good oral intake for health maintenance
	Severe aspiration in any patient
	Any aspiration in an elderly patient or patients with compromised cardiopulmonary function
	Patients anticipating high-dose radiation

Neck Dissection

Neck dissections are either comprehensive (radical and modified radical) or selective. The radical neck dissection is characterized by unilateral removal of lymph nodes in regions I–V, sacrifice of the spinal accessory nerve, internal jugular vein, and sternocleidomastoid, and is rarely used today.

In patients without palpable neck disease or concerning findings on imaging, elective treatment of the neck is pursued based on the probability of occult metastatic disease. In general, if the risk of metastases is greater than 20%, treatment is considered [20, 21]. In particular, patients with nasopharyngeal, pyriform sinus, and base of tongue lesions with propensity for early lymphatic spread should be considered for elective neck treatment [22, 23]. The neck is managed by surgery or radiation depending on the primary tumor management. Glottic tumors T1-2 are generally safe to defer any neck treatment; however, patients with advanced T3-4 tumors are recommended to undergo neck dissections or radiotherapy. Oropharyngeal, hypopharyngeal, or supraglottic laryngeal tumors T2-4 often spread to the neck without palpable signs and should receive lateral neck dissections or radiation.

Patients with clinically positive neck disease are recommended to undergo comprehensive dissection. Those without adenopathy in level V can be considered for selective neck dissection as level V involvement is often rare. If extracapsular extension is present, adjuvant radiotherapy is delivered concurrently with chemotherapy. Individualized neck management will be discussed for each tumor type separately.

Cutaneous Malignancies

Basal Cell Carcinoma (BCC)

Low-risk BCC are categorized by primary tumors of nodular or superficial subtype, less than 10 mm on the cheek, forehead, scalp, or neck, without perineural invasion, and without history of radiation [24–26]. Resection involves 4 mm margins and Mohs micrographic salvage for positive margins. Curettage and electrodesiccation is an in-office alternative, but cannot evaluate for histologic margins.

High-risk BCC are of the morpheaform, basosquamous, sclerosing, mixed infiltrative, or micronodular subtype, are greater than or equal to 10 mm, and involve the periorbita, eyebrows, nose, lips, chin, mandible, peri-auricular region, or temple and recurrent or history of immunosuppression/radiation. High-risk disease is managed upfront with Mohs surgery, which boasts lower recurrence rates and increased tissue sparing than traditional resection.

Squamous Cell Carcinoma (SCC)

SCC arise from premalignant actinic keratosis and are further stratified into low- and high-risk categories [27]. Low-risk SCC is a primary disease; less than 10 mm diameter on the cheek, forehead, scalp, or neck; less than 2 mm in depth; and is Clark levels I–III, with well-defined border, without structural invasion, and in patients without prior radiation. Actinic keratosis and SCC in situ can be treated with in-office cryotherapy, topical 5-FU, imiquimod, and other topicals. Lesions with a diagnosis of low-risk SCC is generally recommended for surgial excision with 4–6 mm margins, with Mohs micrographic surgery reserved for positive margins.

A diagnosis of high-risk SCC includes lesions that are recurrent, are poorly defined, have more than 2mm in depth, Clark levels IV-V, demonstrate rapid growth, show structural invasion, involve the periorbita, eyebrows, nose, lips, chin, mandible, peri-auricular region, or temple, and are histologically aggressive. High-risk SCC is initially treated with Mohs surgery or can receive standard surgical excision.

Melanoma

Following standard punch or incisional biopsies, head and neck melanomas are managed standardly with wide local excision [24, 25]. These include 1 cm margins for tumors with Breslow depth less than 1 mm, 1–2 cm margin for lesions 1–2 mm thick, and 2 cm margins for tumors more than 2 mm thick.

Special considerations exist based on anatomic location. In general, melanomas of the face are resected to the facial muscles, barring invasion of muscle and underlying bone. Melanomas of the ear are considered for partial or total auriculectomy, while those of the ear canal may require resection of temporal bone. Scalp melanomas are resected to the periosteum, and those that abut the periosteum may indicate outer table resection.

Neck Dissection

BCC has very low rates of neck metastases and dissection is reserved for positive nodal disease [25–27]. SCC, on the other hand, can be considered for sentinel node biopsy in high-risk disease. Lesions that (i) are larger than 2 cm, (ii) have a depth greater than 4 mm, (iii) are on the lip or ear, (iv) have presence of perineural invasion or poor differentiation, or (v) are in immunosuppressed patients have an increased risk of metastasis. Palpable disease warrants therapeutic neck dissection. Posterior scalp and neck SCC warrants posteriolateral neck dissection, involving suboccipital and retroauricular nodes.

Melanomas are relatively more complex to manage [24]. Patients with T2-3 tumor, Clark levels IV–V, or ulcerative melanomas are treated with a sentinel node biopsy. Therapeutic neck dissection is indicated for palpable neck disease or positive sentinel nodes. Anterior scalp, temple, ear, and facial melanomas with positive sentinel nodes indicate superficial parotidectomy, as disease commonly metastasizes to the parotid nodes. Posterior scalp and retroauricular melanomas also indicate suboccipital and retroauricular dissection.

Oral Cavity

Surgery is the primary modality of oral cancer ablation. Adjuvant radiation or chemoradiation supplements resection of advanced tumors. Early-stage oral tumors T1-2 often undergo transoral resection. Access to advanced or posterior tumors generally can be performed through a combined transcervical and transoral approach and is rarely facilitated by mandibulotomy.

Lip

While basal cell carcinomas are most prevalent in the lip, SCC comprise 30% [28, 29]. The lip is the most common site for cancer of the oral cavity. Lip resection poses an obvious cosmetic challenge, and concurrent reconstruction is always required.

In situ lesions are managed more conservatively with shave excision, topical 5-fluorouracil, or imiquimod. Invasive lesions generally require formal excision, with exception to select early stage commissure lesions that may be managed with radiation only, due to the complexity of reconstructing the oral commissure. All lesions should be assessed for mandibular or mental nerve involvement prior to excision. Neck metastases are rare (10%) and elective neck dissections for node negative disease are generally not recommended in T1-2 tumors; however should be considered in T3-4 disease [30].

Tongue

Cancers of the tongue are not limited by anatomical barriers and are often more invasive, requiring comprehensive resection with 1 cm margins [31]. T1-2 lesions can be ablated with transverse wedge excisions or wide local excision with frozen sections [32, 33]. Large T2 lesions and posterior lesions classically mandated pull-through or mandibulotomy, particularly for segmental resections. Extensive local disease mandates near-total or total glossectomy.

Resections limited to the oral tongue that encompass less than one quarter of the tongue volume can be closed primarily or skin grafted [34]. When more than one third of the tongue is resected, fasciocutaneous free flap reconstruction should be considered to restore tongue bulk and maintain mobility and is considered mandatory for patients with >50% tongue resection. Reconstruction is also dependent on the degree of floor of mouth involvement which can cause significant tongue tethering. Unfortunately for large T3-4 lesions, even with reconstruction, total glossectomies are complicated by chronic aspiration and breathing difficulties, and laryngectomy is occasionally indicated.

Mandible

SCC can invade directly from the oral cavity into the mandible. Tumors extending to the superficial gingiva are resected with periosteum only. Those with periosteal invasion require at least a marginal mandibulectomy [35, 36]. Generally, if a tumor extends from the alveolar ridge below the level of the mandibular canal, a segmental mandibulectomy is required over a marginal mandibulectomy. Discussion of mandibular resection will be elaborated for each type of tumor later in this chapter.

The mandible, even uninvolved, inhibits proper tumor access and may rarely mandate mandibulotomy. Current guidelines are moving towards more mandibular sparing, particularly with the popularity of the pull-through technique for tumors that do not grossly involve the mandible. In general, mandibulotomies for access alone are avoided due to complications such as nonunion, temporomandibular joint disease, ankyloglosis, or even osteoradionecrosis [37, 38].

Floor of the Mouth

Proper resection of these tumors in proximity to the mandible can involve marginal mandibulectomy with 1 cm margins [39]. Early-stage tumors can be treated with transoral resection or pull-through technique [40]. Tumors that abut the mandible without obvious invasion past the periosteum can be limited to marginal mandibu- lectomy. Those tumors that have radiologic cortical involvement will require complete segmental mandibulectomy with bone cuts 1 cm from the malignant margins. Large tumors that are purely soft tissue with appropriate distance from the mandible can be accessed transcervically and resected en bloc with the neck dissection.

Alveolar Ridge

Primary tumors at this site are rare and share subunit management with floor of mouth tumors. Cases where the tumor does not invade the periosteum, a subperiosteal resection is possible [41, 42]. Small tumors can be addressed with marginal mandibulectomy or maxillectomy, while larger ones generally require segmental mandibulectomy or maxillectomy.

Retromolar Trigone

Mucosa of the retromolar trigone abuts the mandible, and even early-stage malignancies often involve mandible resection by L-shaped coronal marginal mandibulectomy, segmental, or hemimandibulectomy [43].

Hard Palate

Although SCC are the majority of hard palate malignancies, one third of tumors in this area arise from minor salivary glands. Resection involves 1 cm margins. Small tumors can be accessed per-orally [44]. Fortunately, the palatal periosteum bars tumor spread. Periosteal involvement requires removal of a portion of the bony palate with an infrastructure maxillectomy. Large tumors that extend into the pterygoid plates and masticator space benefit from superoanterior exposure of the nasal cavity, a maxillary sinus attained via a transverse-vertical Weber-Ferguson approach. In advanced tumors, en bloc maxillary resections may remove the inferior orbital rim. Thus, reconstructions must address separation of the oral and nasal cavities, replacing the nasal lining, and reconstruction of the orbit. Often a dental prosthesis can supplement rehabilitation of speech and swallowing.

Buccal Mucosa

Small superficial lesions with minimal depth of invasion are excised transorally without muscle resection [45, 46]. However, tumor that has any palpable thickness should have resection of the underlying buccinator muscle. If there are concerns about the depth of invasion, an MRI scan can give critical information about the involvement of the buccinator or extension towards the external skin. Tumors that extend posteriorly towards to retromolar trigone should be assessed for involvement of the masticator space. Lip-split incisions are generally avoided with a careful combined transoral and transcervical approach.

Neck Dissection

Oral cancers often metastasize to nodal basins I, II, and III [47]. Elective treatment of the clinical N0 neck is achieved with a supraomohyoid neck dissection including these three levels [48, 49]. Level IIb can generally be spared in elective neck dissections which may decrease the incidence of spinal accessory nerve weakness. Those with clinically apparent nodal disease undergo a comprehensive dissection followed by adjuvant radiation. If extracapsular extension is present in the lymph nodes, chemotherapy is given concurrently with radiation therapy.

Odontogenic Cysts and Tumors

Odontogenic cysts, regardless of histology, are standardly treated by enucleation; unilocular cysts do not require curettage, while multilocular, scalloped, or recurrent cysts are recommended to be curettage [50–52]. The necessity of tooth extraction is dependent on the histology.

Similar principles of enucleation and curettage apply to odontogenic tumors [20]. This strategy includes but is not limited to adenomatoid odontogenic tumors, ameloblastic fibromas, calcifying cystic odontogenic tumors, odontomas, and squamous odontogenic tumors. Notable exception is the keratocystic odontogenic tumor (KCOT) with high recurrence rate and should always be curettage with careful removal of the entire cyst lining [53, 54]. Pindborg tumors (i.e., calcifying epithelial odontogenic tumors) are resected with a small margin of bone. Odontogenic myxomas have a gelatinous appearance and 0.5–1 cm medullary bone should be removed with the specimen.

Ameloblastomas are the most aggressive benign tumor [55]. Treatment is controversial, but generally ameloblastomas in the mandible are often resected with 1 cm bony margins including periosteum [56]. Maxillary ameloblastomas are recommended to have 1–2 cm margins, and particular care should be taken intraoperatively with resection radiographs to ensure clean margins.

Oropharynx

Oropharyngeal cancers are an area of significant research and changing treatment paradigms due to the rapid increase in HPV-associated oropharyngeal cancer. HPV-positive disease has dramatically better outcomes than HPV-negative disease, and new protocols are investigating whether de-escalation of therapy can maintain excellent outcomes while minimizing morbidity. In general, T1 and T2 lesions can be primarily managed with surgery or radiation therapy depending on their ease of resectability and the extent of involvement of the neck [57]. When moving into more advanced T3 and T4 lesions, surgical resection would leave patients with significant morbidity and most institutions pursue upfront chemoradiotherapy.

The transoral approach is the most common surgical approach utilized. Tumors easily accessible with the direct transoral approach include small tumors of the soft palate, tonsils, and pharyngeal walls. Modifications to the transoral approach to reach larger tumors of the tongue base or retromolar trigone include transoral laser microsurgery (TLM) and transoral robotic surgery (TORS), the latter of which is mainly approved for T1-2 lesions [58–60]. Laser microsurgery proceeds with sequential piecemeal resection and is aided by frozen sections for confirmation of margins. TORS is currently under further development, including adaptation with the single port robotic novel robotic da Vinci [61], and many argue that the cost and difficult setup make it inferior to TLM. Research is underway to develop more flexible robotic arms, allowing it to follow the nonlinear anatomic path.

If transoral access is inadequate, often in inferior lesions, a pharyngotomy is the next step. Multiple variations exist with the traditional being the lateral approach sparing the hypoglossal and superior laryngeal nerve. The transhyoid pharyngotomy enters the vallecula medially, with care taken to close the pharyngotomy judiciously to prevent fistulae. Select extensive lesions may warrant a combined transoral and transcervical approach.

Soft Palate

Stage I and II tumors can be treated with radiation and stage III and IV tumor with chemoradiation to limit velopharyngeal insufficiency [62, 63]. Surgery is generally not recommended for tumors in this location given the superior functional outcomes of radiation therapy [64].

Tonsils

Tonsils and tonsillar pillars are the most common primary carcinoma site. Tonsillar tumors follow the typical treatment algorithm for oropharynx cancers described above. Anatomical access is challenging and aided by TLM or TORS for early-stage cancers and mandibulotomy for more extensive invasion [60, 65, 66]. Large tumors involving the mandible and multiple subunits mandate an en bloc resection with posterior mandibulectomy.

Tongue Base

Tongue base tumors are treated as other oropharyngeal cancers. If surgery is indicated, access can be attained from least to most invasive via transoral excision, lateral pharyngotomy, supra-/transhyoid pharyngotomy, lip split, or paramedian mandibulotomy. Small primaries T1-2 are managed with TLM or TORS [67, 68]. Tumors abutting or involving the mandible will be managed with marginal or segmental mandibulectomy. If total glossectomy is necessary in patients at high risk of aspiration, laryngectomy may prevent aspiration [60].

Posterior Wall

While early oropharyngeal wall tumors are treated with surgery or radiation, most late lesions should be treated with radiation with or without chemotherapy [69, 70]. Despite the deep location, appropriate retraction allows for resection of early tumor using transoral, TLM, or TORS. Lateral tumors are proximal to the internal carotid artery, and care must be taken to anatomic orientation particularly if performing micro or robotic surgery to protect it from injury. Unique to posterior wall tumors and soft palate, the retropharyngeal lymph nodes are most common. Dissection is difficult but can be reached via the transoral or transmandibular approach.

Neck Dissection

Oropharyngeal cancers often present at an advanced stage, half of which have nodal involvement. Node metastasis occurs commonly along levels 2–4, with occasional involvement of retropharyngeal nodes [71, 72]. Of note, oropharyngeal SCC which arise from HPV classically present with cystic lymph nodes.

Given the likelihood of early occult metastasis (40–50% of patients without clinical evidence had metastases), elective neck dissection or radiation is recommended. Those with extracapsular lymph node spread should receive primary chemoradiation. Soft palate cancers metastasize bilaterally, and bilateral neck dissections or radiation should be pursued as indicated.

Hypopharynx

Hypopharyngeal cancers report the poorest long-term survival among head and neck cancers, owing to high probability of distant metastases [73]. Anatomically, these tumors are in close proximity to the larynx, and even barring involvement, resection would compromise laryngeal function. While conventional management was total laryngopharyngectomy, recent advances involve chemoradiation in attempts to preserve the larynx, and transoral laser surgery. Due to the rarity of this disease, management guidelines are highly variable per institution (Table 8.3).

Table 8.3 General management guidelines of hypopharyngeal carcinomas

Procedure	T Stage	Reconstruction
Partial pharyngectomy	1, 2	Primary closure
Supracricoid hemilaryngectomy	1, 2, 3	Primary closure
Partial laryngopharyngectomy	1, 2, 3	Regional or free flap
Endoscopic carbon dioxide laser resection/ transoral robotic surgery	1, 2 (possibly 3 and 4)	Secondary intention
Total laryngectomy with partial/total pharyngectomy	3, 4	Primary closure vs regional or free flap
Total pharyngolaryngoesophagectomy	4	Gastric pull-up

Adapted from Cummings Otolaryngology [20]

In general, the majority treat T1 lesions and select T2 lesions with radiation alone or surgical resections [74, 75]. T2 lesions and above are managed with radiation therapy; however if there is significant laryngeal involvement and dysfunction of the laryngeal structures, a radical resection followed by radiation is preferred [76]. Stage III/IV can be considered for chemotherapy and radiation alone to limit laryngeal resection with surgery as secondary salvage.

Early-Stage Tumors

Generally, these patients are consented for a tracheotomy as pharyngeal edema postoperatively can cause airway compromise. Early T1/2 tumors with posterior or lateral extent can be considered for partial pharyngectomy with lateral pharyngotomy [77, 78]. More extensive tumors may necessitate a lateral transthyroid pharyngotomy, and posterior tumors may be approached with an anterior transthyroid pharyngotomy.

Tumors of the medial piriform sinus without involvement of the piriform apex, extension to the postcricoid, vocal cord paralysis, or invasion of the cricopharyngeus can be managed with a partial laryngopharyngectomy [79]. A supracricoid hemilaryngopharyngectomy expands upon this to include the ipsilateral supracricoid hemilarynx and piriform sinus [80].

Outside of the traditional open approaches, the management of early-stage tumors is moving towards tissue preserving surgeries such as transoral laser microsurgery (TLM). Minimized tissue resection translates to better functional swallowing postoperatively. The tumor is removed piecemeal with 1 cm margins, confirmed with frozen sections. This technique may eliminate the need for tracheostomy and significantly shorter perioperative course.

Late-Stage Tumors

In large lesions not suitable for conservation or those that fail chemoradiation, a traditional laryngectomy or total laryngopharyngectomy are necessary, respectively. These are plagued with pharyngocutaneous fistula rates as high as 40% [81, 82].

Those with tumors extending into the cervical esophagus will need a total pharyngolaryngoesophagectomy. This procedure involves bilateral neck dissections, total thyroidectomy, parathyroid autotransplantation, total laryngopharyngectomy, and transhiatal pull-through esophagectomy with gastric pull-through reconstruction [83].

Neck Dissection

Up to 75% of patients have palpable neck metastases upon presentation, owing to the abundant lymphatics in this region. The broad generalization is that elective neck dissections of levels II-IV should be pursued for N0 stages and therapeutic dissections for N+ necks [84].

Larynx

Laryngeal cancer treatment is focused on functional preservation. The larynx is poised for vocal production, swallowing, and breathing. Each of these three must be considered individually when recommending an optimal treatment for patients. Treatment is divided anatomically based on the three sections of the larynx:

Supraglottis

40% of laryngeal cancers originate in the supraglottis. Early-stage tumors are treated with single-modality therapy, and advanced stage disease is treated with multiple modalities. Smaller tumors are eligible for surgical resection [85]; however, as tumors extend to areas outside of the supraglottic region, or more deeply into the vocal cords, non-surgical management is preferred [86, 87]. Surgical resection can be performed by TLM which has largely replaced open partial laryngectomy approaches given the lower morbidity. TORS is limited by narrow exposure through the oral cavity but has similarly reported similar functional and oncologic outcomes to TLM [88, 89].

Stage III/IV tumors can be treated differentially with total laryngectomy and radiation or chemoradiation alone [33]. Tumors that compromise the cartilage or have extralaryngeal spread are favored for resection. Surgery is always the initial option for salvage. Surgically, the traditional option has been total laryngectomy and bilateral neck dissections, which presents significant morbidity. Supracricoid partial laryngectomy preserves the hyoid and cricoid cartilage and resects all true and false vocal cords, paraglottic spaces, thyroid cartilage, and epiglottis. This is often closed with a cricohyoidopexy. Supracricoid partial laryngectomy is indicated for T3 tumors with fixation of the true vocal cords or invasion of the pre-epiglottic space and T4 tumors with minimal involvement of the thyroid cartilage without extension to the extralaryngeal space [90].

Glottis

59% of laryngeal cancers originate in the glottis. Glottic tumors often present early with persistent hoarseness, allowing for better outcomes. T1 glottic tumors have great control rates with surgery and radiation alone, with the former being slightly preferred due to voice outcomes [91–93]. T2 tumors require more extensive resection of the vocal cord, which impairs voice outcomes, and more deeply invasive tumors have a higher risk of recurrence. TLM is the preferred method for resecting tumors over open approaches when feasible [88]. Voice prognosis from early tumors depends directly on muscular invasion. The exception is anterior commissure tumors which often recur. Open surgical resection may be the best option as radiation often underdoses tumors in this location and TLM has poor visualization in this anatomic region [94].

Stage III/IV tumors, similar to supraglottic tumors, can be treated with surgery and radiation or chemoradiation alone, with surgery for salvage. T3/T4 tumors were classically treated with total laryngectomy with adjuvant radiation; however, numerous trials have demonstrated the feasibility of using concurrent chemoradiation therapy for organ preservation and equivalent survival outcomes. Tumors that cause a dysfunctional larynx prior to treatment, in particular due to destruction of the laryngeal cartilage or cricoid invasion, are preferentially treated with an upfront laryngectomy. Tumors with more than 1 cm subglottic extension or palpable thyroid disease warrant hemithyroidectomy for likely invasion.

Subglottis

1% of laryngeal cancers originate in the subglottis [95]. While rare, these tumors are highly invasive, often spreading distally along the trachea and posteriorly towards the esophagus. Unfortunately, resection must be aggressive, yet survival is poor [96, 97]. Similarly, Stage I/II tumors receive radiation alone, while Stage III/IV tumors are treated with surgery or possibly radiation alone in non-surgical candidates. Surgery for all tumors is total laryngectomy to control the spread. Tracheal involvement requires low tracheal resection and manubrium removal.

Neck Dissection

Supraglottic tumors are highly metastatic and often involve bilateral lymph nodes [98]. Early T1 lesions can avoid elective neck dissection. N0/1 disease is recommended for bilateral selective neck dissection of levels 2–4 [99, 100]. Ipsilateral comprehensive neck dissection levels 1–5 and contralateral selective dissection are warranted for N2/3 disease.

Glottic tumors have lower rates of nodal metastasis; thus early T1/2 glottic tumors can exclude elective neck dissection. Majority of T3 tumors do not necessitate neck management, while T4 tumors are recommended to undergo neck management [101]. This includes dissection of paratracheal nodes levels 2–4.

Subglottic tumors often spread via abundant lymphatics to the pretracheal, paratracheal, inferior jugular, and mediastinal nodes. Thus, bilateral neck dissection with paratracheal node dissection is the standard of care.

Nasopharynx

Nasopharyngeal tumors are heavily susceptible to chemoradiation (generally radiation for stage I/II and chemoradiation for stage III/IV); thus surgery is reserved for local or regional disease recurrence [102, 103]. Contraindications to resection include internal carotid artery involvement, skull base erosion, and intracranial extension.

Surgical approaches can be open or endoscopic, depending on the location and extent of tumor. Challenging access is evident from the posterior location of the nasopharynx and the narrow gateway nasal vestibule, and open approaches require significant exposure from a transpalatal, transmaxillary, transcervical approach, extended osteoplastic maxillotomy, or "maxillary swing" [104]. Endoscopic and robotic nasopharyngectomies are becoming more popular for small central recurrences [105]. These approaches can resect the posterior nasal septum, roof of the nasopharynx, and the medial maxillary wall. Regional recurrence in the neck mandates a modified radical or radical neck dissection.

Nasal Cavity

Nasal cavity tumors are generally treated surgically. Resection must take into consideration involvement of the sinuses, nose, orbit, and cranial base.

Paranasal Sinus

Paranasal sinus tumors are particularly challenging given their insidious progression and advanced disease at time of presentation. General management involves surgical resection and postoperative radiation or chemoradiation. Early T1/2 tumors localized to a single region, such as the nasal cavity, septum, or maxillary sinus, can be managed with surgical resection alone. Increased stage tumors are supplemented by postoperative radiation, and chemotherapy is reserved for unresectable tumors.

Surgical Techniques

The choice of open versus endoscopic resection depends upon the intrinsic tumor properties and surgeon training. Open resection enables comprehensive exposure and should be pursued for involvement of the hard palate requiring maxillectomy, involvement of the orbit requiring orbital exenteration, anterior involvement of the nasal bone, and involvement of the external skin.

The endoscopic approach provides higher definition, allowing careful dissection around critical structures such as the orbit, dura, and carotids while avoiding unnecessary bony/soft tissue ablation [106, 107]. For most sinonasal malignancies, the endoscopic approach is now used whenever feasible [108]. Endoscopic endonasal/sinonasal resection occurs segmentally from the inferior nasal floor superiorly towards the skull base until clear margins are secured. Endoscopic partial maxillectomy removes the medial maxilla with inferior tubinate, the uncinate process, and, if involved, the orbital lamina. Endoscopic transcribriform resection expands the partial maxillectomy to include the anterior cranial base. Tumors that spread into the pterygopalatine or infratemporal fossa can be reached with coronal plane extension following medial maxillectomy. Contraindications to endoscopic resection include involvement of the soft tissue of the face or forehead, frontal sinus, palate, dura of the lateral orbit, brain invasion greater than two centimeters, mandible, cavernous sinus, significant orbit involvement requiring exenteration, or internal carotid total encasement.

Salivary Gland

Benign

The focus of this chapter is on resection of head and neck malignancies; however, given the prevalence of benign parotid tumors and their predominant surgical management, we will discuss them briefly. The majority (85%) of benign salivary tumors are parotid [52, 109, 110].

The approach to the majority of benign lesions is surgical excision with a cuff of healthy tissue, including myoepitheliomas, canalicular adenomas, oncocytomas, and lipoadenoma [111]. Large tumors in the superficial lobe can be resected with a superficial parotidectomy. Otherwise, deep tumors indicate total parotidectomy with facial nerve preservation. Facial nerve involvement indicates some degree of nerve sacrifice. If function is preserved, nerve branches can be selectively removed and reconstructed. Total paralysis on presentation requires facial nerve resection.

Pleomorphic adenomas are the most common benign parotid tumor and make up 75% of benign salivary gland tumors [112, 113]. As 90% arise superficial to the facial nerve, they are treated operatively with superficial or total parotidectomy depending on their location with dissection and sparing of the facial nerve. Transoral resection or enucleation leads to unacceptably high recurrence rates. These often have a substantial recurrence rate of 2–7%, often as a complication of incomplete resection. Treatment is reoperation and adjuvant radiotherapy for multinodular recurrence. Repeat resection carries increased risk of facial nerve damage. Patients who are not good surgical candidates can achieve successful local control with neutron radiotherapy.

Warthin tumors are the second most common benign parotid tumor, found almost exclusively within the parotid. These tumors are slow growing, often asymptomatic. Smoking is a notable risk factor [114], and smoking cessation often significantly decreases risk. Treatment is observation, with resection for symptomatic disease – occasionally are painful or inflamed – or cosmetically desired. Parotidectomies are preferred as recurrence is common with inadequate excision.

Benign submandibular gland tumors involve gland removal with preservation of the marginal mandibular and hypoglossal nerve. Similarly, minor salivary gland tumors should be excised with a cuff of normal tissue, and enucleation should be discouraged. Management of malignant submandibular gland tumors is discussed below.

Parapharyngeal salivary gland tumors are resected via a transcervical incision and exposure of the major neurovascular structures of the upper cervical region. Hemangiomas, similar to those of other anatomical sites, are initially treated with steroids or beta-blockers with surgery or laser therapy reserved or select cases.

Malignant

Tumors that arise in the sublingual glands and minor salivary glands are most often malignant, while those in the parotid are more often benign. These include mucoepidermoid carcinomas, adenoid cystic carcinomas, acinic cell carcinomas, and polymorphous adenocarcinoma. Pleomorphic adenomas have a 10% risk for malignant transformation to carcinomas ex pleomorphic adenoma. Squamous cell carcinoma arising in the parotid gland are assumed to arise as metastases from frontotemporal scalp cutaneous carcinoma. Occasionally, skip lesions occur in the upper neck, and treatment of these should still involve a parotidectomy for presumed occult disease. Lymphomas are one exception and are treated by chemoradiation primarily.

Parotid

The parotid is bordered by the masseter anteriorly, sternocleidomastoid muscle posteriorly, zygomatic arch superiorly, and mandibular ramus inferiorly [115, 116]. While not anatomically separate, surgeons tend to refer to the deep (20%) and superficial lobes (80%) of the parotid which are separated by the plane of the facial nerve. Lymph nodes are located intra- and peri-glandular.

Malignant parotid tumors should be managed with a parotidectomy [109, 117]. Current guidelines are moving towards less aggressive resections when indicated. A total parotidectomy is indicated for high-grade tumors with high metastatic profile, tumors with lymph node metastasis, or any primary deep lobe tumors. Small, encapsulated malignancies in the lateral lobe can be managed with a superficial parotidectomy, and larger tumors can be considered for a partial deep lobe resection.

Parotidectomies are approached via the modified Blair incision, taking care to identify the main trunk of the facial nerve laterally, and the marginal mandibular branch inferiorly [118]. Deep lobe and parapharyngeal space tumors can warrant transcervical resection with possible mandibulotomy. If the facial nerve is involved, general principles apply and resection with negative margins should be pursued. Proximal extension may require mastoidectomy to achieve a negative margin. Facial nerve reconstruction can be completed by neurorrhaphy or interposition graft. However, if no nerve invasion is present and a plane can be surgically developed between the parotid tissue and nerve, preservation is important for improved morbidity.

Facial nerve paresis or paralysis may result from manipulation and traction during dissection, fortunately with full recovery in most cases. Approximately 20% of superficial parotidectomies can result in Frey syndrome, or auriculotemporal nerve syndrome. This is classified by gustatory sweating as a result of sympathetic fibers of transected auriculotemporal nerve branches aberrantly reinnervating the parotid. Treatment for refractory cases can be topical scopolamine or Botox injection.

Submandibular Gland

The submandibular gland is bordered superiorly by the mandible and inferiorly by the anterior and posterior bellies of the digastric muscle [119, 120]. Lymph nodes are all located peri-glandular.

Malignancies require gland excision in continuity with the level Ib nodes (submandibular nodes), present at the inferomedial location on the mandible [69]. Care should be taken to identify the marginal mandibular nerve, which should be reflected superiorly for preservation. The hypoglossal nerve should similarly be protected deep to the digastric muscles. The facial artery and vein can be ligated, and the submandibular ganglion and Wharton duct are the final structures to be sacrificed.

Sublingual and Minor Salivary Glands

The sublingual glands are located superior to the mylohyoid muscle, opposite of the lingual frenulum. Malignancies must be resected via a transcervical or, more popularly, a transoral approach, with a wide local excision often involving the tongue, mylohyoid, mandible, and possibly lingual nerve.

Neck Dissection   Palpable or radio-apparent nodes in the neck should undergo ipsilateral radical neck (Levels 1–5) dissection with adjuvant radiation [121, 122]. Such aggressive treatment is necessary as salivary gland cancers often metastasize to any of the nodal basins.

Armstrong and colleagues demonstrated that 3 out of 30 patients (10%) had metastases in level I, 8 of 30 (27%) in level II, 7 of 30 (23%) in level III, 6 of 30 (20%) in level IV, and 1 of 30 (3%) in level V [123, 124]. They showed that dissection of levels I through IV would have detected all occult metastases. The one patient with a positive level V node also had node-positive disease in levels II through IV.

The guidelines for management of the clinically node-negative neck are under investigation. In general, elective neck dissection can be considered for high-grade or stage III/IV disease, extra-glandular extension, or facial nerve involvement.

Conclusion

Head and neck surgery is a formidable field to master. Each cancer type and anatomic location possesses different management algorithms and unique challenges. Proper comprehensive discussion would mandate a textbook for every tumor category. The importance of an involved radiation oncology team cannot be emphasized enough, as management almost always extends past surgical resection alone. There furthermore remains much to innovate in the field of head and neck surgery. Minimal surgical treatment has allowed great improvements in functional morbidity, significantly limiting the need for tracheostomies. As the field continues to grow, we anticipate improved resection outcomes with decreased aesthetic and functional deficits.

References

1. Nelson WR. In search of the first head and neck surgeon. Am J Surg. 1987;154(4):342–6.
2. Folz BJ, Silver CE, Rinaldo A, et al. An outline of the history of head and neck oncology. Oral Oncol. 2008;44(1):2–9.
3. Crile GW. On the surgical treatment of cancer. Transact Southern Surg Gynecol Assoc. 1906;18:108.
4. Crile G. Excision of cancer of the head and neck: with special reference to the plan of dissection based on one hundred and thirty-two operations. JAMA. 1987;258(22):3286–93.
5. Kleinsasser O. Mikrolaryngoskopie und endolaryngeale Mikrochirurgie: Technik und typische Befunde: Schattauer Verlag; 1991.
6. Polanyi TG, Bredemeier H, Davis T. A CO 2 laser for surgical research. Med Biol Eng. 1970;8(6):541–8.
7. Strong MS, Jako GJ. Laser surgery in the larynx early clinical experience with continuous CO2 laser. Ann Otol Rhinol Laryngol. 1972;81(6):791–8.

8. Mork J, Lie AK, Glattre E, et al. Human papillomavirus infection as a risk factor for squamous-cell carcinoma of the head and neck. N Engl J Med. 2001;344(15):1125–31.
9. Gupta K, Mandlik D, Patel D, et al. Clinical assessment scoring system for tracheostomy (CASST) criterion: objective criteria to predict pre-operatively the need for a tracheostomy in head and neck malignancies. J Cranio-Maxillofac Surg. 2016;44(9):1310–3.
10. Crosher R, Baldie C, Mitchell R. Selective use of tracheostomy in surgery for head and neck cancer: an audit. Br J Oral Maxillofac Surg. 1997;35(1):43–5.
11. Adoga AA, Kirfi AM, Bature IF, Bakari AA. Retrospective analysis of tracheostomy in patients with tumors of the aerodigestive tract. Ann Med Health Sci Res. 2018;8(6)
12. Wiggenraad R, Flierman L, Goossens A, et al. Prophylactic gastrostomy placement and early tube feeding may limit loss of weight during chemoradiotherapy for advanced head and neck cancer, a preliminary study. Clin Otolaryngol. 2007;32(5):384–90.
13. Hardy S, Haas K, Vanston VJ, Angelo M. Prophylactic feeding tubes in head and neck cancers# 318. J Palliat Med. 2016;19(12):1343–4.
14. Atasoy BM, Yonal O, Demirel B, et al. The impact of early percutaneous endoscopic gastrostomy placement on treatment completeness and nutritional status in locally advanced head and neck cancer patients receiving chemoradiotherapy. Eur Arch Otorhinolaryngol. 2012;269(1):275–82.
15. Rutter CE, Yovino S, Taylor R, et al. Impact of early percutaneous endoscopic gastrostomy tube placement on nutritional status and hospitalization in patients with head and neck cancer receiving definitive chemoradiation therapy. Head Neck. 2011;33(10):1441–7.
16. Salas S, Baumstarck-Barrau K, Alfonsi M, et al. Impact of the prophylactic gastrostomy for unresectable squamous cell head and neck carcinomas treated with radio-chemotherapy on quality of life: prospective randomized trial. Radiother Oncol. 2009;93(3):503–9.
17. Chen AM, Li B-Q, Lau DH, et al. Evaluating the role of prophylactic gastrostomy tube placement prior to definitive chemoradiotherapy for head and neck cancer. Int J Radiat Oncol Biol Phys. 2010;78(4):1026–32.
18. Silander E, Nyman J, Bove M, Johansson L, Larsson S, Hammerlid E. Impact of prophylactic percutaneous endoscopic gastrostomy on malnutrition and quality of life in patients with head and neck cancer—a randomized study. Head Neck. 2012;34(1):1–9.
19. Strom T, Trotti AM, Kish J, et al. Risk factors for percutaneous endoscopic gastrostomy tube placement during chemoradiotherapy for oropharyngeal cancer. JAMA Otolaryngol–Head Neck Surg. 2013;139(11):1242–6.
20. Flint PW, Haughey BH, Robbins KT, et al. Cummings otolaryngology-head and neck surgery e-book. In: Elsevier health sciences; 2014.
21. Wei WI, Ferlito A, Rinaldo A, et al. Management of the N0 neck—reference or preference. Oral Oncol. 2006;42(2):115–22.
22. D'Cruz AK, Vaish R, Kapre N, et al. Elective versus therapeutic neck dissection in node-negative oral cancer. N Engl J Med. 2015;373(6):521–9.
23. Robbins KT, Clayman G, Levine PA, et al. Neck dissection classification update: revisions proposed by the American Head and Neck Society and the American Academy of Otolaryngology–Head and Neck Surgery. Arch Otolaryngol–Head Neck Surg. 2002;128(7):751–8.
24. Ow TJ, Grethlein SJ, Schmalbach CE, Head ECotA, Society N. Do you know your guidelines? Diagnosis and management of cutaneous head and neck melanoma. Head Neck. 2018;40(5):875–85.
25. Chan Y. KJ Lee's essential otolaryngology head & neck Surgery. 11th ed. New York: McGraw-Hill Education; 2016.
26. National Comprehensive Cancer Network Clinical Practice Guidelines in Oncology: Basal Cell Carcinoma. 2018;V1. www.nccn.org.
27. National Comprehensive Cancer Network Clinical Practice Guidelines in Oncology: Squamous Cell Carcinoma. 2018. www.nccn.org.
28. Raskob GE, Zitsch IIIRP, Park CW, Renner GJ, Rea JRJL. Outcome analysis for lip carcinoma. Otolaryngol–Head Neck Surg. 1995;113(5):589–96.

29. Vukadinovic M, Jezdic Z, Petrovic M, Medenica LM, Lens M. Surgical management of squamous cell carcinoma of the lip: analysis of a 10-year experience in 223 patients. J Oral Maxillofac Surg. 2007;65(4):675–9.
30. Zitsch RP III, Lee BW, Smith RB. Cervical lymph node metastases and squamous cell carcinoma of the lip. Head Neck J Sci Special Head Neck. 1999;21(5):447–53.
31. Goldenberg D, Ardekian L, Rachmiel A, Peled M, Joachims HZ, Laufer D. Carcinoma of the dorsum of the tongue. Head Neck J Sci Special Head Neck. 2000;22(2):190–4.
32. Ganly I, Patel S, Shah J. Early stage squamous cell cancer of the oral tongue—clinicopathologic features affecting outcome. Cancer. 2012;118(1):101–11.
33. Lydiatt DD, Robbins KT, Byers RM, Wolf PF. Treatment of stage I and II oral tongue cancer. Head Neck. 1993;15(4):308–12.
34. Bokhari WA, Wang SJ. Tongue reconstruction: recent advances. Curr Opin Otolaryngol Head Neck Surg. 2007;15(4):202–7.
35. Marchetta FC, Sako K, Murphy JB. The periosteum of the mandible and intraoral carcinoma. Am J Surg. 1971;122(6):711–3.
36. Tei K, Totsuka Y, Iizuka T, Ohmori K. Marginal resection for carcinoma of the mandibular alveolus and gingiva where radiologically detected bone defects do not extend beyond the mandibular canal. J Oral Maxillofac Surg. 2004;62(7):834–9.
37. Dai T-S, Hao S-P, Chang K-P, Pan W-L, Yeh H-C, Tsang N-M. Complications of mandibulotomy: midline versus paramidline. Otolaryngol Head Neck Surg. 2003;128(1):137–41.
38. Eisen MD, Weinstein GS, Chalian A, et al. Morbidity after midline mandibulotomy and radiation therapy. Am J Otolaryngol. 2000;21(5):312–7.
39. Shaha AR, Spiro RH, Shah JP, Strong EW. Squamous carcinoma of the floor of the mouth. Am J Surg. 1984;148(4):455–9.
40. Rodgers LW Jr, Stringer SP, Mendenhall WM, Parsons JT, Cassisi NJ, Million RR. Management of squamous cell carcinoma of the floor of mouth. Head Neck. 1993;15(1):16–9.
41. Eicher SA, Overholt SM, El-Naggar AK, Byers RM, Weber RS. Lower gingival carcinoma: clinical and pathologic determinants of regional metastases. Arch Otolaryngol–Head Neck Surg. 1996;122(6):634–8.
42. Overholt SM, Eicher SA, Wolf P, Weber RS. Prognostic factors affecting outcome in lower gingival carcinoma. Laryngoscope. 1996;106(11):1335–9.
43. Huang CJ, Chao KC, Tsai J, et al. Cancer of retromolar trigone: long-term radiation therapy outcome. Head Neck J Sci Special Head Neck. 2001;23(9):758–63.
44. Yorozu A, Sykes AJ, Slevin NJ. Carcinoma of the hard palate treated with radiotherapy: a retrospective review of 31 cases. Oral Oncol. 2001;37(6):493–7.
45. Jing J, Li L, He W, Sun G. Prognostic predictors of squamous cell carcinoma of the buccal mucosa with negative surgical margins. J Oral Maxillofac Surg. 2006;64(6):896–901.
46. Diaz EM Jr, Holsinger FC, Zuniga ER, Roberts DB, Sorensen DM. Squamous cell carcinoma of the buccal mucosa: one institution's experience with 119 previously untreated patients. Head Neck J Sci Special Head Neck. 2003;25(4):267–73.
47. Lin HW, Bhattacharyya N. Survival impact of nodal disease in hard palate and maxillary alveolus cancer. Laryngoscope. 2009;119(2):312–5.
48. Civantos FJ, Moffat FL, Goodwin WJ. Lymphatic mapping and sentinel lymphadenectomy for 106 head and neck lesions: contrasts between oral cavity and cutaneous malignancy. Laryngoscope. 2006;116(S109):1–15.
49. Montes DM, Carlson ER, Fernandes R, et al. Oral maxillary squamous carcinoma: an indication for neck dissection in the clinically negative neck. Head Neck. 2011;33(11):1581–5.
50. Wendt JR, Gardner VO, White JI. Treatment of complex postoperative lumbosacral wounds in nonparalyzed patients. Plast Reconstr Surg. 1998;101(5):1248–53.
51. Eversole L, Sabes W, Rovin S. Aggressive growth and neoplastic potential of odontogenic cysts. With special reference to central epidermoid and mucoepidermoid carcinomas. Cancer. 1975;35(1):270–82.
52. Regezi J, Kerr D, Courtney R. Odontogenic tumors: analysis of 706 cases. J Oral Surg (American Dental Association: 1965). 1978;36(10):771.

53. Chapelle KA, Stoelinga PJ, de Wilde PC, Brouns JJ, Voorsmit RA. Rational approach to diagnosis and treatment of ameloblastomas and odontogenic keratocysts. Br J Oral Maxillofac Surg. 2004;42(5):381–90.

54. Brøndum N, Jensen VJ. Recurrence of keratocysts and decompression treatment: a long-term follow-up of forty-four cases. Oral Surg Oral Med Oral Pathol. 1991;72(3):265–9.

55. Carlson ER, Marx RE. The ameloblastoma: primary, curative surgical management. J Oral Maxillofac Surg. 2006;64(3):484–94.

56. Gardner D. Critique of the 1995 review by Reichart et al. of the biologic profile of 3677 ameloblastomas. Oral Oncol. 1999;35(4):443–9.

57. Oliver R, Clarkson JE, Conway D, et al. Interventions for the treatment of oral and oropharyngeal cancers: surgical treatment. Cochrane Database Syst Rev. 2007;(4):CD006205.

58. Bhayani MK, Holsinger FC. Lai SY. A shifting paradigm for patients with head and neck cancer: transoral robotic surgery (TORS). Head Neck. 2010;24(11)

59. Haughey BH, Hinni ML, Salassa JR, et al. Transoral laser microsurgery as primary treatment for advanced-stage oropharyngeal cancer: a United States multicenter study. Head Neck. 2011;33(12):1683–94.

60. Grant DG, Salassa JR, Hinni ML, Pearson BW, Perry WC. Carcinoma of the tongue base treated by transoral laser microsurgery, part one: untreated tumors, a prospective analysis of oncologic and functional outcomes. Laryngoscope. 2006;116(12):2150–5.

61. Chan JY, Wong EW, Tsang RK, et al. Early results of a safety and feasibility clinical trial of a novel single-port flexible robot for transoral robotic surgery. Eur Arch Otorhinolaryngol. 2017;274(11):3993–6.

62. Har-El G, Shaha A, Chaudry R, Hadar T, Krespi YP, Lucente FE. Carcinoma of the uvula and midline soft palate: indication for neck treatment. Head Neck. 1992;14(2):99–101.

63. Calais G, Alfonsi M, Bardet E, et al. Stage III and IV cancers of the oropharynx: results of a randomized study of Gortec comparing radiotherapy alone with concomitant chemotherapy. Bull Cancer. 2000;87:48.

64. Parsons JT, Mendenhall WM, Stringer SP, et al. Squamous cell carcinoma of the oropharynx: surgery, radiation therapy, or both. Cancer: Interdisciplin Int J Am Cancer Soc. 2002;94(11):2967–80.

65. Schneider I, Thumfart WF, Eckel HE, Volling P, Ebeling O. Transoral laser surgery for oral carcinoma. Lasers Otorhinolaryngol Head Neck Surg. 1995;49:185–90. Karger Publishers

66. Hicks WL Jr, Kuriakose MA, Loree TR, et al. Surgery versus radiation therapy as single-modality treatment of tonsillar fossa carcinoma: the Roswell Park Cancer Institute experience (1971–1991). Laryngoscope. 1998;108(7):1014–9.

67. Steiner W, Ambrosch P. Endoscopic laser surgery of the upper aerodigestive tract: with special emphasis on cancer surgery. Stuttgart – New York: Thieme; 2000.

68. Steiner W, Fierek O, Ambrosch P, Hommerich CP, Kron M. Transoral laser microsurgery for squamous cell carcinoma of the base of the tongue. Arch Otolaryngol–Head Neck Surg. 2003;129(1):36–43.

69. Spiro RH, Kelly J, Vega AL, Harrison LB, Strong EW. Squamous carcinoma of the posterior pharyngeal wall. Am J Surg. 1990;160(4):420–3.

70. Meoz-Mendez RT, Fletcher GH, Guillamondegui OM, Peters LJ. Analysis of the results of irradiation in the treatment of squamous cell carcinomas of the pharyngeal walls. Int J Radiat Oncol Biol Phys. 1978;4(7–8):579–85.

71. Werner JA, Dünne AA, Myers JN. Functional anatomy of the lymphatic drainage system of the upper aerodigestive tract and its role in metastasis of squamous cell carcinoma. Head Neck J Sci Special Head Neck. 2003;25(4):322–32.

72. Shah MN, Kane AA, Petersen JD, Woo AS, Naidoo SD, Smyth MD. Endoscopically assisted versus open repair of sagittal craniosynostosis: the St. Louis Children's Hospital experience. J Neurosurg Pediat. 2011;8(2):165–70.

73. Wahlberg PC, Andersson KH, Biörklund AT, Möller TR. Carcinoma of the hypopharynx: analysis of incidence and survival in Sweden over a 30-year period. Head Neck J Sci Special Head Neck. 1998;20(8):714–9.

74. Pingree TF, Davis RK, Reichman O, Derrick L. Treatment of hypopharyngeal carcinoma: a 10-year review of 1, 362 cases. Laryngoscope. 1987;97(8):901–4.
75. Hoffman HT, Karnell LH, Shah JP, et al. Hypopharyngeal cancer patient care evaluation. Laryngoscope. 1997;107(8):1005–17.
76. CHEEVER DW. Cancer of the tonsil: removal of the tumor by external incision (a second case). Boston Med Surg J. 1878;99(5):133–9.
77. CRACOVANER AJ, CHODOSH PL. The lateral approach to the larynx and hypopharynx. AMA Arch Otolaryngol. 1960;71(1):8–15.
78. Holsinger FC, Motamed M, Garcia D, Brasnu D, Ménard M, Laccourreye O. Resection of selected invasive squamous cell carcinoma of the pyriform sinus by means of the lateral pharyngotomy approach: the partial lateral pharyngectomy. Head Neck J Sci Special Head Neck. 2006;28(8):705–11.
79. Ogura JH, Jurema A, Watson RK. Partial laryngopharyngectomy and neck dissection for pyriform sinus cancer: conservation surgery with immediate reconstruction. Laryngoscope. 1960;70(10):1399–417.
80. Laccourreye H, St Guily JL, Fabre A, Brasnu D, Menard M. Supracricoid hemilaryngopharyngectomy: analysis of 240 cases. Ann Otol Rhinol Laryngol. 1987;96(2):217–21.
81. Laccourreye O, Garcia D, Ishoo E, Kania R, de Mones E, Hans S. Supracricoid hemilaryngopharyngectomy in patients with invasive squamous cell carcinoma of the pyriform sinus: part I: technique, complications, and long-term functional outcome. Ann Otol Rhinol Laryngol. 2005;114(1):25–34.
82. Kraus DH, Harrison LB, Zelefsky M, et al. Salvage laryngectomy for unsuccessful larynx preservation therapy. Ann Otol Rhinol Laryngol. 1995;104(12):936–41.
83. Harrison DF. Surgical management of hypopharyngeal cancer: particular reference to the gastric pull-up operation. Arch Otolaryngol. 1979;105(3):149–52.
84. Buckley M, Tulloch J, White R Jr, Tucker M. Complications of orthognathic surgery: a comparison between wire fixation and rigid internal fixation. Int J Adult Orthodon Orthognath Surg. 1988;4(2):69–74.
85. Mcdonald TJ, Desanto LW, Weiland LH. Supraglottic larynx and its pathology as studied by whole laryngeal sections. Laryngoscope. 1976;86(5):635–48.
86. Scola B, Fernández-Vega M, MartÍNez T, Fernández-Vega S, Ramirez C. Management of cancer of the supraglottis. Otolaryngol Head Neck Surg. 2001;124(2):195–8.
87. Sessions DG, Lenox J, Spector GJ. Supraglottic laryngeal cancer: analysis of treatment results. Laryngoscope. 2005;115(8):1402–10.
88. Ambrosch P. The role of laser microsurgery in the treatment of laryngeal cancer. Curr Opin Otolaryngol Head Neck Surg. 2007;15(2):82–8.
89. Ambrosch P, Kron M, Steiner W. Carbon dioxide laser microsurgery for early supraglottic carcinoma. Ann Otol Rhinol Laryngol. 1998;107(8):680–8.
90. Brasnu DF. Supracricoid partial laryngectomy with cricohyoidopexy in the management of laryngeal carcinoma. World J Surg. 2003;27(7):817–23.
91. Myers EN, Wagner RL, Johnson JT. Microlaryngoscopic surgery for T1 glottic lesions: a cost-effective option. Ann Otol Rhinol Laryngol. 1994;103(1):28–30.
92. Fein DA, Mendenhall WM, Parsons JT, Million RR. T1–T2 squamous cell carcinoma of the glottic larynx treated with radiotherapy: a multivariate analysis of variables potentially influencing local control. Int J Radiat Oncol Biol Phys. 1993;25(4):605–11.
93. Thomas JV, Olsen KD, Neel HB, DeSanto LW, Suman VJ. Early glottic carcinoma treated with open laryngeal procedures. Arch Otolaryngol–Head Neck Surg. 1994;120(3):264–8.
94. Cellai E, Frata P, Magrini SM, et al. Radical radiotherapy for early glottic cancer: results in a series of 1087 patients from two Italian radiation oncology centers. I. The case of T1N0 disease. Int J Radiat Oncol Biol Phys. 2005;63(5):1378–86.
95. Stell P, Tobin K. The behavior of cancer affecting the subglottic space. Can J Otolaryngol. 1975;4(4):612–7.

96. Hong WK, Lippman SM, Wolf GT. Recent advances in head and neck cancer—larynx preservation and cancer chemoprevention: the Seventeenth Annual Richard and Hinda Rosenthal Foundation Award Lecture. Cancer Res. 1993;53(21):5113–20.

97. Goguen LA, Posner MR, Tishler RB, et al. Examining the need for neck dissection in the era of chemoradiation therapy for advanced head and neck cancer. Arch Otolaryngol–Head Neck Surg. 2006;132(5):526–31.

98. Chiu RJ, Myers EN, Johnson JT. Efficacy of routine bilateral neck dissection in the management of supraglottic cancer. Otolaryngol Head Neck Surg. 2004;131(4):485–8.

99. Yang CY, Andersen PE, Everts EC, Cohen JI. Nodal disease in purely glottic carcinoma: is elective neck treatment worthwhile? Laryngoscope. 1998;108(7):1006–8.

100. Brentani RR, Kowalski LP, Soares JF, et al. End results of a prospective trial on elective lateral neck dissection vs type III modified radical neck dissection in the management of supraglottic and transglottic carcinomas. Head Neck. 1999;21(8):694–702.

101. Greene RM, DeWitt AI, Otto RA. Management of T3 N0 and T4 N0 glottic carcinomas: results of a national survey. Otolaryngol Head Neck Surg. 2003;128(2):191–5.

102. Wei WI, Sham JS. Nasopharyngeal carcinoma. Lancet. 2005;365(9476):2041–54.

103. Chen MY, Wen WP, Guo X, et al. Endoscopic nasopharyngectomy for locally recurrent nasopharyngeal carcinoma. Laryngoscope. 2009;119(3):516–22.

104. Wei WL, Lam KH, Sham JS. New approach to the nasopharynx: the maxillary swing approach. Head Neck. 1991;13(3):200–7.

105. Wei WI, Ho WK. Transoral robotic resection of recurrent nasopharyngeal carcinoma. Laryngoscope. 2010;120(10):2011–4.

106. Patel MR, Stadler ME, Snyderman CH, et al. How to choose? Endoscopic skull base reconstructive options and limitations. Skull Base. 2010;20(6):397.

107. Lee JY, Ramakrishnan VR, Chiu AG, Palmer J, Gausas RE. Endoscopic endonasal surgical resection of tumors of the medial orbital apex and wall. Clin Neurol Neurosurg. 2012;114(1):93.

108. Lund VJ, Stammberger H, Nicolai P, et al. European position paper on endoscopic management of tumours of the nose, paranasal sinuses and skull base. Rhinol Suppl. 2010;(22):1–143.

109. Witt RL. The significance of the margin in parotid surgery for pleomorphic adenoma. Laryngoscope. 2002;112(12):2141–54.

110. Pogrel MA. Benign non odontogenic lesions of the jaws. Peterson's Principles Oral Maxillofac Surg. 2004;1:597–616.

111. Avelar RL, Antunes AA, Carvalho RW, Bezerra PG, Neto PJO, Andrade ES. Odontogenic cysts: a clinicopathological study of 507 cases. J Oral Sci. 2009;51(4):581–6.

112. Jansisyanont P, Blanchaert R Jr, Ord RA. Intraoral minor salivary gland neoplasm: a single institution experience of 80 cases. Int J Oral Maxillofac Surg. 2002;31(3):257–61.

113. Tanimoto H, Kumoi K, Otsuki N, Hirayama Y. Multiple primary pleomorphic adenomas in a single parotid gland: report of a new case. Ear Nose Throat J. 2002;81(5):341–5.

114. Pinkston JA, Cole P. Cigarette smoking and Warthin's tumor. Am J Epidemiol. 1996;144(2):183–7.

115. Berg DH. Working memory and arithmetic calculation in children: the contributory roles of processing speed, short-term memory, and reading. J Exp Child Psychol. 2008;99(4):288–308.

116. Thackray AC, Lucas RB. Tumors of the major salivary glands. Washington, DC: Armed Forces Institute of Pathology; 1974.

117. Beahrs OH, Woolner LB, Carveth SW, Devine KD. Surgical management of parotid lesions: review of seven hundred sixty cases. AMA Arch Surg. 1960;80(6):890–904.

118. Terris DJ, Tuffo KM, Fee WE. Modified facelift incision for parotidectomy. J Laryngol Otol. 1994;108(7):574–8.

119. Bhattacharyya N. Survival and prognosis for cancer of the submandibular gland. J Oral Maxillofac Surg. 2004;62(4):427–30.

120. Da-Quan M, Guang-Yan Y. Tumours of the minor salivary glands: a clinicopathologic study of 243 cases. Acta Otolaryngol. 1987;103(3–4):325–31.

121. Gold DR, Annino DJ. Management of the neck in salivary gland carcinoma. Otolaryngol Clin N Am. 2005;38(1):99–105.
122. Terhaard CH, Lubsen H, Rasch CR, et al. The role of radiotherapy in the treatment of malignant salivary gland tumors. Int J Radiat Oncol Biol Phys. 2005;61(1):103–11.
123. Armstrong JG, Harrison LB, Thaler HT, et al. The indications for elective treatment of the neck in cancer of the major salivary glands. Cancer. 1992;69(3):615–9.
124. Kelley DJ, Spiro RH. Management of the neck in parotid carcinoma. Am J Surg. 1996;172(6):698–700.
125. Schoeff SS, et al. Nutritional management for head and neck cancer patients. Pract Gastroenterol Series 121. 2013;37(9):43–51.

Chapter 9
Conventional Reconstructive Approaches Following Resection of Head and Neck Cancer

David Perrault and Karl C. Bruckman

General Principles of Reconstructive Surgery

In general, reconstruction of the head and neck is challenging. Primarily because the head and neck anatomy is compact and highly functional. Therefore, similar to the hand, you can imagine that disturbing even a relatively small area of anatomy can have a large impact on function and overall form. Reconstructing the head and neck begins with defining the tissue defect. The size, composition of the tissue loss, and complexity of the defect are variable. On the most severe side of the spectrum, oncologic defects can be large, have complex topology, and involve loss of all tissue components, including skin, adipose, muscle, bone, vessels, and nerve. On the other side of the spectrum, defects can involve isolated skin loss and may just require primary closure of the wound. Given the complex and variable nature of reconstruction in general, the approach has been simplified into principles. Therefore, this chapter reviews the principles of reconstructive surgery, how they are applied, and provides a brief review of the many reconstructive options for the head and neck.

The goals of reconstruction at any anatomic site are restoration or maintenance of form, structural integrity, and function [1, 2]. In practice, this means maintaining a cosmetically normal appearance and preserving the many functions of the head and neck, such as facial animation, intelligible speech, mastication, nasal/oral breathing, vision, and protection of the intracranial contents. These goals are intended to maximize the patient's quality of life and minimize the impact of the disease process and medical interventions on morbidity and mortality.

The reconstructive ladder is a principle that prioritizes the simplest reconstructive option first, then moves up the ladder of increasingly complex interventions.

D. Perrault · K. C. Bruckman (✉)
Division of Plastic & Reconstructive Surgery, Department of Surgery, Stanford University School of Medicine, Stanford, CA, USA
e-mail: Bruckman@stanford.edu

© Springer Nature Switzerland AG 2021
R. El Assal et al. (eds.), *Early Detection and Treatment of Head & Neck Cancers*, https://doi.org/10.1007/978-3-030-69859-1_9

The reconstructive ladder includes (i) healing by secondary intention, (ii) primary closure, (iii) negative pressure wound therapy, (iv) grafts, (v) local and regional flaps, (vi) tissue expansion, and (vii) free tissue transfer, also referred to as free flaps. This concept is valuable in conceptualizing the options for reconstruction in rank of complexity and risk; however, in practice it is less often employed. Rather, the priority is to choose the surgical option that best addresses the goals of reconstruction as outlined above, even if a more simple option is possible [2].

Special Considerations in Head and Neck Cancer Reconstruction

Reconstruction after head and neck cancer resection comes with some special considerations, relating to both the anatomy and the cancer. In the head and neck specifically, larger margins often significantly affect nearby vital structures. This means that small resections can have a large impact on form and function. Even more so, defects are frequently large, involve multiple tissue types (e.g., bone, vessels, soft tissue, and skin), and have been exposed to radiation as a component of treatment of the primary cancer. Therefore, it is not uncommon to have a large complex radiated wound with loss of both soft tissue and bone.

Radiation therapy commonly precedes resection of head and neck tumors. Radiation exposure increases vessel wall fibrosis and decreases vascular smooth muscle density, practically, this impairs postoperative wound healing and leads to increased risk for wound infections, head and neck fistula formation, postoperative hematomas, and overall all postoperative local complications [3–7]. Moving up the reconstructive ladder, all modalities are negatively impacted by radiation therapy. However, free flaps appear to be the most resilient, since they bring healthy nonradiated tissue into the radiated field [1]. As a result, free flaps offer this as a major benefit in head and neck reconstruction. Although the most reliable option for reconstruction in radiated wounds, free flaps are also negatively affected by radiation. The exact effects of radiation on free flap complications has previously been controversial. However, a recent large metanalysis has shown that preoperative radiation increases the risk of flap failure by 1.82 times and increases the risk of wound infection [8].

Changes in nutritional status in head and neck cancer patients is also an important consideration. These patients often have limited oral intake because of pain with eating or generally feeling unwell. Additionally, having cancer and undergoing radiation and chemotherapy further impairs adequate nutrition. For example, it has been shown that despite sufficient oral intake, patients with head and neck cancer often fail to maintain their nutritional status [9]. This malnutrition leads to decreased muscle and fat mass, decreased strength, poor immune function, and ultimately poor wound healing [10, 11].

Therefore, as previously mentioned, in head and neck cancer reconstruction especially, free flaps are commonly employed. They provide well-vascularized tissue, can provide a large bulk of both bone and soft tissue, and bring healthy non-radiated tissue into the defect.

Head and Neck Reconstruction

There are many surgical options for reconstruction in the head and neck. Selecting the best option depends on the defect location, size, the tissues missing, functional goals, and history of previous surgeries or radiation. The following is an overview of the surgical options for reconstruction of the head and neck, organized by the anatomic site. Specifically, below is an overview of the reconstructive options for the scalp and calvarium, eyelid and periorbital region, midface/maxilla, mandible, and pharynx/esophagus.

Scalp Reconstruction

The scalp includes the soft tissue that covers the cranium and its borders including the face and the neck [10, 11]. The scalp and calvarium physically protect the intracranial contents and are an integral component of maintaining a normal appearance [12]. The goals of scalp and calvarial reconstruction include providing bony continuity to protect the intracranial contents and avoiding exposure of the calvarial bone [2]. Cosmetically, it is important to maintain the hair line and to limit hair loss. Scalp reconstruction typically follows the reconstructive ladder.

Secondary Intention

Healing by secondary intention involves local wound care and leaving the wound to heal without surgical intervention. The advantages of secondary intent are potentially avoiding a more invasive operation and a donor site. This is most efficacious when there is a clean wound bed, on a concave surface, and intact vascularized tissue at the base of the wound, pericranium in the case of the scalp [13]. Unfortunately, this approach significantly delays time to a healed wound and results in alopecia at the wound site.

Primary Closure

Primary closure is the simplest option to achieve a closed wound. If possible, primary closure is preferred since the wound is closed in a single stage and there is no donor site morbidity. Unfortunately, in the scalp, primary closure is typically only possible with tissue defects less than 3 cm [14].

Negative Pressure Wound Therapy

Negative Pressure Wound Therapy (NPWT), also referred to as wound Vacuum-Assisted Closure (wound VAC), can be used to both temporize wounds until definitive reconstruction and speedup healing by secondary intention. It functions by contracting the wound mechanically with suction, optimizing the wound environment by removing excess fluid, and facilitating granulation tissue formation at the microcellular level [15–17]. Contraindications to NPWT include a poor wound bed with necrotic tissue, active infection, and a malignant wound. NWPT has classically been discouraged in malignant wounds thinking that the same mechanism of negative pressure that promotes wound healing would also increase local malignant growth; however, this has been recently brought into question [18].

Skin Grafting

Skin grafting is reliable, quick, and technically simple. The disadvantages of skin grafting on the scalp include contour deformity, donor site morbidity, and hair loss at the defect [13]. Both split-thickness and full-thickness skin grafting are possible in the scalp. However, split thickness tends to have better take, as with other parts of body. In general, for skin grafts to take, there must be a vascularized wound bed that is clean. In the scalp, this means that there is intact periosteum, in the case of full-thickness defects [14]. Radiation can often complicate skin graft take; therefore, more recently, artificial dermal substitutes have been used to reconstruct radiated wounds, in conjunction with skin grafting [13, 19].

Local Flaps

There are many local flaps that may be used for scalp reconstruction. A local flap is defined as utilizing the tissue directly adjacent to the defect as the donor site. Local flap types include advancement, rotation, and transposition flaps. These terms refer to how the donor tissue is moved to cover the defect. There are many named flaps that can be used in the scalp. Describing every example would be beyond the scope of this review. It is worth noting the Orticochea technique, since this was initially described for scalp reconstruction in particular, in 1967 [20]. This flap utilized either three or four large skin flaps to cover the central defect [20, 21]. The advantages of local flaps include good color match and relative ease of harvest. However, in the case of oncologic reconstruction, using local flaps is limited since the tissue adjacent to the wound has often been exposed to radiation in the treatment for the primary cancer.

Regional Flaps

Regional flaps are close in proximity to the tissue defect and are transferred with an intact vascular pedicle. Unfortunately, regional flaps are often limited in the amount of tissue and the reach of the flap. Free tissue transfer is far more versatile and more reliable than pedicled flaps for scalp reconstruction. In head and neck reconstruction, since free tissue transfer is preferred for defects that are large enough to need a regional flap, regional flaps are usually limited to those who are unable to tolerate larger operations or are performed in the context of palliative care [14]. Options for regional flaps for scalp reconstruction include the trapezius flap, latissimus dorsi flap, and the temporoparietal fascia flap [13].

The trapezius flap (Fig. 9.1) was first described by Mathes and Nahai in 1979 [22]. The trapezius muscle can be harvested either just as the muscle alone or with a skin paddle. The trapezius muscle and the overlying skin in that area receive their blood supply from the superficial and deep descending branches of the transverse cervical artery [23]. The main advantages of the trapezius flap include the reliable anatomy and robust perfusion [23, 24]. Unfortunately, however, this flap has limited reach and inset into a more distally located defect can be difficult [13].

The latissimus dorsi flap (Fig. 9.2) was first described by Tansini in 1906 for breast reconstruction [25]. The latissimus muscle is broad and can provide good muscle bulk. The muscle can be harvested alone or can be raised with an overlying skin paddle. The trapezius muscle receives its blood supply from the thoracodorsal artery. The primary advantages include the large volume of available muscle and a long pedicle. The main disadvantage includes the need for lateral decubitus positioning intraoperatively for flap harvest [26]. The donor site morbidity associated with harvesting a major muscle is also a concern. Given its reliability, this flap is often saved as a last resort, after free tissue transfer has failed [26].

The temporoparietal flap system (Fig. 9.3) will be described in detail below (section "Temporalis System"), for its use in maxillary reconstruction. However, briefly, it is particularly useful in scalp reconstruction because of its long pedicle and the ability to harvest it with bone, muscle, fascia, and skin.

Tissue Expansion

Tissue expansion is an option in scalp reconstruction, in general. It works by inducing biologic and mechanical creep to increase the amount of skin available [13, 27]. However, there is a high rate of complications when used in the scalp, a recent large systematic review cited an overall complications rate of 27.3%. This high complication rate is made even worse in radiated fields or unstable wounds [28]. As a result, tissue expansion is not commonly used in oncologic scalp reconstruction [13].

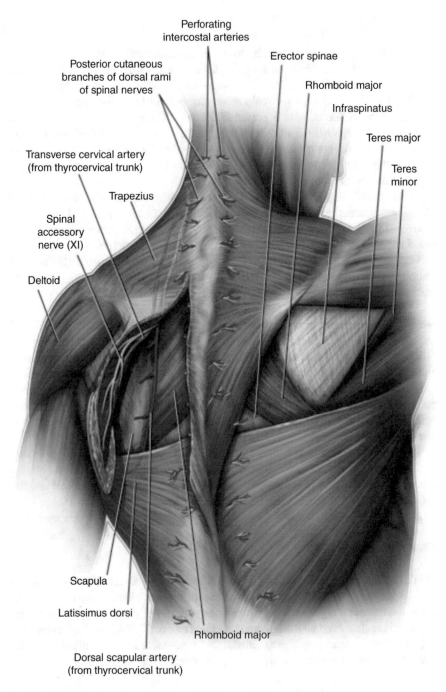

Fig. 9.1 Trapezius flap. (Reprinted by copyright permissions from [99])

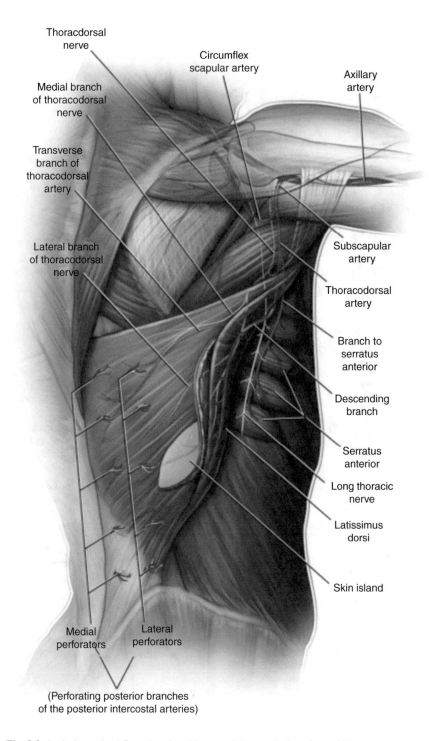

Fig. 9.2 Latissimus dorsi flap. (Reprinted by copyright permissions from [99])

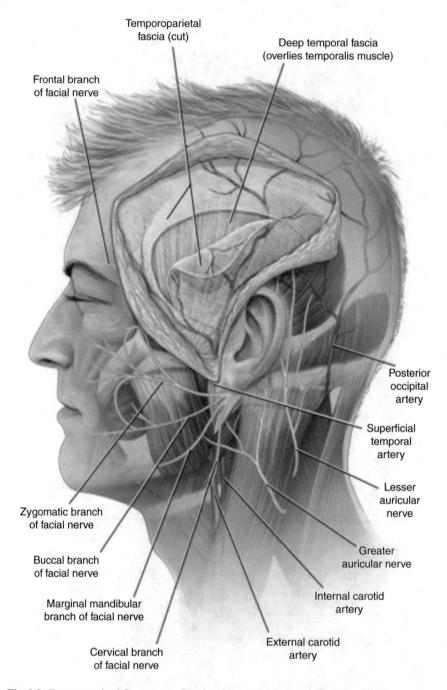

Fig. 9.3 Temporoparietal flap system. (Reprinted by copyright permissions from [99])

Free Tissue Transfer

Free tissue transfer, or free flaps, provide a highly versatile and reliable option for coverage of the scalp. It has the capacity to provide a large amount of healthy tissue that is taken from outside the radiated field. Unfortunately, free flaps are not typically cosmetically appealing because of color mismatch, poor contour, and alopecia of the flap. In the scalp, the superficial temporal artery is the workhorse recipient vessel. The choice of flap depends on the defect characteristics and surgeon's preference. Some of the most commonly used flaps for scalp reconstruction include latissimus dorsi, anterolateral thigh, radial forearm, and rectus abdominus [13, 29, 30].

The anterolateral thigh flap (Fig. 9.4) was first described by Song et al. in 1984 [31]. It provides skin, fascia, and adipose tissue. Furthermore, this flap can be harvested with the vastus lateralis muscle, if greater soft tissue bulk is required [29]. The ALT flap receives is blood supply from of the descending branch of the lateral circumflex femoral artery. The main advantages include good soft tissue bulk, versatility in practice, and a low donor site morbidity [32]. The main disadvantages are that the ALT is a relatively thick flap compared to muscle flaps, resulting in a poor cosmetic appearance of the reconstruction [32].

The latissimus dorsi flap can also be harvested as a free flap. This greatly increases its versatility. The latissimus dorsi flap was reviewed above as a pedicled/regional flap in section "Regional Flaps".

The radial forearm flap is a thin, pliable, and reliable free flap for head and neck reconstruction. It will be reviewed in section "Radial Forearm Free Flap".

The rectus abdominus flap provides substantial soft tissue bulk and affords reliable anatomy. This flap has been reviewed in section "Rectus Abdominis Free Flap".

Calvarial Reconstruction

The calvarium protects the intracranial contents and provides an esthetically pleasing contour. Options for calvarial reconstruction include both alloplastic and autologous materials. Alloplastic options, include titanium mesh, methyl methacrylate, calcium hydroxyapatite, and polyether ether ketone [33]. Alloplastic materials tend to be easy to manipulate, structurally strong, do not resorb, and have the added benefit of avoiding a donor site [34]. The disadvantage of these materials is the risk for infection and exposure of the implant [33, 34]. Autologous options include split calvarial grafts, rib grafts, and iliac bone graft [35, 36]. Autologous bone osteointegrates into the apposed bone and revascularizes, and hence provides durable coverage with a low chance of infection and graft loss [33]. The disadvantage of

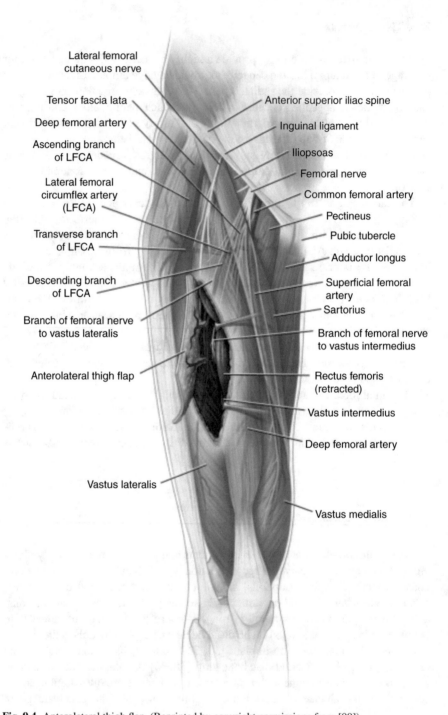

Fig. 9.4 Anterolateral thigh flap. (Reprinted by copyright permissions from [99])

autologous bone are the obligate donor site and the relatively small amount of bone available. In general, autologous reconstruction is preferred over alloplastic reconstruction, for the reasons listed above.

Eyelid and Periorbital Reconstruction

The upper and lower eyelids are exceptionally delicate structures. The goals of eyelid reconstruction are to cover the globe, preserve the tear film, maintain an unobstructed visual field, maintain good closing mechanics, and to restore a normal appearing eye [37]. Therefore, using donor skin of adequate size, similar color and pliability, and minimal donor site morbidity is even more important. Eyelid and periorbital reconstruction tend to follow the reconstructive ladder, with some caveats.

Secondary intention is best for small superficial lesions that located near the medial canthus. The nearby nasal bones resist scar contracture. In contrast, central and lateral eyelid defects carry a high risk of cicatricial ectropion with healing by secondary intent [38]. Moreover, healing by secondary intention in the periorbital area is very rarely done, since significant contour deformity and contracture often result [39].

Primary closure can be attempted for small lesions that do not involve the eyelid margin. Both upper and lower lid defects that involve less than 25–30% of the eyelid margin can be directly closed [37].

Skin grafting is possible for both the upper and lower eyelid. In particular, this is suited for defects of anterior lamella [37]. First choice of donor site is full-thickness graft taken from the contralateral upper eyelid [40]. Full-thickness skin grafts are preferred, to limit contracture.

Full-thickness defects larger than one-third the eyelid margin are repaired with rotation flaps, semicircular flaps, or pedicled flaps [38]. Flap choice is determined by the lid component tissue missing and these reconstructions are truly elegant. Full-thickness defects of the upper lid can be repaired with a modified Tenzel semicircular flap or a Cutler-Beard procedure [38]. Both these options rely on moving components of the lower lid to fill defects in the upper lid. The paramedian forehead flap can also be used for very severe defects. For the lower lid, the Tripier flap uses pedicled skin from the upper lid to reconstruct lower lid defects [37]. The Hughes flap (tarsoconjunctival pedicle flap) takes pedicled conjunctiva, tarsus, and skin from the upper lid to fill large full-thickness lower lid defects [38]. Notably, though, the Hughes flap requires division of the conjunctival pedicle at a later date [41]. The Mustarde flap is a large rotation flap that moves skin from the cheek to cover the lower lid [42].

Generally, free flaps are not used for eyelid reconstruction, since the eyelids are relatively small structures and the priority is good tissue match, which is best obtained from the local anatomy [37, 38].

Midface, Maxilla, and Mandibular Reconstruction

The midface is the central third of the face and includes the maxilla, which is structurally integral to the entire face. In fact, the maxilla is often referred as "keystone" of the midface [43]. It provides the occlusal plane, houses the maxillary dentition, supports the skull base, supports the orbital contents, and serves as the attachment for muscles of mastication and facial expression [44, 45]. There are a number of maxillary defect classification systems, but no unified system is routinely used [46–49]. The lack of a unified classification is likely a result of the complexity of maxillary reconstruction [50]. Although, different classification systems can be employed to direct maxillary reconstruction, the same general principles of reconstruction can be applied. Including replacing like-with-like, restoring structural support, and maintaining a cosmetic appearance. The goals of maxillary reconstruction, in particular, are to achieve separation of the oral and nasal cavities, support the orbital contents, provide functional dentition, and maintain facial contour [44, 45]. With any oncologic reconstruction, but with maxillary defects in particular, there is concern that the reconstruction may interfere with surveillance for recurrent disease. The maxilla especially so, since the defect can be deep, and the margin of resection would be obscured by the reconstruction. However, it appears that free flap and bone reconstruction are not independently associated with worse outcomes in head and neck reconstruction in general [51].

Historically, large maxillary defects were treated with prosthetic devices. The advent of free tissue transfer greatly decreased the use of prosthetics, since free tissue transfer has resulted in better satisfaction scores than prosthetic devices [52, 53]. Prosthetic obturation remains a good option for those who cannot tolerate or have a contraindication to a reconstructive procedure [54].

Midface and maxillary oncologic resections will result in loss of soft tissue, bone, or both. Loss of soft tissue and bone can be replaced with local, regional, and free flaps. The reconstructive ladder in maxillary reconstruction can be applied, but is in general less helpful. Specifically, because maxillary defects are not amenable to healing by secondary intent, primary closure, and skin grafting is less of a viable option given the concern for contracture at the recipient site [50]. Therefore, the reconstructive ladder in maxillary reconstruction usually starts with local flaps. Loss of bone specifically, can be replaced with bone grafts or free vascularized bone flaps. Small bone defects that do not compromise the structural architecture of the midface can be obliterated with soft tissue. However, if the structural support of the midface is compromised (e.g., resection of the orbital floor, nasal sidewall, or a tooth bearing segment of the maxilla), rigid reconstruction is needed to provide structural support and bone stock for osteointegrated dental implants [50]. Additionally, if multiple components are missing, composite flaps can be used.

The goals of mandibular reconstruction include (i) providing structural support of the soft tissues of the oral cavity and lower face, (ii) achieve proper occlusion, (iii) supply bone stock for dental implants, (iv) restore sensation when able, and (v) achieve tongue palate contact for swallowing and speech [55]. Mandibular defects are classified based on location, size, and degree of soft tissue loss. Mandibular reconstruction is distinct from maxillary reconstruction in that prosthetics are never an option [55]. Additionally, although nonvascularized bone grafts have been used in mandibular reconstruction, in a radiated field there is a greater risk of reabsorption of the graft and nonunion [56]. As a result, vascularized bone free flaps have become the standard of care in mandibular reconstruction [55]. The most commonly used donor sites for mandibular reconstruction include the fibula, iliac crest, and the scapula [57].

A review of the options for reconstruction of the midface, maxilla, and mandible follows.

Local Flaps

Local flaps can be used for small defects that do not require bone reconstruction.

Buccal Fat Pad

The buccal fat pad (Fig. 9.5) was first described for head and neck reconstruction by Egyedi in 1977, where he used to tissue to close oral-antral and oro-nasal fistulae [58]. It provides specialized fat that is located between the buccinator muscle and

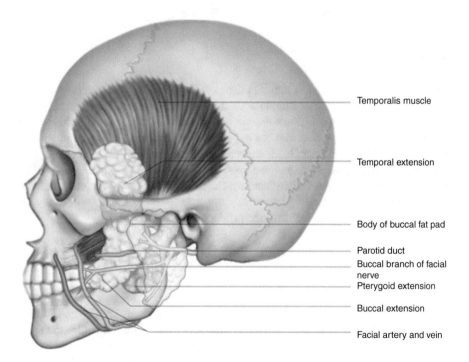

Temporalis muscle

Temporal extension

Body of buccal fat pad

Parotid duct
Buccal branch of facial nerve
Pterygoid extension

Buccal extension

Facial artery and vein

Fig. 9.5 Buccal fat pad. (Reprinted by copyright permissions from [100])

the mandibular ramus [59]. The fat pad is easily accessed and has a rich blood supply from the branches from the maxillary artery, superficial temporal artery, and facial artery [60]. It can be harvested as a pedicled flap to cover small oral defects. In general, it can be used to fill palatal defects up to 4 cm in diameter [60]. However, the size of the buccal fat pad is highly variable and changes with age [59]. Because of the limited reach of the flap, it is best suited for small maxillary defects that do not pass midline [60]. Buccal fat can also be used in combination with other reconstructive techniques to provide extra tissue volume.

Palatal Mucoperiosteal Island Flap

The palatal mucoperiosteal island flap was first described for reconstruction of intra-oral defects by Gullane and Arena in 1977 [61]. It utilizes the soft tissue over the hard palate, raised on a pedicle, and can then be rotated to cover adjacent defects. The blood supply is robust, and includes supplying vessels from the greater and lesser palatine arteries, ascending branch of the facial artery, and palatine branch of the ascending pharyngeal artery [61]. The main advantage of this flap is the large amount of soft tissue available from a local flap, which is approximately 15 cm^2 [62]. The main disadvantages are the short reach of the tissue, limiting the extent of the defects that it can fill, and the lack of bony tissue availability for osseus reconstruction. Notably, in contrast to most flaps, the donor site defect is typically left open, to heal by secondary intention/granulation [62].

Regional Flaps

There are a limited number of regional flaps available for maxillary reconstruction. These include the submental island flap, temporalis flap, and vascularized calvarial bone flap. Unfortunately, regional flaps in the head and neck are often limited by the length of the vascular pedicle and can be insufficient in reconstructing complex and broad defects [50]. For example, deltopectoral, latissimus dorsi, sternomastoid, and trapezius pedicled muscle flaps have been described; however, these were either unreliable, did not provide significant reach, or were too bulky for most defects [43]. Additionally, in oncologic reconstruction, many of these flaps will likely be radiated as part of the treatment for the primary tumor.

Temporalis System

The temporalis muscle flap was described as early as 1961, for reconstruction of a radical mastoidectomy [63]. Since then the flap has been widely applied and further described to include more than just the muscle. This flap system includes the temporalis muscle, temporoparietal galea, coronoid process, and underlying calvarial bone [64, 65]. Flaps using these structures are based of the superficial temporal artery. It can be taken as a pedicled or free flap and as a muscle, fascial, or composite flap. The temporalperietal galea or muscle flap can be used to obliterate oral and orbital defects, reconstruct the upper lip, and in the case of maxillary reconstruction needing bone stock for dental implants, the temporoparietal system can be harvested with calvarial bone as a vascularized bone flap [64]. Advantages of this flap system include reliable anatomy, tissue bulk, and the ability to take vascularized bone [64, 66]. Disadvantages include an unsightly donor site and possible involvement in the radiated field.

Submental Island Flap

The submental island flap was first described by Martin et al. in 1991 for orofacial defects, as an alternative to previously used cervical flaps [67]. The blood supply is the submental artery. Advantages include good color match to the face and a large amount of soft tissue available, originally described as 7 × 18 cm of tissue [67]. As such, it has been used for coverage of range of midface and lower face defects. Unfortunately, if level I lymph nodes are involved, this is a relative contraindication to using this flap [50].

Free Tissue Transfer

There are many options for maxillary reconstruction with free tissue transfer. As mentioned, if appropriate, free tissue transfer is an excellent option. Free tissue transfer enables bringing healthy nonradiated tissue into a poorly healing, likely radiated field. Additionally, it can provide reconstruction for complex defects missing multiple tissue types, and usually be performed in a single stage. Additionally, free flap reconstruction after oral and oropharyngeal cancer can improve patients' quality of life, in part by restoring their ability to speak and swallow [68].

Radial Forearm Free Flap

The radial forearm free flap (Fig. 9.6) was developed Goufan, Baoqui, and Yuzhi in 1978 [69]. It provides a large amount of soft tissue from the forearm. If bone reconstruction is needed, a segment of vascularized radius can also be harvested. Alternatively, autologous bone can be taken as a graft from the iliac crest, calvarium, or rib, which would save the radius as a donor site [46]. The blood supply is the radial artery. Since its development, because of its reliability, it has become widely used in head and neck reconstruction, to the point of being known as a workhorse flap [70]. The advantages of the forearm flap include a thin pliable flap with a long vascular pedicle. Disadvantages include a poorly appearing donor site, which may require a skin graft to close if a large amount of tissue is harvested [71].

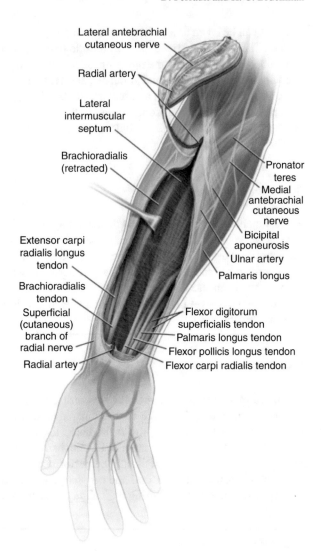

Fig. 9.6 Radial forearm free flap. (Reprinted by copyright permissions from [99])

Lateral antebrachial cutaneous nerve

Radial artery

Lateral intermuscular septum

Brachioradialis (retracted)

Pronator teres

Medial antebrachial cutaneous nerve

Bicipital aponeurosis

Ulnar artery

Palmaris longus

Extensor carpi radialis longus tendon

Brachioradialis tendon

Superficial (cutaneous) branch of radial nerve

Radial artey

Flexor digitorum superficialis tendon

Palmaris longus tendon

Flexor pollicis longus tendon

Flexor carpi radialis tendon

Rectus Abdominis Free Flap

The rectus abdominus free flap (Fig. 9.7) was first described by Pennington et al. in 1980 [72]. It provides a large amount of muscle and can be taken with an overlying skin paddle. If bone graft is needed, it can be taken from the rib or calvarium [46, 73, 74]. It is based off the inferior epigastric artery. Advantages include a long vascular pedicle and large amount of soft tissue [50]. Disadvantages include abdominal wall donor site and the risk of an abdominal bulge or a hernia [75].

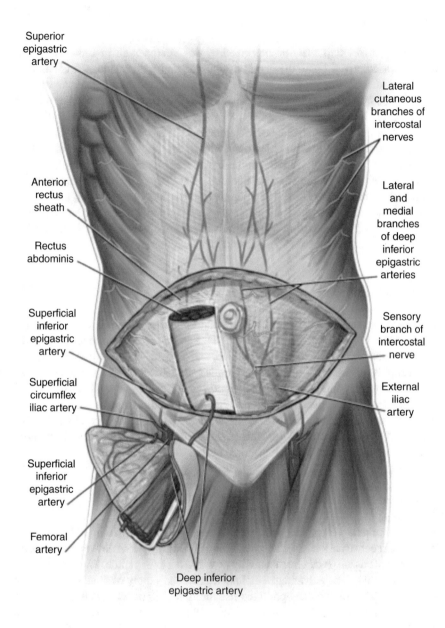

Fig. 9.7 Rectus abdominis free flap. (Reprinted by copyright permissions from [99])

Latissimus Dorsi and the Scapular Free-Flap System

The scapular free flap was first described by dos Santos et al. in 1984 [76]. It can provide vascularized bone, the overlying muscle, and a skin paddle. It is based off either the angular branch from the thoracodorsal artery or the cutaneous scapular artery [76, 77]. The scapular osteocutaneous free flap can also be raised as a bipedicled flap [77]. Meaning that the flap is harvested with two pedicles that allow for two independent vascularized bone segments, which could be useful in special cases. In the case of a total maxillectomy, which requires a large amount of tissue to obliterate the defect, the scapula can be harvested in combination with latissimus dorsi muscle off the same vascular pedicle, providing a customizable flap with a large bulk of muscle and bone [78]. Those who routinely use this flap find it to be highly versatile, have consistent anatomy, and good quality bone and soft tissue for head and neck reconstruction [79]. Disadvantages include difficult intraoperative positioning to harvest the flap for head and neck reconstruction.

Iliac Crest Free Flap

The iliac crest free flap (Fig. 9.8) was first described both experimentally and in a clinic setting by Taylor et al. in 1979 [80, 81]. The flap can be raised with iliac crest as bone stock, the attached internal oblique, and an overlying skin paddle [79]. The blood supply is based off the deep circumflex iliac artery (DCIA). The composite iliac crest internal oblique osteomusculocutaneous free flap is particularly suited to extensive maxillary defects. Advantages include providing a large amount of bone stock that can address the vertical component of the maxillary defect and support placement of osteointegrated implants [82]. Disadvantages include a short vascular pedicle, donor site morbidity, and limited soft tissue pliability [83].

Fibula Free Flap

The free fibula flap (Fig. 9.9) was first described by Taylor et al. in 1975, for lower extremity reconstruction [84]. The free fibula is a highly versatile flap that provides bone and soft tissue. It can be taken with or without a skin paddle. The blood supply is the peroneal artery. Advantages include a generous supply of bone stock that can support dental implants, the option to raise multiple skin paddles, and reliable anatomy [85]. The primary disadvantage of this flap is a relatively short pedicle and the added level of complexity in attempting to change a straight bone into a rigid curved structure [85].

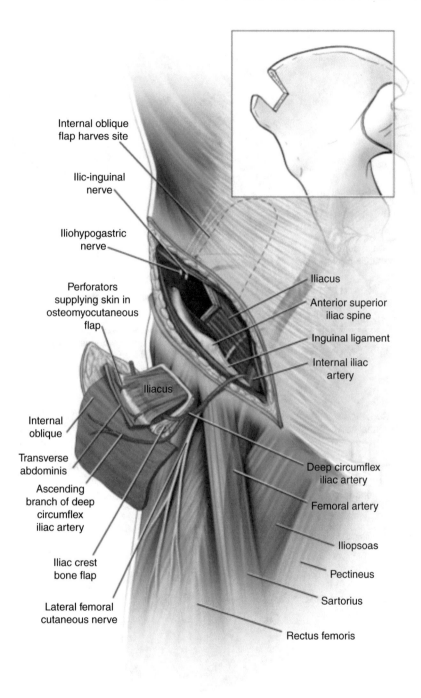

Fig. 9.8 Iliac crest free flap. (Reprinted by copyright permissions from [99])

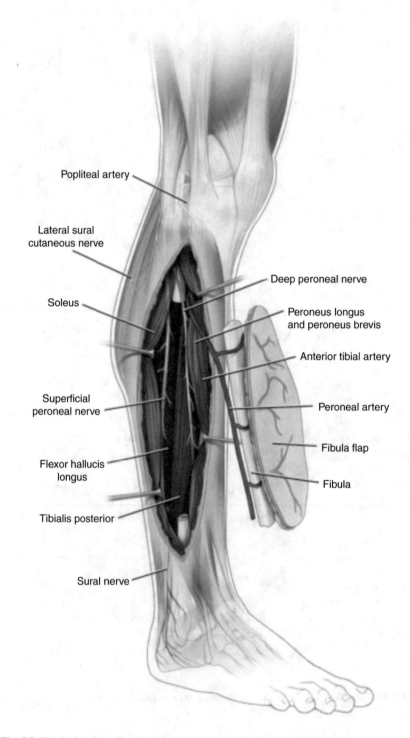

Fig. 9.9 Fibula free flap. (Reprinted by copyright permissions from [99])

Pharyngoesophageal Reconstruction

The pharynx and esophagus are essential components of the aerodigestive system. Dysfunction in these structures impairs speech, ventilation, and oral nutrition intake. Therefore, the goals of pharyngoesophageal reconstruction include restoring speech, normal swallowing, and protecting the airway [86]. Reconstruction of near circumferential or total circumferential defects of the pharynx and esophagus require reconstruction. Pedicled flap options include pectoralis major, supraclavicular artery island, latissimus dorsi, and trapezius pedicled flaps [87]. Free flap options are numerous, such as the anterolateral thigh and radial forearm flap. Additionally, enteric flaps are an option, most commonly the free jejunum flap. Other enteric flaps have been used for pharyngoesophageal reconstruction, but less commonly and typically in special cases.

Pedicled Flaps

Pedicled flaps in pharyngoesophageal reconstruction tend to be reserved as a backup option after free tissue transfer. The pectoralis major flap in particular is highly reliable and considered a workhorse flap for both initial pharyngoesophageal reconstruction and for correcting pharyngocutaneous fistula after reconstruction [87]. The supraclavicular artery island, latissimus dorsi, and trapezius pedicled flaps are also good options; however, these flaps are not nearly as commonly utilized as the pectoralis flap.

Pectoralis Flap

The pectoralis flap (Fig. 9.10) was described as early as 1917 and has been used in head in neck reconstruction since the 1920s [88]. The pectoralis flap can be taken with muscle, rib, and skin. The blood supply originates from the thoracoacromial artery and the perforating branches of the internal mammary artery [88]. Advantages include a single stage reconstruction, reliable pedicle, and providing healthy muscle for radiated and contaminated wounds [89]. Disadvantages include a relatively short reach and a large muscle bulk which can limit ease of creating a tube from of the flap [89, 90].

The trapezius flap and latissimus dorsi flap are already reviewed in this chapter. In pharyngoesophageal reconstruction in particular, the latissimus is a reliable option but tends to provide more tissue thickness than required and tends to be challenging to make into a tube [87].

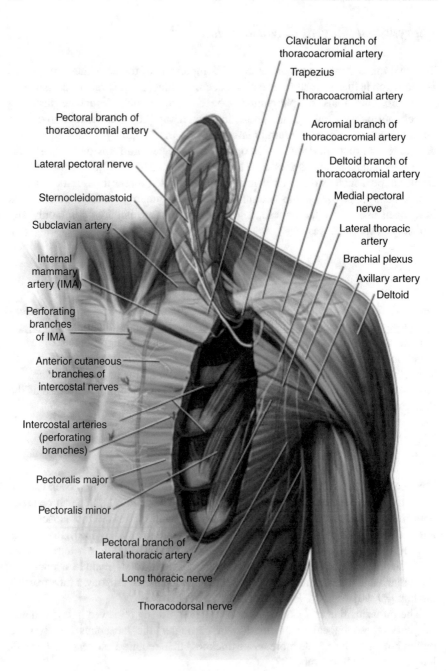

Clavicular branch of
thoracoacromial artery

Trapezius

Thoracoacromial artery

Pectoral branch of
thoracoacromial artery

Acromial branch of
thoracoacromial artery

Lateral pectoral nerve

Deltoid branch of
thoracoacromial artery

Sternocleidomastoid

Medial pectoral
nerve

Subclavian artery

Lateral thoracic
artery

Internal
mammary
artery (IMA)

Brachial plexus

Axillary artery

Deltoid

Perforating
branches
of IMA

Anterior cutaneous
branches of
intercostal nerves

Intercostal arteries
(perforating
branches)

Pectoralis major

Pectoralis minor

Pectoral branch of
lateral thoracic artery

Long thoracic nerve

Thoracodorsal nerve

Fig. 9.10 Pectoralis flap. (Reprinted by copyright permissions from [99])

Free Tissue Transfer

Using jejunum as a pedicled flap (Fig. 9.11) for esophageal reconstruction was first reported in the early 1900s [89]. Its use as a free flap was first reported by Seidenbert et al. in 1959, specifically for pharyngoesophageal reconstruction [91]. The jejunal blood supply originates from the superior mesenteric artery. This flap is unique in the types of flaps reported in this chapter, in that it provides small bowel tissue. All other flaps reported here provide a combination of skin, adipose, fascia, muscle, and/or bone. This makes it particularly suited for pharyngoesophageal reconstruction, since you are transferring a functional tubular structure. Other advantages include a lower rate of fistula formation compared to cutaneous reconstruction of the pharynx/esophagus [92]. As a result, the free jejunum has become the first-line

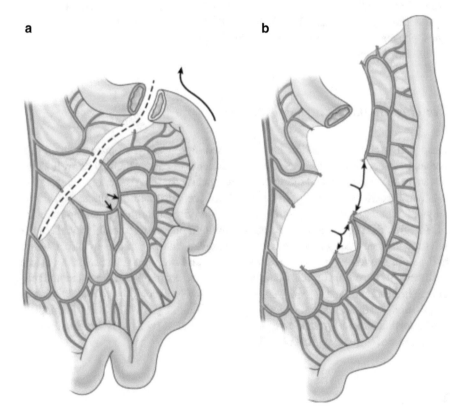

Fig. 9.11 Jejunum as a pedicled flap. (**a**) For esophageal reconstruction, a distance jejunum is better for a pedicled flap. (**b**) To retain the length for supercharging, the third jejunal artery is ligated and divided close to its origin from the superior mesenteric artery. (Reprinted by copyright permissions from [99])

workhorse flap for circumferential pharyngoesophageal reconstruction for many surgeons [92, 93]. Notably, however, there is evidence suggesting that pharyngo-esophageal reconstruction with cutaneous flaps, specifically the anterolateral thigh flap, offers better speech and swallowing function [94]. Disadvantages of free jeju-nal transfer include the need for a laparotomy, abdominal complications, and the relatively high risk of ischemia from the high metabolic demand of jejunum [92].

The radial forearm flap and anterolateral thigh flap have been reviewed else-where in this chapter. Notably, in pharyngoesophageal reconstruction, both of these flaps need to be formed into tubes to provide a pharyngoesophageal conduit. Unfortunately, this means that the conduit will involve an additional suture line along the length of the entire conduit. Exposure of a greater length of suture line to saliva presumably is one of the reasons these flaps tend to have higher rates of fis-tula formation and stricture compared to free Jejunal flaps [89, 95]. It should be noted, however, that there are few studies directly comparing outcomes of free jejunal transfer, anterolateral thigh flap, and radial free forearm flap use for pharyn-goesophageal reconstruction [96]. Choice of flap is typically surgeon- and institution-dependent.

Conclusion and Future Prospective

Head and neck reconstruction has progressed significantly. Improvement in out-comes has been largely affected by advancements in cancer therapy as well as the advent of microsurgery and the subsequent capacity for free tissue transfer. Another relatively recent advancement in head and neck reconstruction is the use of virtual surgical planning and rapid prototype modeling. Virtual surgical planning relies on 3D imaging data obtained from computed tomography scans to build models of the relevant anatomy for intraoperative use, surgical cutting guides to direct tumor extirpation as well as the bony reconstruction, and even mold or 3D print custom hardware [97]. Virtual surgical planning as a tool offers improved precision and reli-ability in head and neck reconstruction. It will likely become more widely used as acquisition costs and logistic challenges are limited [98]. The most immediate future advancements in head and neck reconstruction will likely be based in the application of virtual surgical planning.

References

1. Chim H, Salgado CJ, Seselgyte R, Wei F-C, Mardini S. Principles of head and neck recon-struction: an algorithm to guide flap selection. Semin Plast Surg. 2010;24(2):148–54.
2. Patel SA, Chang EI. Principles and practice of reconstructive surgery for head and neck can-cer. Surg Oncol Clin N Am. 2015;24(3):473–89.
3. Alberdas JL, Shibahara T, Noma H. Histopathologic damage to vessels in head and neck micro-surgery. J Oral Maxillofac Surg Off J Am Assoc Oral Maxillofac Surg. 2003;61(2):191–6.

4. Arinci A, Topalan M, Aydin I, Solakoglu S, Olgaç V, Merla R, et al. Effects of early pre- and postoperative irradiation on the healing of microvascular anastomoses. J Reconstr Microsurg. 2000;16(7):573–6.

5. Watson JS. Experimental microvascular anastomoses in radiated vessels: a study of the patency rate and the histopathology of healing. Plast Reconstr Surg. 1979;63(4):525–33.

6. Benatar MJ, Dassonville O, Chamorey E, Poissonnet G, Ettaiche M, Pierre CS, et al. Impact of preoperative radiotherapy on head and neck free flap reconstruction: a report on 429 cases. J Plast Reconstr Aesthetic Surg JPRAS. 2013;66(4):478–82.

7. Paderno A, Piazza C, Bresciani L, Vella R, Nicolai P. Microvascular head and neck reconstruction after (chemo)radiation: facts and prejudices. Curr Opin Otolaryngol Head Neck Surg. 2016;24(2):83–90.

8. Mijiti A, Kuerbantayi N, Zhang ZQ, Su MY, Zhang XH, Huojia M. Influence of preoperative radiotherapy on head and neck free-flap reconstruction: systematic review and meta-analysis. Head Neck. 2020;42:2165.

9. Jager-Wittenaar H, Dijkstra PU, Vissink A, Langendijk JA, van der Laan BFAM, Pruim J, et al. Changes in nutritional status and dietary intake during and after head and neck cancer treatment. Head Neck. 2011;33(6):863–70.

10. Palmieri TL, Taylor S, Lawless M, Curri T, Sen S, Greenhalgh DG. Burn center volume makes a difference for burned children. Pediatr Crit Care Med J Soc Crit Care Med World Fed Pediatr Intensive Crit Care Soc. 2015;16(4):319–24.

11. Soeters PB, Reijven PLM, van Bokhorst-de van der Schueren MAE, Schols JMGA, Halfens RJG, Meijers JMM, et al. A rational approach to nutritional assessment. Clin Nutr Edinb Scotl. 2008;27(5):706–16.

12. Grimalt R. A practical guide to scalp disorders. J Investig Dermatol Symp Proc. 2007;12(2):10–4.

13. Desai SC, Sand JP, Sharon JD, Branham G, Nussenbaum B. Scalp reconstruction: an algorithmic approach and systematic review. JAMA Facial Plast Surg. 2015;17(1):56–66.

14. Iblher N, Ziegler MC, Penna V, Eisenhardt SU, Stark GB, Bannasch H. An algorithm for oncologic scalp reconstruction. Plast Reconstr Surg. 2010;126(2):450–9.

15. Borgquist O, Ingemansson R, Malmsjö M. The influence of low and high pressure levels during negative-pressure wound therapy on wound contraction and fluid evacuation. Plast Reconstr Surg. 2011;127(2):551–9.

16. Kairinos N, Solomons M, Hudson DA. Negative-pressure wound therapy I: the paradox of negative-pressure wound therapy. Plast Reconstr Surg. 2009;123(2):589–98; discussion 599–600.

17. Orgill DP, Manders EK, Sumpio BE, Lee RC, Attinger CE, Gurtner GC, et al. The mechanisms of action of vacuum assisted closure: more to learn. Surgery. 2009;146(1):40–51.

18. Cai SS, Gowda AU, Alexander RH, Silverman RP, Goldberg NH, Rasko YM. Use of negative pressure wound therapy on malignant wounds – a case report and review of literature. Int Wound J. 2017;14(4):661–5.

19. Tufaro AP, Buck DW, Fischer AC. The use of artificial dermis in the reconstruction of oncologic surgical defects. Plast Reconstr Surg. 2007;120(3):638–46.

20. Orticochea M. Four flap scalp reconstruction technique. Br J Plast Surg. 1967;20(2):159–71.

21. Orticochea M. New three-flap reconstruction technique. Br J Plast Surg. 1971;24(2):184–8.

22. Mathes SJ, Nahai F. Clinical atlas of muscle and musculocutaneous flaps. St. Louis: Mosby; 1979.

23. Uğurlu K, Ozçelik D, Hüthüt I, Yildiz K, Kilinç L, Baş L. Extended vertical trapezius myocutaneous flap in head and neck reconstruction as a salvage procedure. Plast Reconstr Surg. 2004;114(2):339–50.

24. Urken ML, Naidu RK, Lawson W, Biller HF. The lower trapezius island musculocutaneous flap revisited. Report of 45 cases and a unifying concept of the vascular supply. Arch Otolaryngol Head Neck Surg. 1991;117(5):502–11.

25. Rose J, Puckett Y. Breast reconstruction free flaps. In: StatPearls [Internet]. Treasure Island: StatPearls Publishing; 2020. [cited 2020 Jun 22]. Available from: http://www.ncbi.nlm.nih. gov/books/NBK541048/.
26. Har-El G, Bhaya M, Sundaram K. Latissimus dorsi myocutaneous flap for secondary head and neck reconstruction. Am J Otolaryngol. 1999;20(5):287–93.
27. Cox AJ, Wang TD, Cook TA. Closure of a scalp defect. Arch Facial Plast Surg. 1999;1(3):212–5.
28. Newman MI, Hanasono MM, Disa JJ, Cordeiro PG, Mehrara BJ. Scalp reconstruction: a 15-year experience. Ann Plast Surg. 2004;52(5):501–6; discussion 506.
29. Fowler NM, Futran ND. Achievements in scalp reconstruction. Curr Opin Otolaryngol Head Neck Surg. 2014;22(2):127–30.
30. Sokoya M, Misch E, Vincent A, Wang W, Kadakia S, Ducic Y, et al. Free tissue reconstruction of the scalp. Semin Plast Surg. 2019;33(1):67–71.
31. Song YG, Chen GZ, Song YL. The free thigh flap: a new free flap concept based on the septocutaneous artery. Br J Plast Surg. 1984;37(2):149–59.
32. Fischer JP, Sieber B, Nelson JA, Kovach SJ, Taylor JA, Serletti JM, et al. A 15-year experience of complex scalp reconstruction using free tissue transfer-analysis of risk factors for complications. J Reconstr Microsurg. 2013;29(2):89–97.
33. Badhey A, Kadakia S, Mourad M, Inman J, Ducic Y. Calvarial reconstruction. Semin Plast Surg. 2017;31(4):222–6.
34. Goldstein JA, Paliga JT, Bartlett SP. Cranioplasty: indications and advances. Curr Opin Otolaryngol Head Neck Surg. 2013;21(4):400–9.
35. Artico M, Ferrante L, Pastore FS, Ramundo EO, Cantarelli D, Scopelliti D, et al. Bone autografting of the calvaria and craniofacial skeleton: historical background, surgical results in a series of 15 patients, and review of the literature. Surg Neurol. 2003;60(1):71–9.
36. Açikgöz B, Ozcan OE, Erbengi A, Bertan V, Ruacan S, Açikgöz HG. Histopathologic and microdensitometric analysis of craniotomy bone flaps preserved between abdominal fat and muscle. Surg Neurol. 1986;26(6):557–61.
37. Alghoul MS, Kearney AM, Pacella SJ, Purnell CA. Eyelid reconstruction. Plast Reconstr Surg Glob Open [Internet]. 2019 [cited 2020 Jun 22];7(11). Available from: https://www. ncbi.nlm.nih.gov/pmc/articles/PMC6908339/.
38. Chang EI, Esmaeli B, Butler CE. Eyelid reconstruction. Plast Reconstr Surg. 2017;140(5):724e–35e.
39. Mathijssen IMJ, van der Meulen JC. Guidelines for reconstruction of the eyelids and canthal regions. J Plast Reconstr Aesthetic Surg JPRAS. 2010;63(9):1420–33.
40. Shorr N, Goldberg RA, McCann JD, Hoenig JA, Li TG. Upper eyelid skin grafting: an effective treatment for lagophthalmos following blepharoplasty. Plast Reconstr Surg. 2003;112(5):1444–8.
41. Rohrich RJ, Zbar RI. The evolution of the Hughes tarsoconjunctival flap for the lower eyelid reconstruction. Plast Reconstr Surg. 1999;104(2):518–22; quiz 523; discussion 524–526.
42. Mustardé JC. New horizons in eyelid reconstruction. Int Ophthalmol Clin. 1989;29(4):237–46.
43. Muzaffar AR, Adams WP, Hartog JM, Rohrich RJ, Byrd HS. Maxillary reconstruction: functional and aesthetic considerations. Plast Reconstr Surg. 1999;104(7):2172–83; quiz 2184.
44. O'Connell DA, Futran ND. Reconstruction of the midface and maxilla. Curr Opin Otolaryngol Head Neck Surg. 2010;18(4):304–10.
45. Futran ND, Mendez E. Developments in reconstruction of midface and maxilla. Lancet Oncol. 2006;7(3):249–58.
46. Cordeiro PG, Santamaria E. A classification system and algorithm for reconstruction of maxillectomy and midfacial defects. Plast Reconstr Surg. 2000;105(7):2331–46; discussion 2347–2348.
47. Brown JS, Rogers SN, McNally DN, Boyle M. A modified classification for the maxillectomy defect. Head Neck. 2000;22(1):17–26.

48. Okay DJ, Genden E, Buchbinder D, Urken M. Prosthodontic guidelines for surgical reconstruction of the maxilla: a classification system of defects. J Prosthet Dent. 2001;86(4):352–63.
49. Yamamoto Y, Kawashima K, Sugihara T, Nohira K, Furuta Y, Fukuda S. Surgical management of maxillectomy defects based on the concept of buttress reconstruction. Head Neck. 2004;26(3):247–56.
50. Dalgorf D, Higgins K. Reconstruction of the midface and maxilla. Curr Opin Otolaryngol Head Neck Surg. 2008;16(4):303–11.
51. Fancy T, Huang AT, Kass JI, Lamarre ED, Tassone P, Mantravadi AV, et al. Complications, mortality, and functional decline in patients 80 years or older undergoing major head and neck ablation and reconstruction. JAMA Otolaryngol Head Neck Surg. 2019;145:1150.
52. Genden EM, Wallace DI, Okay D, Urken ML. Reconstruction of the hard palate using the radial forearm free flap: indications and outcomes. Head Neck. 2004;26(9):808–14.
53. Hatoko M, Harashina T, Inoue T, Tanaka I, Imai K. Reconstruction of palate with radial forearm flap; a report of 3 cases. Br J Plast Surg. 1990;43(3):350–4.
54. Pool C, Shokri T, Vincent A, Wang W, Kadakia S, Ducic Y. Prosthetic reconstruction of the maxilla and palate. Semin Plast Surg. 2020;34(2):114–9.
55. Likhterov I, Roche AM, Urken ML. Contemporary osseous reconstruction of the mandible and the maxilla. Oral Maxillofac Surg Clin N Am. 2019;31(1):101–16.
56. Foster RD, Anthony JP, Sharma A, Pogrel MA. Vascularized bone flaps versus nonvascularized bone grafts for mandibular reconstruction: an outcome analysis of primary bony union and endosseous implant success. Head Neck. 1999;21(1):66–71.
57. Bak M, Jacobson AS, Buchbinder D, Urken ML. Contemporary reconstruction of the mandible. Oral Oncol. 2010;46(2):71–6.
58. Egyedi P. Utilization of the buccal fat pad for closure of oro-antral and/or oro-nasal communications. J Maxillofac Surg. 1977;5(4):241–4.
59. Samman N, Cheung LK, Tideman H. The buccal fat pad in oral reconstruction. Int J Oral Maxillofac Surg. 1993;22(1):2–6.
60. Arce K. Buccal fat pad in maxillary reconstruction. Atlas Oral Maxillofac Surg Clin North Am. 2007;15(1):23–32.
61. Gullane PJ, Arena S. Palatal island flap for reconstruction of oral defects. Arch Otolaryngol Chic Ill 1960. 1977;103(10):598–9.
62. Moore BA, Magdy E, Netterville JL, Burkey BB. Palatal reconstruction with the palatal island flap. Laryngoscope. 2003;113(6):946–51.
63. Thorburn IB. Experience with pedicled temporal muscle flaps in radical mastoid and tympanoplasty operations. J Laryngol Otol. 1961;75:885–96.
64. Parhiscar A, Har-El G, Turk JB, Abramson DL. Temporoparietal osteofascial flap for head and neck reconstruction. J Oral Maxillofac Surg Off J Am Assoc Oral Maxillofac Surg. 2002;60(6):619–22.
65. Ward BB. Temporalis system in maxillary reconstruction: temporalis muscle and temporoparietal galea flaps. Atlas Oral Maxillofac Surg Clin North Am. 2007;15(1):33–42.
66. Abubaker AO, Abouzgia MB. The temporalis muscle flap in reconstruction of intraoral defects: an appraisal of the technique. Oral Surg Oral Med Oral Pathol Oral Radiol Endod. 2002;94(1):24–30.
67. Martin D, Pascal JF, Baudet J, Mondie JM, Farhat JB, Athoum A, et al. The submental island flap: a new donor site. Anatomy and clinical applications as a free or pedicled flap. Plast Reconstr Surg. 1993;92(5):867–73.
68. You Q, Jing X, Fan S, Wang Y, Yang Z. Comparison of functional outcomes and health-related quality of life one year after treatment in patients with oral and oropharyngeal cancer treated with three different reconstruction methods. Br J Oral Maxillofac Surg. 2020;58:759.
69. Soutar DS, Scheker LR, Tanner NS, McGregor IA. The radial forearm flap: a versatile method for intra-oral reconstruction. Br J Plast Surg. 1983;36(1):1–8.

70. Spoerl S, Schoedel S, Spanier G, Mueller K, Meier JK, Reichert TE, et al. A decade of reconstructive surgery: outcome and perspectives of free tissue transfer in the head and neck. Experience of a single center institution. Oral Maxillofac Surg. 2020;24(2):173–9.
71. Fernandes R. Reconstruction of maxillary defects with the radial forearm free flap. Atlas Oral Maxillofac Surg Clin North Am. 2007;15(1):7–12.
72. Pennington DG, Pelly AD. The rectus abdominis myocutaneous free flap. Br J Plast Surg. 1980;33(2):277–82.
73. Browne JD, Burke AJ. Benefits of routine maxillectomy and orbital reconstruction with the rectus abdominis free flap. Otolaryngol--Head Neck Surg Off J Am Acad Otolaryngol-Head Neck Surg. 1999;121(3):203–9.
74. Bianchi B, Bertolini F, Ferrari S, Sesenna E. Maxillary reconstruction using rectus abdominis free flap and bone grafts. Br J Oral Maxillofac Surg. 2006;44(6):526–30.
75. Patel NP, Matros E, Cordeiro PG. The use of the multi-island vertical rectus abdominis myocutaneous flap in head and neck reconstruction. Ann Plast Surg. 2012;69(4):403–7.
76. dos Santos LF. The vascular anatomy and dissection of the free scapular flap. Plast Reconstr Surg. 1984;73(4):599–604.
77. Coleman JJ, Sultan MR. The bipedicled osteocutaneous scapula flap: a new subscapular system free flap. Plast Reconstr Surg. 1991;87(4):682–92.
78. Uglesić V, Virag M, Varga S, Knezević P, Milenović A. Reconstruction following radical maxillectomy with flaps supplied by the subscapular artery. J Cranio-Maxillo-fac Surg Off Publ Eur Assoc Cranio-Maxillo-fac Surg. 2000;28(3):153–60.
79. Urken ML, Bridger AG, Zur KB, Genden EM. The scapular osteofasciocutaneous flap: a 12-year experience. Arch Otolaryngol Head Neck Surg. 2001;127(7):862–9.
80. Taylor GI, Townsend P, Corlett R. Superiority of the deep circumflex iliac vessels as the supply for free groin flaps. Plast Reconstr Surg. 1979;64(5):595–604.
81. Taylor GI, Townsend P, Corlett R. Superiority of the deep circumflex iliac vessels as the supply for free groin flaps. Clinical work. Plast Reconstr Surg. 1979;64(6):745–59.
82. Genden EM, Wallace D, Buchbinder D, Okay D, Urken ML. Iliac crest internal oblique osteomusculocutaneous free flap reconstruction of the postablative palatomaxillary defect. Arch Otolaryngol Head Neck Surg. 2001;127(7):854–61.
83. Brown JS. Deep circumflex iliac artery free flap with internal oblique muscle as a new method of immediate reconstruction of maxillectomy defect. Head Neck. 1996;18(5):412–21.
84. Taylor GI, Miller GD, Ham FJ. The free vascularized bone graft. A clinical extension of microvascular techniques. Plast Reconstr Surg. 1975;55(5):533–44.
85. Futran ND, Wadsworth JT, Villaret D, Farwell DG. Midface reconstruction with the fibula free flap. Arch Otolaryngol Head Neck Surg. 2002;128(2):161–6.
86. Sokoya M, Bahrami A, Vincent A, Inman J, Mourad M, Sawhney R, et al. Pharyngeal reconstruction with microvascular free tissue transfer. Semin Plast Surg. 2019;33(1):78–80.
87. Welkoborsky H-J, Deichmüller C, Bauer L, Hinni ML. Reconstruction of large pharyngeal defects with microvascular free flaps and myocutaneous pedicled flaps. Curr Opin Otolaryngol Head Neck Surg. 2013;21(4):318–27.
88. Krag C, Kirkby B. The deltopectoral flap: a historical review with comments on its role in neurovascular reconstruction. Scand J Plast Reconstr Surg. 1980;14(2):145–50.
89. Patel RS, Goldstein DP, Brown D, Irish J, Gullane PJ, Gilbert RW. Circumferential pharyngeal reconstruction: history, critical analysis of techniques, and current therapeutic recommendations. Head Neck. 2010;32(1):109–20.
90. Ariyan S, Cuono CB. Myocutaneous flaps for head and neck reconstruction. Head Neck Surg. 1980;2(4):321–45.
91. Seidenberg B, Rosenak SS, Hurwitt ES, Som ML. Immediate reconstruction of the cervical esophagus by a revascularized isolated jejunal segment. Ann Surg. 1959;149(2):162–71.
92. Walker RJ, Parmar S, Praveen P, Martin T, Pracy P, Jennings C, et al. Jejunal free flap for reconstruction of pharyngeal defects in patients with head and neck cancer-the Birmingham experience. Br J Oral Maxillofac Surg. 2014;52(2):106–10.

93. Jones AS, Roland NJ, Husband D, Hamilton JW, Gati I. Free revascularized jejunal loop repair following total pharyngolaryngectomy for carcinoma of the hypopharynx: report of 90 patients. Br J Surg. 1996;83(9):1279–3.
94. Yu P, Lewin JS, Reece GP, Robb GL. Comparison of clinical and functional outcomes and hospital costs following pharyngoesophageal reconstruction with the anterolateral thigh free flap versus the jejunal flap. Plast Reconstr Surg. 2006;117(3):968–74.
95. Azizzadeh B, Yafai S, Rawnsley JD, Abemayor E, Sercarz JA, Calcaterra TC, et al. Radial forearm free flap pharyngoesophageal reconstruction. Laryngoscope. 2001;111(5):807–10.
96. Razdan SN, Albornoz CR, Matros E, Paty PB, Cordeiro PG. Free jejunal flap for pharyngoesophageal reconstruction in head and neck cancer patients: an evaluation of donor-site complications. J Reconstr Microsurg. 2015;31(9):643–6.
97. Hoang D, Perrault D, Stevanovic M, Ghiassi A. Surgical applications of three-dimensional printing: a review of the current literature & how to get started. Ann Transl Med. 2016;4(23):456.
98. Largo RD, Garvey PB. Updates in head and neck reconstruction. Plast Reconstr Surg. 2018;141(2):271e–85e.
99. Wei F, Mardini S. Flaps and reconstructive surgery. 2nd ed. Livingston: St Johns's Hospital/Elsevier. 2018.
100. Kim M-K, Han W, Kim S-G. The use of the buccal fat pad flap for oral reconstruction. Maxillofac Plast Reconstr Surg. 2017;39(1):5. https://doi.org/10.1186/s40902-017-0105-5.

Chapter 10
Rehabilitation of Oral Cancer Patients using Dental Implants and Maxillofacial Prosthetics

Rafiullah Bashiri, Maryam Khalili, and Saul Weiner

Introduction

Dental implantology has revolutionized the practice of dentistry. This technology has provided an opportunity to replace teeth that are "worn out" biomechanically, or lack osseous support, with structures that are mechanically sound and anchored in the bone. Implants provide support for prostheses that restore functional activities, such as mastication and speech. One of the significant positive aspects of dental implants is that dental caries, one of the primary oral diseases, is not a consideration [1].

Dental implantology is today a far cry from the early days when this treatment, driven by clinicians, had little scientific background. Professor Branemark, one of the pioneers of the scientific era for dental implantology, included orthopedic surgical techniques in the treatment protocol for dental implantology [2]. One of the important changes which he instituted was the use of slow speed and water irrigation during preparation of the osteotomy for insertion of the implant. This reduced the damage to the bone and allowed formation of a bony interface adjacent to the implant. Previously when ultraspeed was employed for creating the osteotomy, the interface of the implant with the bone was unpredictable and often composed of

R. Bashiri
Department of Prosthodontics, Division of Comprehensive Oral Health, The University of North Carolina, Adams School of Dentistry, Chapel Hill, NC, USA

M. Khalili
Department of Restorative Dentistry, Temple University Maurice H. Kornberg School of Dentistry, Philadelphia, PA, USA

S. Weiner (✉)
Department of Restorative Dentistry, Rutgers School of Dental Medicine, Newark, NJ, USA

Department of Biomedical Engineering, Stevens institute of Technology, Hoboken, NJ, USA
e-mail: forasaul@aol.com

© Springer Nature Switzerland AG 2021
R. El Assal et al. (eds.), *Early Detection and Treatment of Head & Neck Cancers*, https://doi.org/10.1007/978-3-030-69859-1_10

connective tissue which frequently did not allow sufficient stability during functional activities [3].

Continuing research over the past 50 years has significantly improved the biological stability of the implant and biomechanical designs of both the implant and the associated prosthodontic reconstructions. A current development, in parallel with advances in biomaterials, is the introduction of zirconia implants [4]. It has been suggested that this material is more biocompatible and may have a reduced potential for immunological rejection. Other improvements in surface treatments and technology are currently under development as well. What follows is an overview of the current scientific and clinical applications of dental implants to a group of people who have suffered much from the ravages of a debilitating and disfiguring disease. Their use has allowed the development of new strategies in maxillofacial rehabilitation. The reader is encouraged to consult the periodical literature for more detailed information.

Osseointegration

Osseointegration has been defined as the firm anchoring of a surgical implant by the growth of bone around it without fibrous tissue formation at the interface [5]. It has been extensively studied. The process involves initial mechanical stability of the implant in the osseous bed and, secondarily, bone remodeling and apposition along the implant surface. Mechanical stability is initially achieved as the implant is slightly wider in diameter (0.5–1.0 mm) than the diameter of the drill that creates the osteotomy. The implant threads are generally self-cutting as the implant advances into the osteotomy during insertion [6]. The remodeling process begins almost immediately after insertion. It is critical that fibrin and platelets adhere to the implant surface in the first 72 hours post-insertion. This allows the precursor pre-osteoblast cells and cytokines released from the platelets to begin forming a bone on the external surface of the implant. Although implants can support a prosthesis immediately after insertion, particularly if splinted to other adjacent implants or teeth, the remodeling process is generally considered to be completed in 2–3 months. However, once the prosthesis is inserted onto the implants and a functional occlusion exists, some further remodeling of the peri-implant bone continues for some months. The remodeling process requires an adequate blood supply as it is cell-mediated. Specifically stem cells and monocytes differentiate into osteoblasts and osteocytes. Osteoclasts and inflammatory cells, such as polymorphonuclear cells (PMNs) and macrophages, remove the debris from the drilling of the bone and allow new bone apposition. These cells and platelets release cytokines that mediate cell differentiation, matrix formation, and calcification of the newly formed collagen matrix of the bone to provide support for the implant. A number of cytokines are associated with the process of osseointegration. These include platelet-derived growth factor (PDGF), vascular endothelial growth factor (VEGF), fibroblast growth factor (FGF), bone morphogenic protein 6 (BMP 6), osteopontin, and osteocalcin. This process requires an adequate blood supply since these cytokines are cell and platelet derived [7].

Cancer Treatment

One of the most powerful aspects of implant-based rehabilitation is the possible creative strategy in both implant placement and prosthesis design. This is demonstrated clearly in individuals with a significant deficit in the dentition, jaws, or associated maxillofacial structures either congenitally or as a result of accident or disease. The designs of fixed and removable prostheses take advantage of the available dentition and remaining skeletal structures for stability of the prosthesis. This is nowhere truer than in the case of patients with cancer diseases of the head and neck, where treatment includes ablative surgery of soft and bony tissues, radiation, and chemotherapy. These treatments often result in loss of soft and bony anatomic structures, reduction in blood supply and salivary output, and mucositis of the intraoral soft tissues. The management of these patients presents unique challenges [8].

As a result of cancer therapy, the blood supply to the treated region is frequently compromised. Head and neck dissections during ablation of the tumor remove vascular and lymphatic vessels and reduce the blood supply through the mandible, maxilla, and walls of the maxillary sinus. Radiation to bone causes sclerosis of the capillary bed of Haversian systems that supply the osteocytes encased in canaliculi. The overall blood supply to the trabecular bone and the marrow space is reduced as well [9].

Administration of chemotherapeutic agents for treatment has significant secondary effects on connective tissue and bone metabolism which often results in a decrease in bone density post-chemotherapy. A well-recognized class of drugs that cause disruption of bone metabolism are the bisphosphonates [10]. These drugs (e.g., Zometa, Boniva, Fosamax) interrupt the secondary remodeling of the bone by preventing osteoclastic activity. Tumor cells release the polypeptide receptor activator for nuclear factor κ B ligand (RANKL) that interact with receptor activator of nuclear factor κ B (RANK) receptors on the cell membrane of the osteoclast, which trigger excessive activation of osteoclasts. Increased osteoclastic activity allows expansion of the tumor. Bisphosphonates are taken up by progenitor cells and block the formation of multinucleated osteoclasts, as well as inhibiting their function, which results in osteoclastic apoptosis. These drugs have long-lasting effects since their half-life is approximately 10 years. However, a new generation of chemotherapeutic drugs, the monoclonal antibodies, such as Denosumab (Xgeva) have a much shorter half-life (i.e., 6 months) allowing a return of normal bone metabolism [11]. Xgeva targets the RANKL polypeptide and by binding to it prevents the activation of RANK receptors on the osteoclast cells, which in turn prevents the formation, survival, and function of the osteoclast. However, patients with exposure to any of these medications (e.g., Zometa or Xgeva) are at risk for development of osteonecrosis; thus extreme caution needs to be employed in patient management [12].

Intraoral Cancers and Implant-Supported Prostheses

These prostheses are an important modality in the rehabilitation of the oral cancer patient. Implants can serve as replacements for portions of the resected skeleton and can provide stability for intraoral and extraoral prostheses by allowing secure attachment to the underlying skeleton. Previously, these prostheses, as for example, complete dentures, relied solely on adhesives to stabilize them in place. Today the option of mechanical attachment of the prosthesis to the implant provides greater security and functional stability. Options exist for the prosthesis to be securely attached to the implant such that it can only be removed by the clinician. The patient is required to utilize oral physiotherapy devices in addition to tooth brush and dental floss to daily remove food debris and accumulated biofilm. Other options allow the patient to remove the prosthesis and more readily remove food debris and oral biofilm accumulation [13].

However, as discussed above, the integration of dental implants in the head and neck skeleton requires an adequate blood supply to allow the metabolic activity associated with bone modeling and remodeling for the implants for osseointegration. The treatment for the cancer often involves ablative surgery, radiation, and/or chemotherapy, all of which affect the bone and soft tissues of the orofacial skeleton. Debate exists among maxillofacial surgeons and prosthodontists as to the time of implant placement relative to the cancer therapy. The general consensus today appears that dental implant treatment can be predictable (i.e., the implants achieved osseointegration) if inserted before the initiation of radiation and/or chemotherapy. An organized treatment plan must be in place so that maxillofacial rehabilitation can be appropriately sequenced [14].

As described previously in the section on Osseointegration, healing requires formation of de novo bone in apposition to the implant surface particularly within the threads as these provides a configuration and increased surface area for stability and retention of the implant during functional activities as speech, mastication, and swallowing. The healing time until a clinical acceptable plateau for function is generally several months. The term plateau is used as it is possible to measure the stability of the implant. Studies are available to correlate the required stability of the implant with the magnitude of functional loads. The analysis that is most often employed is resonance frequency analysis (RFA) [15]. In this test, a vibratory force is applied to the implant and the resultant movement of the implant is measured. The order of magnitude of movement observed is in the micron and submicron range.

These considerations are of significance for the cancer patient. Timing is very important in patient management and initiation of the treatment plan for management of cancer treatment. The routine 2–3-month waiting period for the implant to heal is not practical for these patients. Frequently surgical placement of the implants is followed by initiation of chemotherapy or radiation within 1–3 weeks [16]. In these circumstances, implants with accelerated healing times as measured by RFA are preferred. Currently, in parallel, there is significant research underway to facilitate more rapid osseointegration. These activities have focused on modifications to the implant surface. One of those that is most widely accepted is to increase the surface roughness of the implant [17]. This allows increased numbers of platelets and proteins to attach to the implant surface. Another approach is to spray the surface with calcium phosphate or fluoride during manufacture combined together with modification of surface roughness. This has been demonstrated as allowing more rapid mineralization of the de novo bone [18]. A third approach that has met with considerable success is depositing a positive charge on the implant surface that will attract greater quantities of proteins to the implant surface [18]. Using these strategies, the RFA values have been reported to plateau at functional levels within 4–6 weeks after insertion [19]. Other strategies not as yet well validated are also being researched. Generally, the effects of the cancer therapies, radiation, and chemotherapy, on the bone, take 2–4 weeks to have maximum effect. Thus much of the osseointegration process can be completed before the effects of the cancer therapies reach maximum. A number of cancer centers have reported successful osseointegrated implants using a similar protocol [20].

The most common type of cancer occurring in the oral and maxillofacial regions is squamous cell carcinoma. The lip and buccal mucosa are the most frequent sites. Resection of the lesion and repair of the oral soft tissues, if identified early, is self-limited. In more advanced cases, the use of intraoral and extraoral pedicle flaps is required. These generally do not affect implant placement as they do not involve bone. However, the use of these flaps frequently results in scar tissue that can limit the mobility of the mandible and reduce the buccal vestibule. Management of the prosthesis in these cases, particularly if there is a lack of attached gingiva, is more problematical and complex [21]. Although controversial, the literature suggests that implants surrounded by attached gingiva seem to have less soft tissue inflammation [22]. A lack of buccal vestibule limits the denture flange allowing food accumulation during meals [21].

Squamous cell carcinoma also occurs in the gingiva and soft tissues of the floor of the mouth, alveolar processes, and palate. Spread to the bone from these soft tissue locations is more likely. Once the tumor has invaded, the bone more complex surgical and prosthodontic management is required. Resection and stabilization of the fragments to restore mandibular continuity and allow implant placement in the mandible are important to restore the patient's quality of life [23].

In the maxilla, often the alveolar ridge and the palate are involved. Invasion of these structures by the tumor will require resection of portions of the palate and exposure of the maxillary sinus. An obturator prosthesis is required to wall off the sinus and nose. The obturator prevents food from entering the nose and sinuses as well as facilitates intelligible speech. This process is carried out in three distinct phases. The first phase is performed on the day of tumor resection during which a surgical obturator is wired onto the remaining teeth or screwed into place to provide stability and retention. The main goal of using a surgical obturator is to act as a bandage for the resection site and allow healing of the soft tissue. Patients' comfort and rehabilitation becomes more convenient with the use of a surgical obturator. The second phase is initiated 21 days post-surgery. The surgical obturator is removed, and an interim or transitional obturator is placed. This prosthesis is designed differently from the surgical obturator as it is not wired around teeth, and it has wrought wire clasps and denture teeth to provide the patient with some means of speech and chewing efficiency as well as aesthetics. Placement of implants in the available portions of the maxilla, the pterygoid complex, or, as a last resort, the zygoma will stabilize the prosthesis and allow an effective seal between the maxilla and the maxillary sinus. As noted previously, this seal is critical for speech and retention. In the third phase, a definitive prosthesis is provided to the patient that follows a similar design to the interim prosthesis, but considerations of esthetics and durability are applied [24].

Mucoepidermoid carcinoma associated with major salivary glands frequently metastasizes to bone and is considered more invasive. As such it usually requires a wider resection, which challenges the creativity of the prosthodontist to design a prosthesis which is stable in the remaining oral and maxillofacial structures for patient comfort and function. Other rare cancers with a lower incidence (1–4%), such as sarcomas and melanomas, require similar surgical and prosthodontic protocols [25].

Maxillofacial Prostheses

Rehabilitation of cancer patients using maxillofacial prosthetics follows classical principles of prosthodontics that are secondarily modified due to structural and morphological changes as a result of treatment of the disease [26]. The support is achieved by modifying the prosthesis, especially in cases where some of the retentive anatomic structures are missing. The use of implants to provide stability for the prosthesis, aid in retention to avoid dislodgement, and allow functional activities, such as speech and mastication, is a major step forward in post-treatment rehabilitation of patients with cancer. In addition, for removable maxillofacial prostheses, it is important to achieve good soft tissue support. In the maxilla, the palate is important for stabilizing the maxillary prosthesis. Therefore, any loss of the palate creates a significant problem. Palatal resection is associated with exposure of the maxillary sinus. Functionally, the palate must be sealed from the oral cavity for speech and swallowing. The surgeon can create a lateral band (scar band) of connective tissue on the resected side within the cheek to provide an undercut to stabilize the prosthesis and create a seal [27]. The prosthesis is then designed to extend above the lateral band to obtain the seal. The contralateral side of the maxilla serves to support the prosthesis by resting on the remaining palate and alveolar ridge. Implants placed strategically can improve the stability of the prosthesis. At times, splints of teeth and/or implants are employed. Prostheses are often designed in creative ways to take advantage of the remaining osseous structures. Angling and placing the implants in atypical positions with the use of attachments (such as snaps or clip attachments with bar frames) can be considered to provide stability and retention for prostheses, Fig. 10.1. Remote regions, such as the pterygoid complex and the zygoma, can be utilized as sites for implants to stabilize intraoral and extraoral prostheses. Special implant-supported prosthesis designs are available for use in these situations.

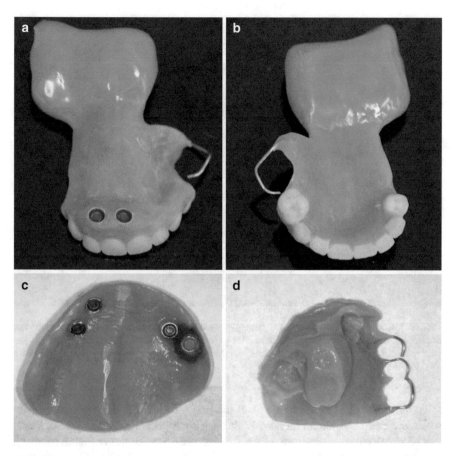

Fig. 10.1 Maxillary obturators. (**a, b**) Maxillary pharyngeal obturator supported by two anterior locator attachments supported by implants and one unilateral wrought wire clasp supported by a contralateral molar are utilized. The posterior bulb, sealing the palatal defect, is hollowed to reduce weight and increase the retention of the prosthesis. (**c**) Dental implant-retained maxillary obturator fabricated for a patient with fibula reconstruction of the palatal defect. The prosthesis is supported by locator attachments supported by bilateral dental implants that had been inserted in the fibula graft. (**d**) Conventional maxillary obturator with wrought wire clasps around natural teeth for retention on one side and a lateral scar band as previously described on the contralateral side

Methods of plate fabrication of surgical reconstruction

Traditional hand bending		Full CAD-CAM	
Advantages	Disadvantages	Advantages	Disadvantages
Inexpensive	Increased surgical	Reduced surgical	Expensive
Minimal	time	time	Extensive planning and
preplanning	Risk of non-bony	Reduced	coordination
	union	complications	Manufacturing and
	Metal weakening	Surgical cutting	turnaround
		guides	
		Rate of bony union	
		Strength of metal	

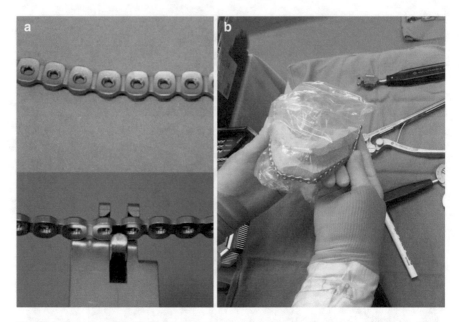

Fig. 10.2 Conventional mandibular reconstruction plates. (**a**) The notches between the holes are predefined bending points that allow the plates to be bent as required. This photo represents the external surface of a 2.5 mm Synthes Matrix Mandible Reconstruction plate. (**b**) Bending pliers are used to bend the plate at a notch between two-screw holes

In the mandible, resection of part of the jaw is commonly done in treatment of squamous cell carcinoma that has invaded the bone [28]. The remaining segments can be stabilized in several ways [29]. First, a stock bar can be contoured to match the defect and screwed to the remaining segments for stability of the mandible (Fig. 10.2). This is usually performed in the operating room. Today more sophisticated approaches are available in which the resection is planned digitally prior to the surgery, and a custom bar is fabricated (Fig. 10.3). In this case, a surgical guide is prepared for the resection to properly position the implants and, subsequently, to screw the custom stabilizing bar to the remaining mandibular segments. In this approach, implants are placed in the segments adjacent to the resection. In a more advanced protocol, a vascularized fibula graft is inserted between the remaining mandibular segments and attached to the stabilizing bar (Fig. 10.4). In this protocol, a computer-aided design (CAD) is used to plan the resection of the diseased section of the mandible, called the fibula-harvesting guide. A second guide is used to plan the location of the implants and the custom titanium supporting bar that will support both the mandibular segments and the fibula graft in position. Upon completion and approval of the design, the two guides and supporting bar are CAM fabricated. On the day of the surgery the fibula bone is exposed, the three-dimensional (3D)

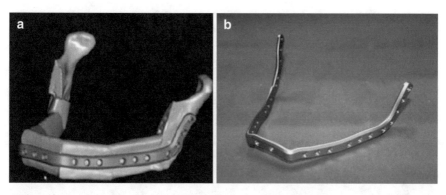

Fig. 10.3 Computer-aided planning of a patient-specific mandibular reconstruction plate. (**a**) The plate was virtually contoured to the virtually planned model of the patient's jaw. The digital image of the jaw was obtained from a cone beam radiographic image. The number, position, and angle of each screw were determined as well. (**b**) A patient-specific mandibular reconstruction plate milled from titanium

custom-fabricated fibular resection guide is placed and stabilized using surgical screws. Once the cuts are made on the fibula bone as desired through the cutting guide slots, the osteotomies are prepared and the implants inserted. The implants are either placed fully guided through the same fibula-harvesting guide, or they are inserted freehand once the guide is removed and the surgeon orients and places the titanium-milled mandibular supporting bar stabilized with surgical screws. At this point, the fibula bone is ready to be harvested, and the blood supply is terminated. Virtual technology allows for planning and design of (i) the quantity of bone required for grafting and, (ii) more importantly, the design of the prosthesis to restore the continuity of the dental occlusion (Fig. 10.5).

Soft Tissue Management

The soft tissue used to cover the surgical defect is either a mucosal or a skin graft, neither of which is ideal to support a prosthesis [30]. It is important that the prosthesis should not rest on these tissues. This can be prevented by utilizing the teeth or implants for prosthesis support. In the case of a removable prosthesis, one of the design strategies is to utilize support only from soft tissues that are not affected by radiation or chemotherapy. The denture should rest on the non-irritated mucosa with or without support from the reconstructed area. Occlusal contacts should be restricted to areas overlying stable, non-reconstructed sites. To gain support from the reconstructed area, a cantilevered bar attached to the remaining teeth or implants can be utilized without loading the soft tissue. This approach has the advantage of

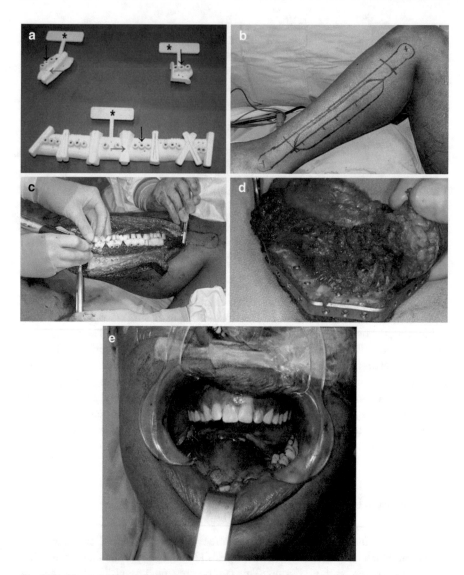

Fig. 10.4 The digital CAD CAM protocol associated with a fibula replacement of the body of the mandible following resection of an intraosseous squamous cell carcinoma. (**a**) The three-dimensional (3D) custom-fabricated fibular resection and implant placement guide. (**b**) An outline on the leg of the incision and flap design for retrieval of the fibula graft. (**c**) The flap reflected, the guide attached, and the implants placed prior to removal of the fibula graft from the leg and wound closure. (**d**) The fibula graft has been cut, retrieved and segments attached to the patient-specific mandibular reconstruction plate. Note the implants positioned in the right, central and left segments of the bone graft. (**e**) Insertion of the fibula graft-reconstruction plate unit and stabilization to the distal mandibular segments (rami) with surgical screws

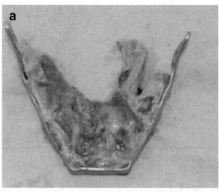
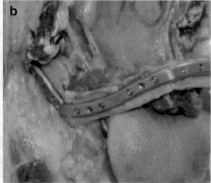

Fig. 10.5 Example of a fibula graft attached to a reconstruction plate. (**a**) Six fibula segments were harvested using a cutting guide and attached to the reconstruction plate. (**b**) Completion of the mandibular reconstruction with a fibula flap and a patient-specific reconstruction plate

permitting the patient to remove the prosthesis. For many of these patients, removable prostheses are preferred as it is easier to clean and maintain implants, teeth, and prostheses free of biofilm and debris. This becomes very important especially at annual or quarterly follow-ups of patients with their head and neck surgical oncologists or plastic surgeons. These patients require evaluation of the surgical sites for recurrence of disease. Removable prostheses allow ready access for these examinations [31].

Mucositis

In addition to the surgical issues discussed above, radiation and chemotherapy treatments result in inflammation of the oropharyngeal soft tissues (Fig. 10.6) [32]. More recently, mucositis associated with immunotherapy has been reported [33]. Mucositis is a problem that can interfere with the use of prostheses that have extensive soft tissue support. These tissues are often friable with little tolerance for loading with removable prostheses. For these patients, it is often preferable to support the prosthesis with implants, taking the pressure off of the mucosa [32]. In the case of radiation therapy, the determinants of the severity of mucositis are the (i) total radiation dose, (ii) fractionation size and scheme, (iii) total volume of tissue that is irradiated, and (iv) type of ionizing radiation that is administered. There are strategies that can reduce the degree of mucositis without loss of therapeutic effect. Intensity-modulated proton therapy (IMPT, also known as proton therapy) reduces the dose to specific sites and structures thereby lessening the incidence of mucositis and adverse events compared to previous generations of radiation therapy, such as intensity-modulated radiotherapy (IMRT) [34].

Fig. 10.6 A clinical presentation of oral mucositis with mixed ulceration and pseudomembrane formation

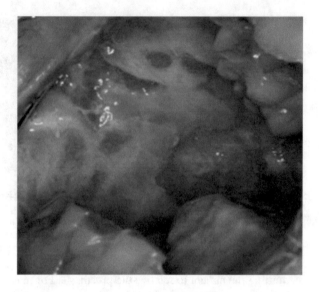

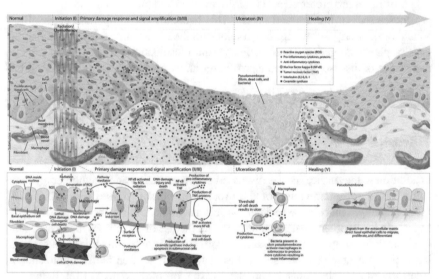

Fig. 10.7 Pathobiology of oral mucositis. This is a five-stage model, which incorporates a complex interaction that includes primary damage to basal epithelial cells from cancer treatment and secondary insult to surrounding tissues as a result of proinflammatory mediators. (Figure reproduced with permission from Ref. [36].)

The pathogenesis of mucositis has been well characterized. Initially, radiation and/or chemotherapy induce damage to the epithelial cell layers (Fig. 10.7). In particular, damage to the basal layers reduces the thickness of the epithelium resulting in a lessened resistance to physical stress as from a prosthesis pressing on soft tissue as well as bacterial invasion from the oral microbiota. The breakdown of reactive oxygen species and free radicals from intracellular proteins by radiation and/chemotherapy is also believed to be important in the initiation of mucosal injury. These small, highly reactive molecules are by-products of oxygen metabolism and can cause significant intracellular damage. Second messengers that transmit signals from receptors on the cellular surface to the inside of the cell are also important factors in mucositis. The second messengers IP3 and DAG are cleaved by phospholipase 3 intracellularly in the PMNs that are part of the inflammatory response. These, in turn, upregulate release of inflammatory cytokines including TNF-α and substance P. These inflammatory cytokines are important in the pathogenesis of mucositis. In addition as noted before, weakening of the epithelial barrier allows the infiltration of the oral microbiota into the epithelium. The metabolic products of these bacteria are significant in the maintenance of oral mucositis [35].

The steps in the development of oral mucositis. Generation of reactive oxygen species (ROS) triggers release of inflammatory cytokines and transcription factors leading to mucosal cell death, ulceration, and pseudomembrane formation [36].

Clinically, the development of mucositis varies between patients. In the initial stage, the oral mucositis presents as erythema of the oral mucosa, which then often progresses to erosion and ulceration. Typically, the ulcerations are covered by a white pseudomembrane. It takes approximately 2–4 weeks for the healing to occur after the last dose of chemotherapy or radiation therapy. The length of time of the radiation or chemotherapy treatment and amount of time after completion of the treatment for the stem cells to mature are important factors in the healing process. In chemotherapy-induced oral mucositis, lesions are usually limited to non-keratinized surfaces (i.e., lateral and ventral surfaces of the tongue, buccal mucosa, and soft palate) [37].

The clinical signs and symptoms of oral mucositis can exacerbate with infection from the local flora, particularly in immunosuppressed patients. Viral infections with herpes simplex virus (HSV) or fungal infections, such as candidiasis, can superimpose on the oral mucositis lesion and complicate the process of diagnosis and treatment of such lesions [35].

To date, the management process of oral mucositis is largely palliative. The Multinational Association for Supportive Care in Cancer and the International Society of Oral Oncology (MASCC/ISOO) have developed clinical practice guidelines for the management of oral mucositis [38].

A. *Nutritional support:* Severe pain and altered taste sensation compromise the patients' intake of nutrients and liquids. Patients should be monitored by a dietician or professional caregiver to prevent any weight loss. Although it varies from center to center, prophylactic feeding gastrostomy tubes are placed for patients with severe mucositis.

B. *Pain control:* Oral pain resulting from mucositis significantly affects patients' nutritional intake, quality of life, and ability to practice oral care. Each cancer center has its own strategy to manage oral mucositis. The table below presents a wide range of modalities that are available according to the need of patients (Table 10.1). Viscous 2% lidocaine local anesthetic is used commonly to reduce

Table 10.1 Common oral mucositis rinses

Bland rinse
Magic ,mouthwash
0.9% saline
Sodium bicarbonate solution
Topical anesthetic: Sprays, ointment, gel, and rinse
Lidocaine or benzocaine
Dicyclomine
Capsaicin
Mucosal protectant
Gelclair (EKR therapeutics)
Cellulose
Kaolin
Sucralfate (Carafate, Axcan Pharma)
Aluminum hydroxide
Analgesics
Benzydamine rinse (not available in United States)
Opioids (nonsteroidal anti-inflammatory drugs contraindicated)
Others
Baking soda salt rinses
Pentoxifylline
Chlorhexidine mouthwash
Allopurinol rinse

pain from oral mucositis. Mixtures of lidocaine with diphenhydramine and a soothing covering agent, such as Maalox (Novartis Consumer Health, Inc., Fremont, MI) or Kaopectate (Chattem, Inc., Chattanooga, TN), in equal volumes provide a longer-lasting analgesic effect. Sucralfate is the most common topical agent that is used as a mucosal bioadhering agent to provide a longer-lasting analgesic effect.

C. *Oral decontamination:* Microbial colonization of oral mucositis lesions complicates the management of the mucositis, exacerbating the pain. A decontamination regime provides a significant positive outcome helping to reduce the progression of the mucositis and reduces the time for healing.

D. *Palliation of dry mouth:* A side effect of cancer treatment is a thickening of the saliva resulting from a decrease in the serous component. Temporary or permanent xerostomia can further aggravate the inflamed tissue in these patients and increases the risk of fungal, viral, and bacterial superinfection upon the mucositis resulting from radiation or chemotherapy. Dry mouth also makes mastication and swallowing difficult. Patients should be counseled and made aware of the likelihood of these problems as well as the importance of keeping their mouth moist and free of food debris.

The following measures can be taken for palliation of a dry mouth [39], Table 10.1:

- Carry a bottle of water and sip water as needed to alleviate mouth dryness. In addition, artificial saliva or other supportive agents that keep the mouth moist during the day are available over-the-counter at pharmacies.
- Rinse with a solution of ½ teaspoon baking soda (and/or ¼ or ½ teaspoon of table salt) in a cup of warm water, several times per day to clean and lubricate the oral tissues and to buffer the oral environment.
- Chew sugarless gum to stimulate salivary flow.
- Use cholinergic agents as necessary.

Conclusion

Dental implants are becoming an increasingly important modality in maxillofacial rehabilitation of the head and neck cancer patient. They serve to stabilize prostheses that replace portions of the dentition, the maxilla and mandible that are removed as part of the patient's treatment for the disease. The technologies illustrated in this chapter that are being currently employed continue to improve. They are allowing the cancer patient to live and function with an improved quality of life. New developments and research particularly in the field of tissue engineering hold promise to continue to improve the delivery of much needed health care to patients recovering from debilitating maxillofacial disease.

References

1. McKinney RV, Steflick DE, Koth DL, et al. The scientific basis for dental implant therapy. J Dent Educ. 1988;52:696–705.
2. Branemark PI, Adell R, Breine U, et al. Intra-osseous anchorage of dental prostheses. Experimental studies. Scand J Plast Reconstr Surg. 1969;3:81–100.
3. Albrektsson T. Direct bone anchorage of dental implants. J Prosthet Dent. 1983;50:255–61.
4. Depprich R, Naujoks C, Ommerborn M, et al. Current findings regarding zirconia implants. Clin Implant Dent Relat Res. 2014;16:124–37.
5. Albrektsson B, Chrcanovic B, Östman PO, et al. Initial and long-term crestal bone responses to modern dental implants. Periodontol 2000. 2017;73:41–50.
6. Berglundh T, Abrahamsson I, Lang NP, et al. De novo alveolar bone formation adjacent to endosseous implants. Clin Oral Implants Res. 2003;14:251–62.
7. Kuzyk PRT, Schemitsch EH. The basic science of peri-implant bone healing. Indian J Orthop. 2011;45:108–15.
8. Ueda M, Hibino Y, Niimi A. Usefulness of dental implants in maxillofacial reconstruction. J Long Term Effects Med Implants. 1999;9:349–66.
9. Verdonck HW, Meijer GJ, Laurin T, et al. Assessment of vascularity in irradiated and nonirradiated maxillary and mandibular minipig alveolar bone using laser doppler flowmetry. Int J Oral Maxillofac Implants. 2007;22:774–8.
10. Bagan JV, Murillo J, Jimenez Y, et al. Avascular jaw osteonecrosis in association with cancer chemotherapy: series of 10 cases. J Oral Pathol Med. 2005;34:120–3.

11. Taylor KH, Middlefell S, Mizen KD. Osteonecrosis of the jaws induced by anti-RANk ligand therapy. Br J Oral and Maxillofacial Surg. 2010;48:221–3.

12. Diz P, Lopez-Cedrun JL, Aranez J, et al. Denosumab-related osseous necrosis of the jaw. J Amer Dent Assn. 2012;143:981–4.

13. de F Oliveria H, Panzer H, Celia R. Capacity of denture plaque/biofilm removal and antimicrobial action of a new denture paste. Braz Dent J. 2000;11:97–104.

14. Okay DJ, Genden E, Buchbinder D, et al. Prosthetic guidelines for surgical reconstruction of the maxilla. A classification system for defects. J Prosthet Dent. 2001;86:352–63.

15. Chen MH, Lyons KM, Tause-Smith A. Clinical significance of the use of resonance frequence analysis in assessing implant stability. A systematic review. Int J Prosthodont. 2019;32:51–8.

16. Schoen PJ, Reintsema H, Raghoebar GM, et al. The use of implant-retained mandibular prostheses in the oral rehabilitation of head and neck cancer patients. A review and rationale for treatment planning. Oral Oncol. 2004;40:862–71.

17. Ivanoff CJ, Hallgren C, Widmark G, et al. Histological evaluation of the bone integration of (TiO$_2$) blasted and turned titanium microimplants in humans. 2001;12:128–34.

18. Buser D, Broggini N, Wieland M, et al. Enhanced bone apposition to a chemically modified SLA titanium surface. J Dent Res. 2004;83:529–33.

19. Ersanli S, Karabuda C, Beck F, et al. Resonance frequency analysis of one stage dental implant stability during the osseointegration period. J Periodontol. 2005;76:1066–71.

20. Curi MM, Condezo EFB, Ribeiro KDCB, et al. Long-term success of dental implants in patients with head and neck cancer after radiation therapy. Int J Oral Maxillofac Surg. 2018;47:783–8.

21. Shifman A, Lepley JB. Prosthodontic management of post-surgical soft tissue deformities associated with partial mandibulectomy. Part 1: Loss of the vestibule. J Prosthet Dent. 1982;48:178–83.

22. Bouri A Jr, Bissada N, Al-Zahrani MS, et al. Width of keratinized gingiva and the health status of the supporting tissues around dental implants. Int J Oral Maxillofacial Implants. 2008;23:323–6.

23. Judy KW, Robertson E, Chabra D, et al. Prosthetic rehabilitation with HA-coated root form implants after restoration of mandibular continuity. Int J Oral Implantol. 1990;8:25–8.

24. Borlase G. Use of obturators in rehabilitation of maxillectomy defects. Ann Royal Australian Coll Dental Surg. 2000;15:75–9.

25. Olsen KD, Devine KD, Weiland LH. Mucoepidermoid carcinoma of the oral cavity. Otolaryngol Head Neck Surg. 1981;89:783–91.

26. Curtis TA. Treatment planning for intraoral maxillofacial prosthetics for cancer patients. J Prosthet Dent. 1967;18:70–6.

27. Aramany MA, Myers EN. Prosthetic reconstruction following resection of the hard and soft palate. J Prosthet Dent. 1978;40:174–8.

28. Deepanandan L, Narayanan V, Baig MF. Mandibular invasion of squamous cell carcinoma: factors determining surgical resection of mandible using computerized tomography and histopathologic study. J Maxillofacial Oral Surg. 2010;9:48–53.

29. Yap YL, Lim J, Ong WC. Stabilization of mobile mandibular segments in mandibular reconstruction: Use of a spanning reconstruction plate. Craniomaxillofac Trauma Reconstr. 2012;5:123–6.

30. Karfage A, Schoen PJ, Raghoebar GM, et al. Five year followup of oral functioning and quality of life in patients with oral cancer with implant-retained mandibular overdentures. J Sci Special Head Neck. 2011;33:831–9.

31. Shaw R, Sutton D, Brown J, et al. Further malignancy in field change adjacent to osseointegrated implants. Int J Oral Maxillofacial Surg. 2004;33:353–5.

32. Sonis ST. Mucositis: the impact, biology and therapeutic opportunities of oral mucositis. Oral Oncol 2009. 2009;45:1015–20.

33. Jackson LK, John DB, Sosman JA, et al. Oral health in oncology: impact of immunotherapy. Support Care Cancer. 2015;23:1–3.

34. Chu KP, Le QT. Intensity-modulated and image-guided radiation therapy for head and neck cancers. Front Radiation Oncol. 2011;43:217–54.
35. Hong CH, Napenas JJ, Hodgson BD, Stokman MA, et al. A systematic review of dental disease in patients undergoing cancer therapy. Support Care Cancer. 2011;18:1007–21.
36. Lalla RV, Saunders DP, Peterson DE. Chemotherapy or radiation-induced mucositis. Dent Clin N Am. 2014;58:341–9.
37. Chen YK, Hou HA, Chow JM, Chen YC, Hsueh PR, Tien HF. The impact of oral herpes simplex virus infection and candidiasis on chemotherapy-induced oral mucositis among patients with hematological malignancies. Eur J Clin Microbiol Infect Dis. 2011;30:753–9.
38. Lalla RV, Bowen J, Barasch A, et al. MASCC/ISOO clinical practice guidelines for the management of mucositis secondary to cancer therapy. Cancer. 2014;120:1453–61.
39. Villa A, Connell CL, Abati S. Diagnosis and management of xerostomia and hyposalivation. Ther Clin Risk Manag. 2015;11:45–51.

Index

Printed in the United States
by Baker & Taylor Publisher Services